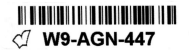

W9-AGN-447

VALUING HEALTH
FOR REGULATORY COST-EFFECTIVENESS ANALYSIS

Wilhelmine Miller, Lisa A. Robinson, and Robert S. Lawrence, Editors

Committee to Evaluate Measures of Health Benefits for
Environmental, Health, and Safety Regulation

Board on Health Care Services

INSTITUTE OF MEDICINE
OF THE NATIONAL ACADEMIES

THE NATIONAL ACADEMIES PRESS
Washington, D.C.
www.nap.edu

THE NATIONAL ACADEMIES PRESS   500 FIFTH STREET, N.W.   Washington, DC 20001

NOTICE: The project that is the subject of this report was approved by the Governing Board of the National Research Council, whose members are drawn from the councils of the National Academy of Sciences, the National Academy of Engineering, and the Institute of Medicine. The members of the committee responsible for the report were chosen for their special competences and with regard for appropriate balance.

This study was supported by Contract No. 282-99-0045 between the National Academy of Sciences and Department of Health and Human Services. Any opinions, findings, conclusions, or recommendations expressed in this publication are those of the author(s) and do not necessarily reflect the view of the organizations or agencies that provided support for this project.

Library of Congress Cataloging-in-Publication Data

Valuing health for regulatory cost-effectiveness analysis / Wilhelmine
    Miller, Lisa A. Robinson, and Robert S. Lawrence, editors ; Committee
    to Evaluate Measures of Health Benefits for Environmental, Health,
    and Safety Regulation, Board on Health Care Services.
        p. ; cm.
    Includes bibliographical references and index.
    ISBN 0-309-10077-1 (casebound book)
    1. Medical care—Cost effectiveness—Research—Methodology. 2. Cost
effectiveness.   I. Miller, Wilhelmine. II. Robinson, Lisa A.
III. Lawrence, Robert S., 1938-   . IV. Institute of Medicine (U.S.).
Committee to Evaluate Measures of Health Benefits for Environmental,
Health, and Safety Regulation.
    [DNLM: 1. Cost-Benefit Analysis—methods—United States. 2. Health
Policy—economics—United States. 3. United States Government Agencies
—United States.   WA 540 AA1 V215 2006]
    RA410.5.V35 2006
    362.1068'1—dc22
                                                    2006001486

Additional copies of this report are available from the National Academies Press, 500 Fifth Street, N.W., Lockbox 285, Washington, DC 20055; (800) 624-6242 or (202) 334-3313 (in the Washington metropolitan area); Internet, http://www.nap.edu.

For more information about the Institute of Medicine, visit the IOM home page at: **www.iom.edu.**

Copyright 2006 by the National Academy of Sciences. All rights reserved.

Printed in the United States of America.

The serpent has been a symbol of long life, healing, and knowledge among almost all cultures and religions since the beginning of recorded history. The serpent adopted as a logotype by the Institute of Medicine is a relief carving from ancient Greece, now held by the Staatliche Museen in Berlin.

"Knowing is not enough; we must apply.
Willing is not enough; we must do."
—Goethe

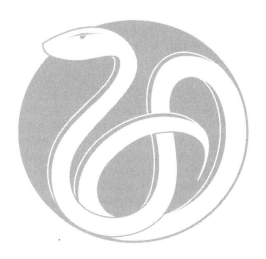

INSTITUTE OF MEDICINE
OF THE NATIONAL ACADEMIES

Advising the Nation. Improving Health.

THE NATIONAL ACADEMIES
Advisers to the Nation on Science, Engineering, and Medicine

The **National Academy of Sciences** is a private, nonprofit, self-perpetuating society of distinguished scholars engaged in scientific and engineering research, dedicated to the furtherance of science and technology and to their use for the general welfare. Upon the authority of the charter granted to it by the Congress in 1863, the Academy has a mandate that requires it to advise the federal government on scientific and technical matters. Dr. Ralph J. Cicerone is president of the National Academy of Sciences.

The **National Academy of Engineering** was established in 1964, under the charter of the National Academy of Sciences, as a parallel organization of outstanding engineers. It is autonomous in its administration and in the selection of its members, sharing with the National Academy of Sciences the responsibility for advising the federal government. The National Academy of Engineering also sponsors engineering programs aimed at meeting national needs, encourages education and research, and recognizes the superior achievements of engineers. Dr. Wm. A. Wulf is president of the National Academy of Engineering.

The **Institute of Medicine** was established in 1970 by the National Academy of Sciences to secure the services of eminent members of appropriate professions in the examination of policy matters pertaining to the health of the public. The Institute acts under the responsibility given to the National Academy of Sciences by its congressional charter to be an adviser to the federal government and, upon its own initiative, to identify issues of medical care, research, and education. Dr. Harvey V. Fineberg is president of the Institute of Medicine.

The **National Research Council** was organized by the National Academy of Sciences in 1916 to associate the broad community of science and technology with the Academy's purposes of furthering knowledge and advising the federal government. Functioning in accordance with general policies determined by the Academy, the Council has become the principal operating agency of both the National Academy of Sciences and the National Academy of Engineering in providing services to the government, the public, and the scientific and engineering communities. The Council is administered jointly by both Academies and the Institute of Medicine. Dr. Ralph J. Cicerone and Dr. Wm. A. Wulf are chair and vice chair, respectively, of the National Research Council.

www.national-academies.org

COMMITTEE TO EVALUATE MEASURES OF HEALTH BENEFITS FOR ENVIRONMENTAL, HEALTH, AND SAFETY REGULATION

ROBERT S. LAWRENCE *(Chair)*, Associate Dean for Professional Practice and Programs and Edyth Schoenrich Professor of Preventive Medicine, Bloomberg School of Public Health, Johns Hopkins University, Baltimore, Maryland

HENRY A. ANDERSON, Chief Medical Officer, Environmental and Occupational Disease Epidemiologist, Wisconsin Division of Public Health, Madison

RICHARD T. BURNETT, Senior Research Scientist, Healthy Environments and Consumer Safety Branch, Health Canada, Ottawa, Ontario, Canada

CARL F. CRANOR, Professor of Philosophy, University of California, Riverside

MAUREEN L. CROPPER, Professor, University of Maryland, and Lead Economist, The World Bank, Washington, DC

NORMAN DANIELS, Professor of Ethics and Population Health, Harvard School of Public Health, Boston, Massachusetts

DENNIS G. FRYBACK, Professor of Population Health Sciences and Industrial Engineering, Department of Population Health Sciences, University of Wisconsin, Madison

ALAN M. GARBER, Staff Physician, Veterans Affairs Palo Alto Health Care System; Henry J. Kaiser, Jr. Professor and Professor of Medicine, Director, Center for Health Policy, and Director, Center for Primary Care and Outcomes Research, Stanford University, Stanford, California

MARTHE R. GOLD, Arthur C. Logan Professor and Chair, Department of Community Health and Social Medicine, City University of New York Medical School, New York

JAMES K. HAMMITT, Professor of Economics and Decision Sciences and Director, Harvard Center for Risk Analysis, Harvard University, Boston, Massachusetts

LISA I. IEZZONI, Professor of Medicine, Harvard Medical School, and Co-Director of Research, Division of General Medicine and Primary Care, Beth Israel Deaconess Medical Center, Boston, Massachusetts

PETER D. JACOBSON, Professor of Health Law and Policy and Director, Center for Law, Ethics, and Health, University of Michigan School of Public Health, Ann Arbor

EMMETT KEELER, Senior Mathematician and Professor of Health Economics, RAND, Santa Monica, California

WILLARD G. MANNING, Professor, Harris School of Public Policy Studies, The University of Chicago, Chicago, Illinois

v

CHARLES POOLE,* Associate Professor, Department of Epidemiology, University of North Carolina School of Public Health, Chapel Hill
DAVID A. SCHKADE, Jerome Katzin Professor, Rady School of Management, University of California, San Diego

ADVISERS TO THE COMMITTEE

ALAN KRUPNICK, Senior Fellow and Director, Quality of the Environment, Resources for the Future, Washington, DC
JUDITH L. WAGNER, Scholar-in-Residence, Institute of Medicine, Washington, DC
MILTON C. WEINSTEIN, Henry J. Kaiser Professor of Health Policy and Management, Harvard School of Public Health and Center for Risk Analysis, Boston, Massachusetts

IOM Staff

Wilhelmine Miller, Project Director
Ryan L. Palugod, Research Assistant

Principal Consultant

Lisa A. Robinson, Independent Consultant

---

*Served from March 2004 to June 2005.

Reviewers

This report has been reviewed in draft form by individuals chosen for their diverse perspectives and technical expertise, in accordance with procedures approved by the National Research Council's (NRC's) Report Review Committee. The purpose of this independent review is to provide candid and critical comments that will assist the institution in making its published report as sound as possible and to ensure that the report meets institutional standards for objectivity, evidence, and responsiveness to the study charge. The review comments and draft manuscript remain confidential to protect the integrity of the deliberative process. We wish to thank the following individuals for their review of this report:

ELENA ANDRESEN, Professor of Epidemiology, University of Florida, College of Public Health and Health Professions, and Research Health Scientist, North Florida/South Georgia VA Medical Center, Gainesville

DAVID A. ASCH, Eilers Professor of Health Care Management and Economics, Executive Director, Leonard Davis Institute of Health Economics, The Wharton School, University of Pennsylvania, Philadelphia

TRUDY A. CAMERON, Professor of Economics, University of Oregon, Eugene

LELAND B. DECK, Senior Economist, U.S. Environmental Protection Agency (retired) and Vice President, Abt Associates (retired), Rockville, Maryland

AMY D. KYLE, Research Scientist and Lecturer, Environmental Health Sciences Division, School of Public Health, University of California, Berkeley

JOSEPHINE MAUSKOPF, Global Director, Health Economics, RTI-International, Research Triangle Park, North Carolina

THOMAS O. MCGARITY, Professor, University of Texas School of Law, Austin

RICHARD D. MORGENSTERN, Senior Fellow, Resources for the Future, Inc., Washington, DC

CHARLES E. PHELPS, Provost, University of Rochester, Rochester, New York

MICHAEL STOTO, Senior Statistical Scientist and Associate Director for Public Health, Center for Domestic and International Health Security, The RAND Corporation, Arlington, Virginia

CASS SUNSTEIN, Karl N. Llewellyn Distinguished Service Professor of Jurisprudence, School of Law, The University of Chicago, Chicago, Illinois

PETER UBEL, Associate Professor of Internal Medicine, Director, Program for Improving Health Care Decisions, and Staff Physician, Ann Arbor Veterans Affairs Medical Center, University of Michigan, Ann Arbor

ROBERT WACHBROIT, Professor of Philosophy, Maryland School of Public Policy, University of Maryland, College Park

JONATHAN B. WIENER, Professor of Law, Environmental Policy, and Public Policy Studies, Duke University, and Founding Director, Center for Environmental Solutions, Durham, North Carolina

Although the reviewers listed above have provided many constructive comments and suggestions, they were not asked to endorse the conclusions or recommendations nor did they see the final draft of the report before its release. The review of this report was overseen by **John C. Bailar III, Professor Emeritus, The University of Chicago,** and **Louise B. Russell, Research Professor, Institute for Health, Health Care Policy and Aging Research, Rutgers, The State University of New Jersey.** Appointed by the NRC and Institute of Medicine, they were responsible for making certain that an independent examination of this report was carried out in accordance with institutional procedures and that all review comments were carefully considered. Responsibility for the final content of this report rests entirely with the authoring committee and the institution.

Preface

Valuing Health for Regulatory Cost-Effectiveness Analysis responds to several important analytical and policy challenges. These include how to estimate the health-related effects of regulatory interventions to reduce environmental, health, and safety risks; how to conduct informative cost-effectiveness analyses (CEAs) of such interventions prospectively; and how to use the results of CEAs and of other kinds of economic analyses in public policy decisions about regulating risks to human health and safety. In 2003 John D. Graham, the Administrator of the Office of Information and Regulatory Affairs in the Office of Management and Budget, asked the Institute of Medicine (IOM) to convene an expert consensus committee to address these questions. A consortium of federal regulatory and health policy offices and agencies supported this effort financially and, equally essentially, with information and analytic expertise generously provided to the study committee throughout the project.

This report of the Committee to Evaluate Measures of Health Benefits for Environmental, Health, and Safety Regulation is the latest in a series by the IOM and the National Research Council (NRC) of The National Academies that have addressed risk assessment and communication; economic evaluation of environmental, health, and safety risks; and measurement of population health. These precursor reports include the NRC reports *Risk Assessment in the Federal Government: Managing the Process* (1983); *Improving Risk Communication* (1989); *Valuing Health Risks, Costs, and Benefits for Environmental Decision Making: Report of a Conference* (1990); and *Estimating the Public Health Benefits of Proposed Air Pollu-*

tion Regulations (2002); and the IOM report *Summarizing Population Health: Directions for the Development and Application of Population Metrics* (1998). We build on the insights of these earlier efforts and cover new ground in this latest work, which offers guidance on the application of summary health measures to the economic analysis of regulations. This report takes as its primary audience regulatory analysts and public-sector decision makers. We have tried to make the text accessible for lay readers also, to help promote public understanding of important governmental functions and processes.

The work of the Committee to Evaluate Measures of Health Benefits has involved multidisciplinary collaborations of a breadth unusual even for IOM committees, which frequently draw on members with diverse expertise. Representing capability in environmental and population health sciences, economics, ethics, law, statistics, and medicine, the Committee worked together over 20 months to develop a sound and feasible approach to incorporating CEA with health-related effectiveness measures into regulatory impact analyses. Committee members, advisers, IOM staff and consultants, and federal agency experts learned together, through undertaking three case studies, the challenges and possibilities for regulatory CEA.

As chair, I have been most impressed by the intellectual openness and generosity of all of the committee in our work together to address an essentially practical problem of public policy. When conflicting convictions and preferences grounded in members' particular disciplines emerged, all made a great effort to see beyond the questions of theory and the ideal to constructive and feasible proposals and methods for analysts and decision makers. The steady hand on the tiller of Wilhelmine Miller, study director, allowed the committee to navigate successfully the many challenging currents of our deliberations, and for this we are all indebted to her. This report is the result of an especially productive collaboration.

Robert S. Lawrence, M.D.
Chair
December 2005

Acknowledgments

Valuing Health for Regulatory Cost-Effectiveness Analysis reflects the contributions of many people. The Committee would like to acknowledge and thank those who so generously participated in the development of this report.

First, we would like to thank the federal sponsors of this project who supported and guided the project, including John Graham, Administrator, Office of Information and Regulatory Affairs (OIRA) in the Office of Management and Budget; John Morrall, III, OIRA; and project officers Joanna Siegel, Agency for Healthcare Research and Quality (AHRQ), and Phaedra Corso, Centers for Disease Control and Prevention (CDC). Financial support was provided by the Environmental Protection Agency (EPA), several agencies and offices of the Department of Health and Human Services and the Department of Transportation, the Consumer Product Safety Commission (CPSC), and the Department of Agriculture.

The Committee's deliberations were informed by presentations and discussions held November 30 and December 1, 2004, at public workshop and meeting sessions. The following experts and scholars made presentations and continued to share advice and expertise with the Committee and project staff over many months: John Brazier, University of Sheffield; Dan Brock, Harvard University; David Feeny, University of Alberta; Peter Franks, University of California–Davis; Amiram Gafni, McMaster University; Daniel Hausman, University of Wisconsin; Robert Kaplan, University of California–Los Angeles; Paul Kind, University of York; Ellen MacKenzie, Johns Hopkins University; Erik Nord, Norwegian Institute of Public Health;

Joshua Salomon, Harvard University; Elizabeth Vigdor, Duke University; and David Wasserman, University of Maryland. Edward Sondik, Director, National Center for Health Statistics, Dave Moriarty, CDC, William Lawrence, AHRQ, and S. "Chris" Haffer, Centers for Medicare and Medicaid Services, provided information on federal data collection and statistical policy and fielded many questions over the course of the project. Reed Johnson, Research Triangle Institute, also presented his research to the Committee at its first meeting in May 2004. Susan Stewart, National Bureau of Economic Research, made her research on statistically inferred health indexes available to the Committee.

Federal agency staff supported this project in several important ways. Randall Lutter, Food and Drug Administration (FDA), Albert McGartland, EPA, and Lawrence Blincoe, National Highway Traffic Safety Administration (NHTSA), introduced current agency practices in presentations at the Committee's May 2004 meeting. Numerous agency staff participated in subsequent interviews supporting the Committee's commissioned paper on current practices (Robinson, 2004). A full list of participants is provided in that paper; however, we would particularly like to thank the following individuals for setting up the interviews and reviewing the draft materials: James DeMocker, Bryan Hubbell, Lyn Luben, and Nathalie Simon, EPA; Clark Nardinelli and Richard Williams, FDA; Clare Narrod, Ronald Meekof, and Charles Williams, Department of Agriculture; Robert Burt and Deborah Aiken, Occupational Safety and Health Administration; Robert Stone, Mine Safety and Health Administration; Lawrence Blincoe and James Simons, NHTSA; Charles Rombro, Federal Motor Carriers Safety Administration; and Gregory Rodgers, CPSC. Without their enthusiastic and extensive support, this report and its evidentiary basis would not exist; the Committee is extremely grateful for their assistance.

The three case studies undertaken by the Committee involved many of the agency staff already mentioned as well as many others. A synopsis of the case studies, included as Appendix A to this report, acknowledges all of the participants; the Committee would especially like to thank the following individuals. The case studies would not have been possible without extended consultations with and help from those involved in the original agency regulatory analyses, particularly Bryan Hubbell, EPA; Clark Nardinelli, FDA; and Lawrence Blincoe and James Simons, NHTSA. Several CDC staff provided important assistance in developing and implementing the approaches used to assess health-related quality of life impacts in each case study. Anne Haddix, Office of the Director, CDC, offered CDC's staff expertise in planning and conducting the case studies. Phaedra Corso, Center for Injury Prevention, CDC, deserves special recognition for initiating the first case study (of the NHTSA child restraints regulation), which provided the basic framework for the subsequent studies and was an important learning experience for the Committee. Sajal Chattopadhyay, Xiangming Fang, Tursynbek Nurmagambetov, Seymour Williams, and Darwin LaBarthe, all of CDC, devoted considerable time and effort to the case studies. Committee consultants Carmen Brauer and Peter Neumann, Harvard School of Public Health, Janel Hanmer, University of Wisconsin, Robert Black, Independent Consultant, Bryce Mason, RAND, and Patrick Sullivan, University of Colorado Health Sciences Center, made indispensable contributions to the case study analyses. William Lawrence, AHRQ, provided data and advice throughout the project.

We were especially fortunate to have three experts serve as advisers and sounding boards throughout the course of the study. Alan Krupnick, Judith Wagner, and Milton Weinstein helped design and critique the case studies, proposed lines of investigation and analysis for the report, and reviewed many drafts of Committee materials; their participation has enriched our work immeasurably. S. Matthew Liao, Greenwall Fellow in Bioethics and Health Policy, Johns Hopkins University, assisted in the development of the Committee's discussion of the ethical implications of economic analysis in regulatory policy during his internship at the Institute of Medicine (IOM), and Andrew Wolman, George Washington University Law School, provided pro bono legal research. Lisa A. Robinson served as principal consultant to the Committee over the course of our study, bringing great expertise, energy, and intelligence to the project. We are indebted to her for contributions that extended well beyond the formal consultancy. Ryan Palugod expertly provided research assistance and general support to the Committee, consultants, and IOM staff.

This study was directed by Wilhelmine Miller, senior program officer of the Board on Health Care Services, which provided overall guidance and support to the study committee.

Contents

VALUING HEALTH
FOR REGULATORY COST-EFFECTIVENESS ANALYSIS

Executive Summary

Regulating risks to human health and safety is an essential responsibility of government. At the federal level, agencies issue a wide range of regulations to protect human health and safety in areas that include improving air and water quality and safeguarding the food supply; reducing the risk of injury on the job, in transportation, and from consumer products; and minimizing exposures to toxic chemicals. Such regulations can substantially improve health and safety and typically impose costs, which may be considerable, to do so.

To ensure that these regulations address hazards to human life and health responsibly, fairly, and efficiently, policy makers and the general public need accurate and reliable information on the likely impacts of government actions. For economically significant rules, agencies are required to present an economic analysis—in the form of a benefit–cost analysis (BCA)—of the national impacts of alternative regulatory strategies and to assess the distribution of the impacts across different segments of society. These BCAs, which involve the monetary valuation of the impacts, are convenient because the index used to aggregate diverse types of improvements—to health and to ecosystems, for example—is money, the same unit in which costs are expressed. Such analyses help to inform analysts, decision makers, and the public at large about the benefits and costs of alternative interventions.

In 2003, the U.S. Office of Management and Budget (OMB) issued new guidance that requires agencies to supplement BCA with cost-effectiveness analysis (CEA) for economically significant health and safety regulations (OMB, 2003a). In CEA, the result is a ratio of monetary costs to a non-monetary benefit measure, which can range from single-dimension measures, such as deaths averted, cases of illness or injury avoided, or tons of pollution reduced, to integrated measures such as health-adjusted life years (HALYs), which combine different types of health impacts in a single number. The single-dimension measures have the advantage of being relatively straightforward, but are of limited usefulness when more than one type of benefit is of interest. To address this problem, integrated measures that reflect both life expectancy and health-related quality of life (HRQL) traditionally have been developed and used in medical and public health studies. Such estimates are available for many more types of health effects than are estimates of the monetary measures used in BCA.

This report of the Institute of Medicine's (IOM's) Committee to Evaluate Measures of Health Benefits for Environmental, Health, and Safety Regulation provides recommendations and guidance regarding the measurement of health and safety improvements using CEA. In response to a request from OMB, the Committee investigated alternative approaches for assessing health-related impacts in CEA by reviewing current federal agency practices; commissioning supporting research; reviewing the available literature; and completing three case studies of agency rulemakings.

Based on its investigations, the Committee concludes that CEA provides useful information for the development of regulatory policies. At the same time, CEA (like BCA) poses significant challenges in this context. Some of these challenges are practical, relating to the time and cost of doing such analyses, while others relate to the strengths and limitations of the available data on the nature of the risk reductions and the measurement of their value.

The magnitude of the impacts of major health and safety regulations argues for careful attention to the development of high-quality, unbiased analyses that include thorough documentation of their limitations. The Committee's recommendations, both for selecting measures to value health outcomes in regulatory CEA and for supplementing these measures with other information, aim to ensure that the analytic results are accurate and reliable, and useful to a variety of audiences. After describing the charge to the Committee, this summary provides an overview of the key concepts and conclusions of this report and presents the Committee's recommendations.

The Charge to the Committee

A consortium of federal sponsors charged the IOM Committee to identify current and proposed measures of health benefits for use in regulatory

CEA, describe and evaluate these measures, recommend a subset of measures for use by federal regulatory agencies, and identify areas of research needed to enhance the use of such measures in regulatory analysis.

Specifically, the Committee was asked to:

- *Describe current practices among federal agencies for evaluating the costs and benefits of regulatory actions.*
- *Review measures for aggregating health improvements currently used in CEA, including specific instruments and assessment techniques for developing composite measures that combine consideration of longevity and HRQL.*
- *Develop criteria for choosing among measures potentially useful in the evaluation of health outcomes in regulatory CEA.*
- *Assess the various health benefit measures in terms of their data requirements, feasibility of application, theoretical validity, appropriateness for special populations (children, ethnic minorities), and ethical implications.*
- *Recommend measures appropriate for federal agency use in evaluating health outcomes in regulatory CEA, given the Committee's criteria.*
- *Construct CEA case studies, using information from published BCAs, to illustrate the application of alternative health benefit measures in CEA and to compare the CEAs and BCAs.*
- *Discuss criteria for identifying regulations for which CEA will be informative.*
- *Recommend research that would improve the measurement of health benefits for regulatory CEAs.*

Regulatory Development and Economic Analysis

Federal agencies are directed by Executive Order 12866 and other authorities to estimate and report the expected benefits of proposed major regulations in conjunction with their estimated costs (EOP, 1993). The current guidance for these analyses is provided in OMB Circular A-4, which addresses the use of both BCA and CEA to assess the effects of economically significant health and safety regulations (OMB, 2003a). The resulting analyses are considered, along with other factors, in determining whether to regulate a particular hazard and to select among regulatory strategies that differ in stringency or types of requirements. Researchers examining regulatory priorities also use the results of these analyses to compare the effectiveness of different types of interventions, for example, to compare the cost per life saved across investments in diverse areas such as reducing air pollution, increasing traffic safety, and applying new medical treatments.

The starting point for assessing the *costs* of a proposed regulatory activity is identical for BCA and CEA; they use the same conceptual framework and estimation practices. On the *benefits* side, both BCA and CEA begin with a risk assessment, which involves estimating the change in the likelihood of illness, injury, or death associated with each regulatory option in comparison to a "without regulation" baseline. Regulations often result in small changes in individual risk, which become substantial when aggregated across all of those who are potentially affected. Most major regulations require the assessment of a variety of different health risks. For example, air pollution regulations reduce the incidence of several types of acute and chronic cardiovascular and respiratory conditions as well as associated mortality. In addition, some health and safety regulations provide nonhealth benefits, such as preserving natural resources.

BCA is based on estimates of the monetary value of all risk reductions and other impacts. CEA, in contrast, uses nonmonetary effectiveness measures. When a regulation reduces the risks of different kinds of illness or injury, or of both fatal and nonfatal effects, analysts may use effectiveness measures that reflect impacts on both HRQL and longevity. These composite measures, referred to as HALYs or (more specifically) quality-adjusted life years (QALYs), convert different types of health effects to an integrated unit so that regulatory costs can be compared to a single measure of health-related effectiveness.

Federal agencies have had substantial leeway in determining their specific approach to economic analysis. This flexibility is needed due to gaps and variability in the underlying research base as well as the substantial variation in the types of impacts associated with different regulations. Such analyses must often be conducted within tight time frames and with limited staff and budgetary resources (Robinson, 2004). The rulemaking schedule usually does not allow time for new valuation research; analysts generally rely on preexisting studies, analytic methods, and/or quantitative models. Some agencies have undertaken long-term efforts to develop approaches applicable across many of their regulations.

Agencies have made substantial progress in implementing the 2003 OMB guidance requiring CEA and have completed HALY-based analyses. Some of these analyses use expert judgment to apply one of the available generic HRQL measurement tools (described later in this summary). Others use HRQL estimates from existing studies of similar health endpoints; this practice is often referred to as *benefits transfer*. Agencies are also conducting new valuation research to a limited extent. Because some agencies have used monetized HALY estimates in their regulatory analyses for many years, they are using the same approaches to develop effectiveness measures for CEA.

Health-Related Effectiveness Measures

While CEA based on integrated measures of effectiveness is just beginning to be more widely applied to regulatory decision making, HALYs and other mortality-based indicators have long been used to evaluate effectiveness in health care policy.[1] Early analyses focused on the number of preventable deaths averted; now such analyses also routinely calculate years of life saved. The life-years approach provides more weight to averting deaths among persons who otherwise would have longer remaining life expectancies; an intervention that prevents deaths among children will generally lead to larger estimates of life years gained than an intervention that prevents deaths among adults.

In recent years, measures have been developed to capture the effects of illness and injury on individual well-being prior to death. These impacts are usually represented with indexed estimates of HRQL, using a scale anchored by death (0) and perfect or optimal health (1.0). Adverse health effects associated with illness and injury can then be arrayed along this scale.

The extent to which HRQL impacts are more or less important than changes in longevity depends on the nature of both the risk and the intervention. While the challenge of calculating composite measures is often attributed to the difficulty of valuing the changes in morbidity, changes in longevity may more significantly affect the results. The Committee's own investigations suggest that the importance of mortality relative to HRQL effects varies substantially among regulatory interventions. Regardless, both mortality and HRQL impacts such as illness and disability are of interest to decision makers.

HALYs address this interest by melding descriptive information about health status and longevity. QALYs are the most extensively developed and widely used HALY measure. As a measure of health, a QALY is a relatively simple building block that can be applied at both individual and population levels.

HALY or QALY estimates for various scenarios are normally constructed in three steps:

- Describe or characterize health states or disease conditions and estimate their expected duration.
- Value the health states in comparison to other health states.
- Multiply the values for different health states by estimates of the duration in each state.

---

[1]See Gold et al. (1996b) for recommendations for best practices in CEA for health and medicine.

When used in policy or regulatory analysis, the resulting values can then be multiplied by the number of averted cases of each type to determine the total impact.

For these estimates to be meaningful and useful, the characterization and valuation of the health states of interest should be part of a consistent set of estimates. Researchers may either survey a sample of individuals directly to elicit values for the health states of concern or use one of several available generic HRQL indexes, which are preference-weighted health state classification systems. The EuroQol-5D, Health Utilities Index, Quality of Well-Being Scale, and the SF-6D are among the most common such instruments. Generic indexes provide established values (based on surveys of general or community populations) for different states of health described in terms of the impacts of an overall condition on aspects of functioning and experience such as mobility, self-care, and pain. Once the characteristics of the health state of interest are matched to the functional and experiential domains used in the specific index, an HRQL index value can be calculated based on the results of the instrument's underlying valuation survey.

Regardless of whether the index used is generic or specially designed for a particular study, the index values for health states derived from valuation surveys are based on information about individuals' relative preferences for different states of health. The three most commonly used elicitation techniques involve asking survey respondents to do the following:

- Trade off the time spent in different health states,
- Consider the trade-off between perfect health and the risks of different adverse health effects (standard gamble methods), or
- Locate different health states on a visual scale.

A fourth, less developed, elicitation approach that attempts to address societal values (rather than the respondent's preferences for own health) is the person trade-off method. This approach asks respondents to make choices between different health improvements for distinct groups of people.

Each of these methods for establishing health state index values has strengths and weaknesses. All of them consider only relative preferences for different health states (not preferences for health compared to other aspects of welfare) and generally assume that the value elicited for a particular health state is the same regardless of its duration.

When estimating HALYs for regulatory assessments, analysts may choose to use existing research or to conduct new primary research. In either case, the research may apply one of the generic indexes or be based on index values estimated specifically for the particular study. If a generic index is used, the research may rely on either patients or experts to describe or characterize the health states of interest using the index's classification scheme. (In either case, however, the *values* attached to the health states characterized should represent those of the population affected by the policy or regulation.)

Related decisions will depend on the nature of the health effects under consideration, as well as on the quality and suitability of available research. Judging the adequacy of a given approach for a particular regulatory application requires considering the match between the risks and population assessed in the study and the effects of the regulatory intervention.

Criteria for Selecting Integrated Measures of Health Impacts for Regulatory Analysis

The Committee developed the following criteria for applying HALYs in regulatory analysis.

- First, the measure should be applicable to the range of health states and conditions considered in regulatory analysis.
- Second, the measure should be sensitive or responsive to change, and not exhibit floor or ceiling effects within the range of measured values.
- Third, values for health states should be derived from a sample of adequate size that is representative of the population affected by the costs and benefits of the regulatory intervention.
- Fourth, the measure should be acceptable to users and to the public, including those involved or interested in the regulatory development process.
- Fifth, the measure should be practical in the regulatory context and as inexpensive to use as is compatible with other objectives.

No single QALY instrument or estimation strategy is clearly superior to others on all of these criteria. Analysts and decision makers must exercise judgment in selecting an approach for a particular regulatory analysis. The Committee concludes that health-related CEA is both feasible and informative in the analysis of any regulation for which health benefits have been estimated.

Ethically Informed Decisions

Both BCA and CEA focus on the efficient allocation of economic resources. Implicit in each approach are value judgments regarding the appropriate weighting of different types of effects. It is important that the users of BCA and CEA understand these ethical assumptions and consider their implications when making decisions. For CEA, ethical considerations include concerns that are inherent in the QALY measure, along with aspects of regulatory impacts that the QALY measure does not capture.

By itself, a QALY-based CEA cannot address an important and difficult set of distributive questions and choices, including how much priority to give to the sickest or the worst off in valuing health effects; when to allow modest benefits to many people to outweigh significant benefits to fewer; and when to allocate resources to produce "best outcomes" as compared with giving more people fair chances to receive some benefit. For example, some health risks subject to regulation disproportionately affect those in poor health already. This raises the question of whether it is appropriate to weight health improvements differently for persons with and without impaired health, given that "postregulatory" health status will be worse for the former than for the latter.

The summary, the aggregate nature of a net benefit estimate or a cost-effectiveness ratio implies that it will not provide information on the distribution of regulatory benefits or costs in a population; such measures sum the effects on those who gain or lose under the regulation. A QALY is valued the same (e.g., at 1.0 if in perfect or optimal health) regardless of who is affected. Therefore, one of the most difficult issues to address in structuring a regulatory CEA is whether and how to disaggregate impacts that occur in different components of the general population.

The basic values embedded in our political system and reflected in federal regulatory guidance require that decision makers consider the distributional implications of regulations. As a result, such considerations must be explicitly introduced into the process of developing and issuing regulations along with the summary analytic results. The most basic normative commitment from using QALYs as an outcome measure in CEA is valuing some form of *life years*, rather than the number of lives saved. This difference between treating all deaths prevented equivalently and estimating losses and gains in longevity across the affected population is illustrated by an example in Table ES-1. The table shows that the use of lives as an impact measure assigns the same value to preventable mortality regardless of whether the individual is middle aged or elderly, while the use of life years shows that such mortality more significantly affects younger individuals. Adjusting for HRQL increases the relative differences between older and younger people slightly, as shown by the ratios in the rows for life year and QALY estimates in Table ES-1. The standard practice of discounting to reflect the timing of the impacts and the general preference for receiving gains sooner and deferring losses, reduces this relative difference considerably, however.

Summary BCA and CEA measures also omit both costs and benefits that cannot be easily expressed in numerical terms, either because the scientific research base is inadequate to support quantified estimates or because

TABLE ES-1 Lives, Life Years, and Quality-Adjusted Life Years (QALYs)

	Preventable Deaths	Life Years[a]	QALYs[b]
Age (in years)			
5	1	73	65
35	1	44	37
75	1	12	9.1
Ratio of values by age			
5/35	1	1.7	1.8
5/75	1	6.1	7.1
35/75	1	3.7	4.1

NOTE: These calculations are undiscounted. Discounting future life years and QALYs diminishes the differences between results for younger and older persons.

[a]Based on age-specific life expectancy for 2002 (NCHS, 2005).
[b]Based on EQ-5D norms for the U.S. population (Hanmer et al., 2006).

values have not been developed for those impacts. For example, it may be difficult to estimate the impact of a regulation on endangered species or to determine the value of reduced species diversity. Similarly, certain aspects of the risks, such as the extent to which individuals dread the prospect of lingering illness, typically are not captured in valuation. QALY-based CEA tracks only impacts on health and longevity, and it cannot account for the nature of the risk itself and societal perceptions and values related to it. Knowledge of risks, degree of personal control over risk exposures, and other features of risks may affect the justification for regulatory action as well as the value placed on the resulting risk reductions. These risk features deserve explicit consideration by decision makers alongside the summary results of economic analyses.

The failure to account for the distinctive features of risks may in some circumstances lead to misinterpretation when cost-effectiveness ratios for different regulations are compared. CEA is a tool for determining the relative efficiency of different interventions to achieve a defined objective, such as maximizing life-year or QALY gains. Ignoring other qualitative features of the risks involved or the contexts of the risks may well produce misleading comparisons of different regulatory options or interventions and lead to poor societal and regulatory decisions.

Conclusions and Recommendations

The Committee's investigations, analyses, and deliberations led to the following overarching conclusions.

- CEA, like BCA, offers a useful tool for the development and assessment of regulatory interventions to promote human health and safety. Different measures of effectiveness, including single-dimension units such as life years and units that combine estimates of HRQL and longevity such as QALYs, each provide useful perspectives on regulatory impacts.
- As in the case of BCA, the results of CEA for regulatory interventions are not by themselves sufficient for informed regulatory decisions. The results of economic analyses are routinely supplemented with other types of research and with information from the public to provide a more comprehensive assessment of the advantages and disadvantages of different regulatory strategies. These other sources of information are a necessary part of the decision-making process.
- Although it is feasible to apply CEA to regulatory interventions today, additional data and methodological improvements would enhance the quality and usefulness of such analyses.
- Federal regulatory agencies rely on disparate types of data and contemplate widely varying interventions and types of impacts. Consequently, they use diverse approaches to value health-related benefits. Greater consistency in the reporting of assumptions, data elements, and analytic methods and in presenting the resulting estimates of costs and benefits and summary measures (net benefits, cost-effectiveness) would increase the transparency and comparability of the results and lead to better informed policy decisions.
- Comparisons of cost-effectiveness ratios for diverse interventions can be misleading if they do not include information that highlights differences in methods, unmeasured effects, and distributional impacts across interventions.

These conclusions led the Committee to develop recommendations in four areas: selecting integrated measures of effectiveness; constructing and reporting cost-effectiveness ratios; presenting information for regulatory decision making; and collecting data and conducting research to improve HRQL measurement for regulatory CEA.

Selecting Integrated Measures of Effectiveness

The QALY is the best measure at present on which to standardize HALY estimation because of its widespread use, flexibility, and relative simplicity. QALY estimates may be based on newly collected information or on previously conducted research. The Committee recognizes that, in the near term, regulatory agencies are likely to rely on published research and to adopt relatively simple approaches for developing QALY estimates.

Recommendation 1: Regulatory CEAs that integrate morbidity and mortality impacts in a single effectiveness measure should use the QALY to represent net health effects.

- QALY estimates should be based, to the greatest possible extent, on research that considers the risk characteristics addressed and the population affected by the regulatory intervention.
- The index values estimated for health conditions or health states of interest should be based on information from the population affected by the costs, benefits, or other impacts of the regulatory intervention, which for most economically significant regulations will be best represented by the general U.S. population.
- In the absence of direct preference elicitation for health conditions of interest from the affected population, QALY estimates should be based on well-developed, generally accepted, and widely used generic HRQL indexes, whose valuation is based on general population samples.
- The characterization of the health states or conditions of interest using generic HRQL indexes should be based on information obtained from people who are familiar with the conditions, such as patients.

Constructing and Reporting Cost-Effectiveness Ratios

A central objective of the Committee's recommendations is to improve the quality and comprehensiveness of the information available to policy makers to promote well-informed regulatory decisions. We believe this objective can be met through the provision of measures of cost-effectiveness that are standardized to the extent practical within and across agencies. Because different measures have particular advantages and limitations, all regulatory CEAs should report more than one measure of effectiveness. Reporting a variety of measures provides decision makers with a more comprehensive understanding of the impacts of different regulatory choices and responds to different questions. It is also important to increase the transparency of the presentation of analytic assumptions, methods, and results in regulatory analyses.

Recommendation 2: Regulatory analyses should report four measures of cost-effectiveness:

- *Compliance cost per death averted* using the net number of deaths averted as the outcome measure.
- *Compliance cost per life year gained* using the net change in years of preventable mortality as the outcome measure.

- A *health-benefits-only ratio* using the net change in QALYs as the outcome measure. This ratio focuses on the value of health benefits. Costs would include those associated with compliance, offset by estimates of the net changes in health care treatment costs associated with the outcomes included in the QALY measure.
- A *comprehensive ratio* using QALYs as the outcome measure and incorporating the value of other benefits as offsets to compliance costs. The cost measure would incorporate both net changes in health care treatment costs and the value of any monetized nonhealth benefits as offsets.

Recommendation 3: The life-year and QALY estimates used in regulatory analyses should reflect actual population health as closely as possible, comparing the predicted HRQL and life expectancy of the affected population in the absence of the intervention (i.e., the regulatory baseline) to the predicted postintervention HRQL and health-adjusted life expectancy.

Recommendation 4: Incremental cost-effectiveness ratios are generally the most useful summary measure for comparing different regulatory interventions. Such ratios are not meaningful, however, for interventions that reduce both costs and risks. Options that are dominated (i.e., have higher costs and lower effectiveness) also should not be included in the incremental comparisons.

Recommendation 5: In addition to reporting effects in the aggregate, regulatory analyses should report QALY impacts separately for each health endpoint. Impacts should also be reported in terms of single-dimension measures such as avoided cases of disease and cause-specific mortality.

Recommendation 6: The reporting of all CEA results should be accompanied by information on related uncertainties and on nonquantified effects.

Recommendation 7: Regulatory analyses should not assign monetary values to estimates of HALYs as a method for valuing health states.

Presenting Information Needed for Regulatory Decision Making

Regardless of whether it relies on BCA or CEA, economic analysis is but one of many inputs into the policy-making process. The Committee endorses the emphasis in current policy guidance on considering the distribution of impacts, the ethical implications of different options, and the implications of nonquantifiable effects, and believes the results of CEA should continue to be one of many elements considered in a deliberative policy development process. Numbers can be very powerful in policy contexts; thus it is important that decision makers not only consider the results of economic analyses but also engage in deliberations with all constituencies and affected parties.

Recommendation 8: The regulatory decision-making process should explicitly address and incorporate the distributional, ethical, and other implications of a proposed intervention along with the quantified results of BCA and CEA. Comparisons of different interventions should highlight these distinctive features of the interventions and also any methodological differences, both in the case of cost-effectiveness ratios and of estimates of net benefits.

Recommendation 9: Because of the many value dimensions encompassed by societal decisions regarding the mitigation of risks to health and safety and the far-ranging impacts of such decisions, policy makers and program administrators should work to ensure the substantive involvement of a broad range of individuals and groups at all stages of policy development for regulating risks.

Collecting Data and Conducting Research to Improve HRQL Measurement and Regulatory CEA

Although useful for regulatory analysis, the data and methods currently available for measuring and valuing health in CEA have limitations that should be addressed by a long-term research agenda. The areas where additional routine data collection and research are most needed and likely to be fruitful include the following.

Recommendation 10: A high research priority should be improving the data used to assess the health risks (effects on incidence of particular types of illness, injuries, and deaths, and the duration and latency of effects) addressed by regulatory actions.

Recommendation 11: The Department of Health and Human Services (DHHS) and other federal agencies should collect HRQL information through routinely administered population health surveys and other major studies and data collection efforts related to risk assessment and monitoring.

Recommendation 12: DHHS should coordinate, with the involvement of federal regulatory offices and agencies, the development of an integrated research agenda to improve the quality, applicability, and breadth of HRQL measures for use in regulatory CEA. The Committee identifies the following areas as priorities for research:

- Methods for eliciting societal values for investments in health (such as person trade-off techniques).
- Methods for measuring children's HRQL, including characterization of the impact of illness and injury and the valuation of these impacts.
- Methods to correlate QALY values based on different generic HRQL indexes so that estimates from different underlying valuation surveys are consistent and can be used in the same analysis.

Given the substantial impact of major health and safety regulations on the national economy and societal welfare, it is imperative that related decisions be based on high-quality analyses, the results and limitations of which are clearly communicated in a form that is understandable by a wide variety of audiences. Because these rules vary significantly in the type of intervention, the characteristics of the affected population, and the characteristics of the risks addressed, benefit measures are needed that can apply to a broad range of health scenarios. These measures should be supplemented by discussion of any attributes of the scenarios that are not captured in the quantitative measures. Furthermore, the substantial uncertainty that accompanies the risk analysis that underlies the calculation of health-related effects, along with the uncertainty about the preference weighting of QALYs, should be conveyed in sensitivity and uncertainty analyses.

Finally, the process of developing and issuing regulations should be publicly accessible and based on information (including that used in BCA and CEA) that is comprehensible and communicated to a wide audience. Policy makers should facilitate the involvement of affected individuals, populations, and organizations in deliberations about health and safety risks and proposed interventions. Presenting the information for regulatory analysis fully and consistently is an important aspect of an accountable policy process.

1

Introduction

Promoting human health and safety by reducing exposures to risks and harms through regulatory interventions is a critical responsibility of government. Such efforts encompass a wide array of activities in many different contexts, such as improving air and water quality; safeguarding the food supply; reducing the risk of injury on the job, in transportation, and from consumer products; and minimizing exposures to toxic chemicals. Estimating the magnitude of the expected health and longevity benefits helps policy makers decide whether particular interventions merit the expected costs associated with achieving these benefits and informs their choices among alternative strategies. The results of such cost-effectiveness analyses (CEAs) can be one important contribution to the regulatory decision-making process.

This report of the Committee to Evaluate Measures of Health Benefits for Environmental, Health, and Safety Regulation provides recommendations and guidance on the valuation of health and safety improvements in CEA. More specifically, it considers how health-adjusted life-year (HALY) measures, which combine morbidity and mortality effects in a single index value, should be used to assess the benefits of regulatory interventions.

This introductory chapter first presents the Committee's charge in the context of recent policy guidance. It then describes the role of economic analysis in the regulatory development process. Next, it introduces CEA in more detail, noting how it differs from benefit–cost analysis (BCA). The chapter concludes with a brief overview of the remainder of the report.

THE CHARGE TO THE COMMITTEE

This report responds to a change in the requirements for economic analysis of major regulations developed by federal agencies. Until recently, agencies were required only to conduct BCAs, assessing both net impacts on the national level and their distribution across different subgroups of concern. In 2003 new government-wide requirements for CEA of major health and safety rules were added, and those are now being implemented by the agencies. The charge of this Committee is to provide advice related to these new requirements.

Background

Federal agencies are directed by executive order (and sometimes by statute) to estimate and report the expected benefits of proposed major regulations in conjunction with their estimated costs.[1] For economically significant health and safety rules, these analyses must generally include both a BCA and a CEA. BCA involves estimating the monetary value of benefits (e.g., improvements in human health or in the natural environment), then subtracting regulatory costs (e.g., related to industry compliance) to determine the net benefits of regulatory options. Ideally, the value of benefits is determined from estimates of willingness to pay (WTP) for the risk reductions or other impacts. In contrast, CEA involves dividing regulatory costs by a nonmonetary benefit measure (e.g., number of lives saved, cases of illness avoided, years of life gained, or tons of pollution reduced) to determine the unit costs of achieving the benefits.

When regulations reduce the risks of different kinds of illness or injury, or of both fatal and nonfatal effects, analysts may use measures that reflect impacts on health-related quality of life (HRQL) and longevity as the indicator of effectiveness. These measures are generally referred to as HALYs; the quality-adjusted life year (QALY) is the most common HALY metric. HALY measures convert different types of health effects to a composite unit so that regulatory costs can be compared to a single measure of health-related effectiveness.

Until recently, guidelines for regulatory analysis focused on the conduct of BCA. In 2003, however, the U.S. Office of Management and Budget (OMB) within the Executive Office of the President (EOP) issued Circular A-4, *Regulatory Analysis*, which instructed executive branch agencies to

---

[1]Not all of the activities of regulatory agencies result in regulations subject to requirements for economic analysis. For example, the Food and Drug Administration's review and approval of new drugs does not involve issuance of regulations and is not subject to requirements for BCA or CEA.

begin conducting CEAs for economically significant health and safety regulations whenever feasible. The guidance also continues to require preparation of a BCA and assessment of the distribution of the impacts. The guidelines explicitly recognize that BCA and CEA provide different perspectives on the economic effects of regulatory interventions, in combination offering complementary and useful information for decision making. An additional rationale for requiring CEA offered by OMB is that it facilitates cross-program comparisons (see Box 1-1).

BOX 1-1
OMB's Rationale for Requiring CEA
as Part of Regulatory Analysis

In remarks to a 2003 conference on Valuing Health Outcomes at Resources for the Future, John Graham, Administrator of the Office of Management and Budget's (OMB's) Office of Information and Regulatory Affairs, gave the following rationale for requiring the conduct of regulatory cost-effectiveness analyses (CEAs) in addition to benefit–cost analyses (BCAs) (Graham, 2003b):

". . . CEA is useful because it provides information about which regulatory alternatives will produce the most health gains per unit of resource investment. It is a 'bang for the buck' exercise, where the payoff is measured in health units rather than dollars. My experience as both a professor and government administrator is that some people who are skeptical of traditional benefit–cost analysis gain insight from the cost-effectiveness perspective. I think it is instructive that the peer-reviewed medical and public health literature is far more dominated by CEA than BCA . . . . Since the CEA only provides relative comparisons, we need BCA to determine whether the benefits of any particular alternative justify the costs."

". . . In order to promote more consistency, OMB will be sponsoring interagency discussions about the most promising and practical effectiveness measures. We will also request that agencies supply OMB their original data on mortality and morbidity. OMB will then be in a position to compare rulemakings across agencies using similar methods and assumptions. The Administration is moving with determination toward more performance-based budgeting, and a greater focus on cost-effectiveness and net benefits should be helpful in budgeting."

"In BCA, the monetary valuation of lifesaving is as important as it is controversial . . . . While these issues are crucial in BCA, they may be considered less important for CEA. In the health field, CEA is often defended partly on a social-contract basis rather than on a pure free-market basis. Here is a version of the social-contract argument. In what the late John Rawls called the 'original position,' where citizens are blinded by a 'veil of ignorance' to their own age, health status and wealth, they might rationally prefer a social contract that would maximize the number of healthy life years saved through public policy, given the resources available. Of course, I am not aware of any interest groups in this town who are prepared to wear this veil of ignorance when they visit Congress or OMB, but that is 'just' a practical problem!"

These remarks suggest that OMB is interested in the use of CEA for two purposes: to inform the decisions regarding the selection of a regulatory approach to a particular problem and to aid in cross-program comparisons of performance. Such comparisons, sometimes referred to as "league tables" or "scorecards," might, for example, involve comparing the cost per life saved across programs that address air pollution, foodborne disease, and automobile accidents. In contrast, the selection of regulatory approaches involves within-program comparisons, such as different options for reducing the emission of a particular air pollutant.

To support these applications of CEA, OMB asked the Institute of Medicine (IOM) to evaluate various cost-effectiveness methodologies and assess their theoretical soundness, feasibility, and ethical underpinnings and implications, as well as to provide recommendations and guidance to federal agencies regarding the use of these measures in regulatory analysis. This report aims to help agencies understand the strengths and weaknesses of various health measures used in CEA, and demonstrates their application. It also provides advice on the appropriate consideration of cost-effectiveness within the larger decision-making context. The report builds on the work of the U.S. Panel on Cost-Effectiveness in Health and Medicine (PCEHM), which published its recommendations in 1996 (Gold et al., 1996b), and on the work of an earlier IOM Committee on Summary Measures of Population Health (IOM, 1998). It also benefits from the work of the National Research Council Committee on Estimating the Health-Risk-Reduction Benefits of Proposed Air Pollution Regulations (NRC, 2002).

The Task

OMB's Office of Information and Regulatory Affairs and a consortium of federal agency sponsors charged the IOM Committee to identify existing and proposed measures of benefits for use in regulatory CEA, to describe and evaluate these measures, to recommend a subset of measures to be considered for use by federal regulatory agencies, and to identify areas of research needed to enhance the development and consistent use of such benefit measures by the agencies.

Specifically, the Committee was asked to:

- *Describe current practices among federal agencies for evaluating the costs and outcomes of regulatory measures.*
- *Review measures of health benefits currently used in CEA, including specific instruments and assessment techniques applied to value health within these composite measures.*
- *Develop criteria for choosing among measures potentially useful in the evaluation of health outcomes of regulatory actions.*

- *Assess the various measures of health benefits in terms of their data requirements and feasibility of application, theoretical validity, appropriateness for special populations (children, ethnic minorities), and ethical implications.*
- *Recommend measures appropriate for use by federal agencies in evaluating the health outcomes of regulatory actions in light of the Committee's criteria.*
- *Construct CEA case studies, using information from published BCAs, to illustrate the impact of alternative measures of health benefits within CEA and to compare the CEAs and BCAs.*
- *Discuss criteria for identifying regulations for which CEA of regulatory impacts would be informative.*
- *Recommend research that would improve the measurement of health benefits in regulatory analyses.*

The sponsors' charge specifically directed that aspects of CEA other than the measurement and valuation of health benefits—discounting, for example—be considered only as they relate to the question of valuing health benefits.[2] The charge also specified that the Committee should refrain from examining methods for assigning a monetary value to HALY measures. The Committee does, however, comment more generally on the practice of using monetized HALY measures in BCA.

To respond to the charge, in March 2004 the IOM constituted a 16-member committee of experts in health services research, environmental health, economics, psychology and survey research, statistics and epidemiology, decision analysis, ethics, law and regulatory policy, and disability policy. This report represents the Committee's findings, conclusions, and consensus recommendations.

THE ROLE OF ECONOMIC ANALYSIS IN REGULATORY DEVELOPMENT

The process for developing major regulations is complex and often spans several years. It involves numerous individuals ranging from technical experts within the agencies to political appointees in the executive branch, and may include members of Congress and the judiciary, as well as a large number of interest groups and individual citizens. The types of

---

[2]Throughout this report, we use the terms "value" and "valuing" in their broader, everyday senses, that is, to represent the worth, importance, or usefulness of something (such as a particular state of health). We do not use these terms in their narrower, economic meaning of monetary equivalent.

information considered are diverse, including factors such as technical feasibility and equity considerations as well as economic effects. Below, we briefly summarize the regulatory development process and the role of economic analyses (BCA and CEA) in related decision making as context for the remainder of this report. Chapter 2 builds on this discussion and provides more information on the types of regulations affected, the requirements for economic analysis, and current agency practices.

Regulatory Development Process

The starting point for the federal regulatory process is usually a statute passed by Congress that requires the development of regulations. These statutes identify, in general terms, the issues and goals that Congress expects the agencies to address and the goals of related regulations. Although the statute may also legislate some specific aspects of the regulations (as discussed in more detail in Chapter 2), executive branch agencies have primary responsibility for determining the detailed requirements.

Although the statute may include deadlines for regulatory action, or deadlines may be established by the courts if the action has been subject to litigation, the executive branch usually has some discretion in setting regulatory priorities. Thus the schedule for regulatory activity is determined by a combination of legal requirements, Presidential priorities, and Administration and individual agency preferences. This schedule is reflected in the regulatory agendas developed by each agency, which are published twice a year in the *Federal Register* and list all recently completed and planned regulatory actions.

Once an agency decides to move ahead with a regulation, it often convenes an internal agency workgroup to study the problem and identify regulatory options (see, e.g., EPA, 2003); generally a particular office has lead responsibility. The workgroup is likely to include personnel with expertise in related technical, scientific, economic, legal, health, and other issues. This workgroup or responsible office commissions related studies; the economic analysis is often one of several research efforts undertaken to support major rules. For example, separate studies may address the technical feasibility or effectiveness of different regulatory requirements, as well as the health risks associated with the hazard. Agency staff also engage in both informal and formal public outreach activities; public involvement may, in some cases, include public hearings or negotiations among directly affected groups and other interested parties. Based on the results of these efforts, agency staff prepare suggested regulatory language and supporting analyses, which are reviewed internally and then by OMB if the regulation is significant. Other agencies are involved in this review if the regulation has implications for their activities.

BOX 1-2
Key Requirements of the Administrative Procedure Act

Under the Administrative Procedure Act, the key process requirements that must be met are to provide notice to the public and to solicit public input. With exceptions only for emergency situations, all regulations must first be issued as a Notice of Proposed Rulemaking and published in the *Federal Register*. As part of the process, agencies establish a time period (often 90 days) during which interested citizens may submit comments. When the final regulation is published in the *Federal Register*, the agency's response to the comments is included. The final regulation is then incorporated into the Code of Federal Regulations.

The proposed regulatory language is then published in the *Federal Register*, along with a preamble that discusses the rationale for the overall regulation and its specific provisions and that summarizes the economic analysis. Related reports, including the complete economic analysis, are placed in a docket (and generally on the agency's website), where they can be reviewed by the general public.

This process is governed by statutory guidelines as well as by agency administrative directives. Under the Administrative Procedure Act (APA, 5 U.S.C. Art. 500 et seq.), agencies are required to provide supporting information and request comment from the public before finalizing the regulation.[3] These requirements are rooted in notions of due process and fairness and, if not strictly followed, the courts will rule that the regulation has not been appropriately issued. The APA requirements are summarized in Box 1-2.

Once the agency receives comments, the workgroup may reconvene to review the comments, determine whether additional analysis or public outreach is needed, and develop the final regulation and supporting analyses. The final regulation is then published in the *Federal Register* after review within the issuing agency as well as by OMB and other agencies. The economic analysis is generally updated to reflect any new information received as well as any changes in the regulatory requirements, and placed in the docket along with other supporting documentation. This documentation includes the comments received by the agency and the agency's detailed responses. The *Federal Register* preamble to the regulation generally summarizes the comments received and the agency's responses, provides information supporting and describing the final regulatory provisions, and sum-

---

[3]See Jacobson and Hoffman (2003) for more detailed information on these requirements.

marizes the economic analysis. The final rule may later be overturned by congressional action, the results of litigation, or new regulatory efforts.

Requirements for Regulatory Analysis and Decision Making

Within the legal framework and administrative process discussed above, the results of economic analyses (including both BCA and CEA) are one of many types of information considered by policy makers. Executive Order 12866, "Regulatory Planning and Review," establishes the Administration's basic approach to regulatory development and decision making. This Executive Order was issued by President Clinton in 1993 and reaffirmed by the current Bush Administration. Box 1-3 provides a brief review of its evolution.

BOX 1-3
History of Administrative Guidance on Regulatory Analysis

According to the Office of Management and Budget, or OMB (1997), requirements for regulatory analysis and centralized review can be traced back to the early 1970s. Initially, assessment efforts were directed narrowly at particular types of impacts. The Nixon Administration concentrated on reducing the burden of environmental regulations on business. Under President Ford, the focus shifted to inflation; ultimately, the members of Ford's Council on Wage and Price Stability concluded that a regulation would not be truly inflationary unless its social costs exceeded its benefits. As a result, benefit–cost analysis was required for major regulations; this requirement has persisted in modified form through today.

President Carter built on the Ford legacy, issuing Executive Order 12044, *Improving Government Regulations* (1978). This Executive Order established general principles for regulatory development and required analysis of regulations with major economic impacts. President Carter also initiated a process for centralized review of significant regulations.

President Reagan then made regulatory relief a cornerstone of his economic program and developed a more centralized system involving OMB review of agencies' major regulatory actions (1981). He issued Executive Order 12291, *Federal Regulation*, which required agencies to prepare benefit–cost analyses for major rules and instructed them to issue only those regulations that maximize net benefits. The first Bush Administration continued to adhere to these requirements.

In 1993, President Clinton issued Executive Order 12866, *Regulatory Planning and Review*. This Executive Order continued the Reagan requirements for centralized OMB review with some modifications, for example, to provide more public information on the review process. This Executive Order retained the requirements for benefit–cost analysis as well as the general principle that regulations should be issued only if their benefits justify the costs. The current Bush Administration has affirmed its commitment to Executive Order 12866, amending it only to change the roles and responsibilities of some of the officials involved in regulatory review.

Executive Order 12866 sets out basic principles for decision making and establishes a regulatory analysis and review process for ensuring that these principles are met. Some of its key provisions include:

- Ensuring that regulations are promulgated only when necessary.
- Establishing a regulatory development process that includes interagency coordination, centralized review, and public involvement.
- Requiring consideration of a wide range of impacts, including both those that can be expressed in quantitative terms and those that cannot.

The general regulatory philosophy supported by the Executive Order is expressed in its first section as follows:

> Federal agencies should promulgate only such regulations as are required by law, are necessary to interpret the law, or are made necessary by compelling public need, such as material failures of private markets to protect or improve the health and safety of the public, the environment, or the well-being of the American people (EOP, 1993, p. 1).

Subsequent sections of the Order implement this philosophy through a variety of requirements for analysis and review, which are further reinforced in OMB's 2003 Circular A-4, *Regulatory Analysis.* (This Circular is included as Appendix C.) The Circular expands the discussion of the types of market failures that may lead to the need for federal regulation, including externalities (e.g., actions that impose uncompensated benefits or costs on others, such as industrial pollution), market power related to imperfect competition or natural monopolies, and inadequate or asymmetric information. Both the Executive Order and the Circular direct that agencies should assess nonregulatory approaches (e.g., economic incentives or information dissemination) as well as a variety of types of regulatory options when considering how to address these problems. They also emphasize the need to consider the impact of regulations on different levels of government.

Much of Executive Order 12866 is focused on establishing a process for centralized review of regulations to ensure they meet the goals of the Order and of the Administration. This process includes interagency review and review by state, local, and tribal governments, as well as by OMB staff. In addition, the Executive Order requires agencies to involve the public in regulatory development, for example, by disseminating information on regulatory plans, providing opportunities for public comment, considering the use of consensual approaches such as negotiated rulemakings, and publishing information on the rationale for the regulation as well as the supporting analyses.

Executive Order 12866 also establishes the basic requirements for economic analysis of major regulations. These requirements concentrate on the comparison of benefits and costs, although the Order also notes that regulations should be designed to meet their goals in a cost-effective manner. More specifically, in its discussion of general principles, it notes:

> In deciding whether and how to regulate, agencies should assess all costs and benefits of available regulatory alternatives, including the alternative of not regulating. Costs and benefits shall be understood to include both quantifiable measures (to the fullest extent that these can be usefully estimated) and qualitative measures of costs and benefits that are difficult to quantify, but nevertheless essential to consider. Further, in choosing among alternative regulatory approaches, agencies should select those approaches that maximize net benefits (including potential economic, environmental, public health and safety, and other advantages; distributive impacts; and equity), unless a statute requires another regulatory approach (EOP, 1993, p. 1).

For economically significant regulations (defined in Box 1-4), the Executive Order establishes a number of specific analytic requirements. Consistent with its overall philosophy, the Order defines both costs and benefits broadly to include both economic impacts and other social welfare concerns such as fairness or equity, and indicates that both quantified and nonquantifiable impacts must be considered. Examples of benefits include "the promotion of the efficient functioning of the economy and private markets, the enhancement of health and safety, the protection of the natural environment, and the elimination or reduction of discrimination or bias"; examples of costs include

> the direct cost both to the government in administering the regulation and to businesses and others in complying with the regulation, and any adverse effects on the efficient functioning of the economy, private markets (including productivity, employment, and competitiveness), health, safety, and the natural environment" (EOP, 1993, p. 7).

BOX 1-4
Definition of "Economically Significant" Regulations

According to Executive Order 12866, regulatory actions are identified as economically significant if the resulting rule is likely to:

> Have an annual effect on the economy of $100 million or more or adversely affect in a material way the economy, a sector of the economy, productivity, competition, jobs, the environment, public health or safety, or State, local, or tribal governments or communities (EOP, 1993, p. 4).

This focus on both quantitative and qualitative benefits and on the distribution of impacts is reinforced by two additional executive orders that require agencies to address risks that disproportionately affect children and to address adverse human health or environmental effects on minority and low-income populations. The provisions of these executive orders are summarized in Box 1-5.

The analytic requirements established by these Presidential executive orders and defined more extensively in OMB Circular A-4 are discussed in more detail in Chapter 2 and in a background paper commissioned by the Committee (Robinson, 2004). Although the requirements apply specifically to significant regulations subject to OMB review, such analyses are often carried out for rulemakings that are not economically significant, as well as

---

BOX 1-5
Executive Orders

Executive Order 13045: Protection of Children from Environmental Health Risks and Safety Risks

In April 1997, President Clinton issued an Executive Order directing all federal agencies to (1) identify and assess health and safety risks that may disproportionately affect children, and (2) ensure that agency activities address such risks (EOP, 1997, p. 1). To meet these goals, the Order establishes a task force to address these issues, requires agencies to coordinate related research, and creates a forum to measure progress. In addition, the Order directs agencies, when proposing and promulgating regulations concerning these types of risks, to submit to the Office of Management and Budget (OMB) an evaluation of the regulation's effects on children and an explanation of why the regulation is preferable to other feasible alternatives considered.

Executive Order 12898: Federal Actions to Address Environmental Justice in Minority Populations and Low-Income Populations

This Executive Order was issued in 1994 by President Clinton, and establishes achieving environmental justice as part of the mission of executive branch agencies. Each agency is required to identify and address "disproportionately high and adverse human health or environmental effects of its programs, policies, and activities on minority populations and low-income populations" (EOP, 1994, p. 1). Specifically, the Order establishes an interagency working group to provide coordination and guidance, requires each agency to develop an environmental justice strategy, and establishes research priorities. Agency activities must include provisions for improving related research and data collection efforts, for ensuring greater public participation, and for identifying differential patterns of natural resource consumption among minority and low-income populations.

by independent federal agencies not subject to OMB review, such as the Consumer Product Safety Commission and the Nuclear Regulatory Commission. In addition, the Circular A-4 requirements are an important source of information on best practices for analysts outside of the federal government, including those working in state and local government, industry associations and public interest groups, and academia.

Both Executive Order 12866 and OMB Circular A-4 focus on choosing among different regulatory and nonregulatory options for meeting a particular policy goal, for example, to reduce exposure to a certain set of hazardous air pollutants or specific types of food contaminants. However, the resulting analyses are often also used for comparisons across different types of interventions (for example, comparing air pollution and food safety rules to other programs) to identify those that may be most cost-effective or produce the greatest net benefits.

Several of these broad comparisons of the cost-effectiveness of policy interventions have been published within the past few decades. An early paper (Morrall, 1986) compared the costs per life saved across 44 different risk-reducing regulations (see also Morrall, 2003). Such cross-program comparisons have also been provided as part of federal budget documents (e.g., EOP, 2002). A broader review was completed by Tengs and colleagues (1995), who considered the cost per year of life saved for 587 regulatory and nonregulatory interventions. Recently, Hahn (2005) provided an in-depth discussion of the advantages and limitations of these types of comparisons, which he refers to as regulatory "scorecards." Such comparisons have been encouraged by Congress. For example, since 1997 OMB has been required to prepare annual reports on the costs and benefits of federal regulations under the "Regulatory Right to Know Act" (Pub. L. No. 106–554) and its predecessors.

Summary

Within the current framework for regulatory development, economic analysis is one of many factors that must be considered by decision makers. Other considerations include the statutory requirements, the justification for regulatory action, the feasibility of nonregulatory as well as regulatory options, the potential effects of nonquantifiable impacts, the distribution and equity of the impacts, and the results of public involvement and comment.

BENEFIT–COST AND COST-EFFECTIVENESS ANALYSIS

Regulatory policy involves difficult and complex decisions about when and how to require changes in behavior to promote improvements in social welfare. By definition, these choices involve imposing costs on some organizations and individuals in order to provide benefits to the same or different groups. Thus determining when the benefits justify the costs is an inherent, important, and unavoidable part of regulatory decision making.

Contemporary approaches to the economic evaluation of the health and safety impacts of public policy actions have roots in several distinct intellectual traditions. Welfare economics, which provides the conceptual foundation for BCA, serves as the predominant framework for informing public decisions about the economic impact of regulatory interventions and resource allocation. Within this tradition, social welfare or well-being is understood as the aggregation of individuals' personal welfare, and personal well-being is defined as the satisfaction of individual preferences, valued in monetary terms. Although such valuation can, in theory, incorporate altruistic concerns for the well-being of others as well as consideration of equity, in practice it has been difficult to account for these types of factors. Traditionally, BCA has focused on economic efficiency—that is, on allocating resources to maximize social welfare—and is accompanied by separate assessment of the distribution of the impacts and equity concerns.

As welfare economics was developing in the mid-20th century, an alternative framework for evaluating technology and programs emerged within the fields of health services research and policy development. With the growth of publicly organized and financed systems of health care and the emergence of costly medical equipment and procedures, analytic tools to guide resource allocation and evaluate alternative technologies were needed. Public health policy analysts and planners adapted CEA to address the allocation of resources for clinical and public health interventions.

In health policy and planning contexts, health itself is often construed as a socially recognized need or essential good. This framework implies that the fulfillment of health needs should be exempt from direct competition with other claims on resources, and that health cannot be measured with the same currency as other goods or services. The perspective of health policy analysts and planners typically is to maximize population health rather than to satisfy individual preferences. Summary measures of population health, such as average life expectancy or, more elaborately, HALYs, serve as the unit of measurement; health outcomes are not translated into market values by monetization. Analytical approaches that take the maximization of population health rather than aggregated individual welfare as their aim have been called "extra-welfarist," although some argue that welfare economics can subsume these considerations (Culyer, 1991; Hurley, 2000; Adler, 2005).

These alternative frameworks offer different strategies for evaluating health and safety improvements. BCA, which monetizes health benefits by estimating individuals' willingness to pay to achieve a particular state of health or to avoid a fatal or nonfatal risk, lies comfortably within welfare economic theory. In contrast, CEA presents a given health outcome in terms of the monetary costs required to achieve it. The health outcome may be expressed either in single-dimension units such as a life year gained, or in terms of a construct such as a HALY measure that integrates longevity and morbidity. The extent to which the health outcome measures used in CEA are consistent with welfare economic theory remains controversial (Pliskin et al., 1980; Kopp et al., 1997; Dolan and Edlin, 2002; Krupnick, 2004), as discussed in more detail in Chapter 3.

The following sections first provide a brief overview of BCA, introducing concepts and practices that are referenced in subsequent sections of this report. This discussion is intended for those readers who are unfamiliar with this type of analysis; readers interested in a more detailed and technical discussion of BCA should reference one of the many available texts. We then turn to the main focus of this report and introduce CEA in more detail, providing the foundation for the extended discussion of related issues provided in the subsequent chapters of this report. We conclude with a summary of the factors that are difficult to capture in economic analysis, regardless of whether BCA or CEA is used.

The discussion is supplemented by a set of three case studies undertaken by the Committee, based on completed regulatory actions. These case studies summarize the BCA and/or CEA developed by the agencies and present the Committee's application of different HALY approaches. Aspects of these cases are used to illustrate more general analytic points throughout this report, and the case studies themselves are summarized in Appendix A.

Benefit–Cost Analysis[4]

In BCA, the desirable effects of policy actions (e.g., improvements in health and reductions in injury and loss of life) are compared with the costs associated with devoting resources to achieve these positive impacts. Both benefits and costs are calculated at the societal level, and measured in monetary terms to the extent possible. Net benefits, the extent to which the total benefits exceed total costs, can be compared across policy options to determine what intervention, if any, will maximize social welfare.

---

[4]Mishan (1971) is generally cited as the seminal work on BCA; Just et al. (2004) and Freeman (2003) provide more recent "state-of-the-art" discussions of related theory and practices. The current guidance on the application of these concepts in the context of regulatory analysis is summarized in Chapter 2 of this report as well as in Robinson (2004).

Valuation Approach

In BCA, valuation is based on the concept of individual utility, which refers to the sense of satisfaction or well-being that individuals derive from the goods and services they consume. Because it is not possible to measure utility directly, analysts generally rely on estimates of individual WTP or similar measures to determine the value of the impacts of regulations or other programs. Simply stated, this approach presumes that the monetary value of an intervention (e.g., a regulation) is equal to the maximum amount of money the affected population would be willing to pay to obtain the intervention, or the minimum amount of compensation it would require to forego the intervention.[5]

This approach is based on the concept of opportunity costs, recognizing that, because resources are limited, any decision to use them for one purpose means that they cannot be used for other purposes. The resulting analysis can help decision makers identify the policy option that provides the largest net gain to society, by investing limited economic resources in a way that maximizes social welfare. In other words, BCA focuses on determining the socially efficient use of economic resources.

In practice, costs are often defined to include the economic impacts of the *requirements* imposed by a regulation or other intervention, and benefits include the *outcomes* or goals associated with imposing the requirements.[6] Both costs and benefits may include offsetting effects; for example, a rule that requires expenditures to decrease hazardous air emissions from engines may lead to fuel cost savings, or a rule that requires treatment to remove a drinking water contaminant may lead to the use of chemicals that pose other risks. Because the end result is the calculation of net benefits (i.e., benefits minus costs), the distinction between costs and benefits does not need to be defined precisely as long as all impacts have the correct sign (positive or negative) and are not double counted.

Several different approaches for estimating monetary values are consistent with the framework that underlies BCA. The preferred method is to rely on observed market prices, as long as the market is reasonably competitive. Regulatory costs, such as those associated with installing pollution controls or administering a new program, often can be estimated

---

[5]The choice between using maximum WTP and minimum willingness to accept (WTA) compensation is often said to depend on whether the affected population has a right to the intervention (e.g., Mitchell and Carson, 1989; Freeman, 2003). Although WTP and WTA are not necessarily equal, in practice WTP is nearly always applied due to problems in the empirical measurement of WTA.

[6]For a more technical discussion that relates these measures to the underlying concepts of consumer and producer surplus, see for example Just et al. (2004) and Freeman (2003).

based on market data. However, the benefits of regulatory requirements, such as improvements in human health, generally reflect outcomes that are not normally bought or sold. Thus analysts must rely on other valuation approaches.

As noted earlier, the starting point for estimating monetary values is typically the concept of individual WTP: the maximum amount of money an individual would voluntarily exchange to obtain the improvement (e.g., reduced health risks or better health status), given his or her budget constraints.[7] For outcomes that are not directly traded in markets, researchers may estimate monetary values by asking individuals what they would be willing to pay for the improvement. These types of approaches, which include contingent valuation surveys, conjoint analyses, and similar research strategies, are generally referred to as "stated preference" methods. Alternatively, researchers may estimate WTP based on market behavior for related goods; these approaches are generally referred to as "revealed preference" methods. Wage-risk studies, which estimate the change in wages required for riskier jobs (using statistical methods to separate out other factors that affect wage levels), are one example of a revealed preference approach.[8]

These methods focus on individual WTP and may not fully capture the value an individual places on risk reductions or other benefits that accrue to fellow members of society. Although WTP studies could, in theory, be designed to include altruistic considerations, the extent to which this is accomplished in practice is debatable and may raise double-counting issues when WTP is summed across individuals (Jones-Lee, 1992; Viscusi et al., 1988). In addition, in some cases it may be appropriate to add components of a cost-of-illness (COI) measure to a WTP estimate to provide a more complete accounting of social welfare impacts, particularly if the WTP measure excludes costs borne by others (e.g., employers and insurers).[9]

---

[7]The application of this concept to the valuation of health impacts was introduced by Schelling (1968) and Mishan (1971).

[8]Wage-risk studies reflect the market equilibrium that results from workers' demands for wages and firms' willingness to supply jobs at these wage rates. See Freeman (2003) for a discussion of the relationship between the resulting estimates and WTP.

[9]In some cases, analysts rely on COI estimates as a substitute for WTP, when WTP studies of reasonable quality are not available for the health effect of concern. However, COI estimates are not a preferred measure of value from the perspective of welfare economics. Such estimates usually include medical expenses (e.g., for doctor visits, prescription medicine, hospital stays) and may also include lost work time (e.g., foregone earnings, decreased household production). However, they tend to understate WTP for risk reductions due, at least in part, to the exclusion of the value of lost leisure time and pain and suffering (EPA, 2000b, Appendix B; EPA, 2005b). This use of COI as a substitute for, or supplement to, estimates of WTP differs from its use in CEA, as discussed later in this chapter.

Calculation of Net Benefits

Once the benefits and costs of regulatory options are estimated, the monetary values can be aggregated and compared as part of the decision-making process. Several kinds of criteria can be applied to determine whether a policy is worth pursuing, given the BCA results. Perhaps the simplest formulation is the Pareto Principle, which states that a project is desirable (or economically efficient) if it makes at least one person better off, and makes no person worse off. Although attractive in theory, few policies meet this criterion because regulations impose costs or otherwise adversely affect at least some individuals or organizations.

To address this limitation, variations on this standard were developed by Kaldor and Hicks (Hicks, 1939; Kaldor, 1939).[10] These variations suggest that a project is desirable if it makes "the winners" (i.e., those who benefit) better off by an amount large enough to compensate "the losers" (i.e., those who are harmed); or, alternatively, that a project should be rejected if the losers could pay the winners to not pursue the policy and not be worse off. These criteria do not demand that actual compensation occur. The Kaldor-Hicks criterion forms the basis of the standard decision framework generally applied in BCA. This framework suggests that policies should not be pursued if costs exceed benefits, and, if more than one policy provides positive net benefits, the preferred choice is the option with the largest net benefits.

In practice, regulatory decisions are rarely, if ever, based solely on the results of a BCA. This type of analysis provides a useful framework for organizing and analyzing information, and increases the comparability of costs and benefits. To the extent that the costs and benefits of regulations can be quantified, it promotes the identification of economically efficient interventions. However, as discussed earlier in this chapter, decision makers must also weigh issues related to distributional impacts and equity and the potential effects of nonquantified factors, and they must respond to concerns raised by the public. As discussed in Chapter 2, statutory and other legal requirements also must be met.

Cost-Effectiveness Analysis

CEA constitutes another major practice for quantitative evaluation of policies for improving human health, safety, and longevity. In CEA, the

---

[10]See Mishan (1988) for a standard treatment of Kaldor-Hicks.

desirable effects of a policy option are not measured in dollars. Instead, they may be accounted for by single-dimension measures (e.g., cases of disease or injury averted, years of preventable mortality avoided, tons of emissions reduced) or with integrated metrics such as HALYs. The costs of each option are then divided by the effect measure to determine the cost per "unit" of benefit provided.

The following section provides general information on CEA and summarizes some of the key differences between CEA and BCA. The subsequent chapters of this report consider the use of CEA and (to a limited extent) BCA in regulatory analysis in more detail.

Valuation Approach

CEA is based on many of the same principles as BCA, reflecting similar concerns with social welfare and individual choice. Because CEA results in a ratio, consistent definition of what is counted as cost (the numerator) and what is counted as effect (the denominator) is of greater importance than in BCA. To promote comparability across analyses, practitioners have defined a "reference case" that includes recommendations for distinguishing between costs and benefits in the CEA context.

Valuation practices for health and safety CEAs have been developed largely in the context of health care policy, not regulation. In 1993, the U.S. Public Health Service appointed a group of 13 experts, the PCEHM, to consider issues related to improving the quality and comparability of CEAs used in health policy and medical decision making. In its 1996 report (Gold et al., 1996b), the PCEHM provides specific recommendations for measuring and distinguishing between costs and benefits. These recommendations, codified as a reference case from the societal perspective, are the current standards for best practices in this field.

The starting point for assessing the costs of an intervention is the same in CEA and BCA; both rely on the concept of opportunity costs as the basis for valuation and generally use the same approaches to estimate these costs. Both types of analysis also attempt to address all (nonnegligible) costs that are attributable to the intervention and its current and future consequences. CEA differs only in that analysts must be careful to exclude those costs that are addressed by the effectiveness measure to avoid double counting.

For health care programs, PCEHM recommends that, in the reference case, costs include changes in the use of health care resources, treatment-related changes in the use of non-health care resources, changes in the use of informal caregiver time, and changes in the use of patient time due to treatment.[11] PCEHM defines these cost components as follows (Gold et al., 1996b, pp. 179–181):

- Direct health care costs include those associated with medical services such as the provision of supplies (including pharmaceuticals) and facilities as well as personnel salaries and benefits.
- Direct non-health care costs include nonmedical resources used to support the intervention; the Panel's examples include the costs of child care while a parent is undergoing treatment, of dietary changes, and of transportation to and from a medical facility.
- Informal caregiver time reflects the unpaid time spent by family members or volunteers in providing home care. (Paid time for nursing and other medical care is included in the direct health care component.)
- Patient time involves the time spent in treatment, but not other changes in time use attributable to the health condition of concern. In particular, lost productivity due to illness is excluded from these costs in the reference case to avoid double counting; ideally the effects of illness on the patient's usual activities should be part of the effectiveness measure.

The first two categories involve goods and services for which payment is generally provided; thus monetary expenditures can be used to estimate related values. The latter two areas involve the use of uncompensated time, which is generally valued at the after-tax wage rate, under the assumption that (at the margin) this rate represents the opportunity cost of not engaging in paid work.

The Panel's recommendations focus on the use of CEA to assess health care interventions; the analysis of costs in a regulatory CEA involves additional considerations. First, the regulation itself imposes costs related to the actions it requires organizations and individuals to undertake. For example, an air pollution regulation may require the installation of emissions control devices to reduce the incidence of respiratory and cardiovascular conditions. Second, because the regulation is *preventing* health effects from occurring, the health care costs listed above accrue as *savings* rather than as expenditures. Third, regulations may have both health- and non-health-related benefits (e.g., reduced damage to ecological systems) that are not taken into account in health-related effectiveness measures and hence could

---

[11]The COI measures used in BCA may differ in some respects from these recommendations for CEA, particularly because they often include the effects of illness on lifetime earnings or productivity, rather than focusing only on the impacts directly associated with medical treatment.

conceivably be included as offsets to costs, as discussed in the Committee's recommendations.

Most health and safety regulations typically lead to more than one type of health benefit, in many cases preventing a range of different types of illnesses or injuries as well as increasing life expectancy. As a result, benefit measurement in regulatory CEAs is likely to rely on integrated HALY measures, such as QALYs, that allow analysts to combine information about various health conditions. These measures provide a common metric for estimating the HRQL impact of different conditions, which includes functioning in domains such as mobility, emotion, social activity, and self-care.

When these measures are applied, health states are assigned index values[12] that reflect their relative desirability or impact on health-related quality of life. These values are usually placed on a zero-to-one scale, where zero corresponds to death and one corresponds to perfect or optimal health. Nonfatal health impairments (disability and morbidity) are assigned intermediate values, with lower numbers representing more severe impacts. (Most indexes can accommodate negative values, representing impaired health states that have been valued as worse than death.) For public policy decisions, PCEHM recommends that these condition weights be based on the preferences of the general population ("community weights"), rather than those of patients or clinicians, to better reflect societal values (Gold et al., 1996b).

These index values are generally based on surveys that are similar in many respects to the stated preference surveys used to estimate WTP. Perhaps the most significant difference is the form of the valuation question. Rather than asking individuals what they would be willing to pay to avert a health risk, HALY surveys ask respondents about the relative desirability of different health states. Chapter 3 discusses the methods for constructing index values and the strengths and weaknesses of alternative approaches.

Once index values are estimated, they can be multiplied by the duration of each condition to determine the associated HALYs, multiplied by the number of cases averted for each health state, then added across conditions to create a single effectiveness measure. As discussed in subsequent chapters, these values are generally discounted to reflect the extent to which the impacts are spread over time.

The idea of using such summary health measures in CEA was introduced four decades ago (Chiang, 1965; Fanshel and Bush, 1970). In 1977,

---

[12]Throughout the report, we use the term "health state index value" for consistency. These index values are also referred to as "utility weights" or "preference weights" in the research literature.

Weinstein and Stason offered theoretical grounding and analytical guidelines for using QALYs to evaluate health and medical practices, noting that they combine information about changes in survival and morbidity in a way that reflects individuals' willingness to trade off between them. First employed to evaluate clinical medical interventions, QALYs compared relatively similar health conditions within an identifiable population, such as alternative surgical techniques to improve blood flow to the heart muscle in patients with coronary artery disease. QALYs have also been applied in assessing interventions that may affect a broader population (including currently healthy individuals), such as disease screening and vaccination programs.

In regulatory analysis, CEA is likely to involve the aggregation and synthesis of diverse health conditions, including, for example, acute and chronic effects that result to varying degrees in preventable mortality. In addition, regulatory analysis usually involves predicting outcomes that include small risk reductions spread throughout a large population. As a result, the assessment often focuses on "statistical" cases representing the aggregation of changes in risks across many individuals.[13]

The most obvious difference between these HALY or QALY measures and the WTP measures used in BCA is that the latter use dollars to represent the value placed on different health outcomes as well as other (non-health) impacts, whereas the former focus on index measures of HRQL and longevity. As a result, an individual's WTP may be constrained by his or her available resources, whereas HALY measures are, by design, independent of individuals' income or wealth. In practice, however, the income or wealth term is not always statistically significant in WTP studies and HALY measures may be influenced by individuals' income or wealth.[14]

These measures also differ in a number of other important respects. One key difference is that WTP indicates the extent to which individuals are willing to make trade-offs between different uses of resources, while HALY measures restrict the trade-offs to alternative health states. As discussed in Chapter 3, some commonly used HALY measures assume that the value placed on a given health state in the abstract does not depend on the duration of that health state; that is, regardless of whether the illness or impairment lasts for one day or several years, the index value is the same. In contrast, WTP studies can be constructed to include duration as one of the attributes addressed in valuation.

---

[13]For example, a regulation that prevents a risk of 1 in 10,000 from affecting a population of 10,000 individuals would prevent one statistical case: $1/10,000*10,000 = 1$.

[14]More extensive discussion of the differences between HALY measures and WTP is provided in Hammitt (2002) and Krupnick (2004).

These and other restrictions mean that, although HALY measures are based on surveys reflecting individual choices, these choices may not fully reflect individual preferences and are not entirely consistent with the tenets of utility theory that underlie welfare economics. Although HALY measures can be constructed in a way that at least partially reflects individual preferences, such measures often do not fully conform to the concept of utility as understood in economic theory.[15]

Calculation of Cost-Effectiveness

In CEA, the result of the analysis of costs and benefits is a ratio: the cost per unit of effect (e.g., the cost per QALY). When multiple strategies achieve the same outcome (e.g., each leads to the same reduction in the number of cases of heart disease per year), the cost-effectiveness ratios can be used to identify the most economically efficient approach, that is, the option that achieves the goal at the lowest cost.

However, regulatory options usually differ in the amount of both costs and benefits, and there is no general agreement on a standard for using CEA to select among the options. The one exception is where an option is *dominated*; that is, at least one other option under consideration is both more effective *and* less costly. In contrast, the decision criteria for BCA suggest that projects with negative net benefits (costs that exceed benefits) should not be pursued, and that the option that leads to the highest net benefits is the most economically efficient.

If the goal of an analysis is to allocate health care or other resources within a fixed budget, CEA can be used to inform the allocation of the budget across health-improving interventions and services. In the context of regulatory programs, there is no "regulatory budget" per se. Instead, decision makers are choosing among different options for pursuing a particular statutory or policy goal.

Some have argued for applying a cost limit as a guide when using CEA to allocate resources or to establish a threshold for policy action. For example, a number of values have been advocated as cost-per-QALY dollar thresholds that differentiate a worthwhile expenditure on a new medical technology or therapy from a poor one. Phelps and Mushlin (1991) have argued that, if such a threshold value is applied, CEA performs similarly to BCA; however, the assumptions necessary for complete equivalence are fairly restrictive. A wide range of limiting or threshold investments per

---

[15]CEAs using HALY metrics as the effectiveness measure are sometimes referred to as cost–utility analyses. This report uses the term "CEA" exclusively so as to not rely on assumptions about the consistency of HALY measures with the basic tenets of utility theory.

QALY have been proposed or cited as implicitly operative: from $50,000 to $160,000 and much higher per QALY (Hirth et al., 2000). There is no sanctioned, widely accepted threshold, however, at this time (Laufer, 2005; Neumann, 2005).

In the regulatory context, the cost-effectiveness ratio is useful in exploring the incremental effects of investing additional resources to address a particular problem or reduce a certain type of risk.[16] In addition to providing insights into the selection of regulatory options, these ratios have been used in the types of league tables and scorecards described earlier to identify the relative cost-effectiveness of different regulatory and nonregulatory interventions, particularly in terms of the costs per life or life year saved.

These ratios can be reviewed by decision makers to determine whether additional increments of investment are worthwhile, and to identify the types of interventions that appear most cost-effective. Subsequent decisions ultimately require the exercise of judgment, due to the lack of consensus on the "worth" of the additional health benefits achieved, and the need to consider factors not included in the quantitative analysis.

CEA is similar to BCA in that it provides a useful framework for collecting, analyzing, organizing, and reporting information on the impacts of regulatory options. It has the advantage of avoiding the need to assign monetary values to health and safety impacts, and thus may be more palatable to those who are uncomfortable with monetization of these types of benefits.[17] However, the decision to implement a regulation ultimately involves commitment to a predicted level of expenditure or cost, implicitly assigning a monetary value to the quantified and nonquantified benefits.

CEA also faces many of the same challenges as BCA. HALY measures are based on survey techniques that use different types of instruments, but otherwise face some of the difficulties encountered in the use of stated preference studies to estimate WTP, as discussed in Chapters 2 and 3. In addition, as traditionally practiced, both CEA and BCA focus on economic efficiency and confront decision makers with the need for supplemental information on distributional effects and equity issues. As with all assessment methods, CEA and BCA both produce somewhat incomplete and uncertain quantitative estimates because of gaps in the underlying research base. However, well-structured economic analyses of both types can help to identify the sources and extent of uncertainties and indicate the types of research that would be most useful.

---

[16]For more detailed discussions of the calculation and interpretation of incremental cost-effectiveness ratios, see Drummond et al. (1997), Hunink et al. (2001), and Fenwick et al. (2004).

[17]For more detailed critiques of BCA, see, for example, Ashford (1980), Lave (1996), and Kopp et al. (1997).

Summary

Prospective analysis of the predicted economic effects of regulatory interventions helps participants in the regulatory development process anticipate and weigh the likely consequences of possible courses of action. Both BCA and CEA provide a structured framework for conducting research on possible impacts and presenting the results. Such research can affect not only the policy decision, but also public perceptions and understanding of both the policy process and the action taken. BCA and CEA both have the potential to improve the accountability of government by presenting information about the costs and benefits of a proposed intervention (and the reasons bearing on the ultimate decision) in comprehensible, transparent, and comprehensive terms.

BCA and CEA provide complementary measures of outcomes. BCA focuses on determining the net benefits of an action, that is, which regulatory option provides the greatest increase in welfare, net of any harm or cost imposed. BCAs generally use estimates of WTP to value both health-related impacts and other effects on welfare, such as environmental effects. In contrast, CEA focuses on the cost per unit of benefit, that is, the ratio of costs relative to a unit of improvement. CEAs based on HALY measures account for both the impacts on HRQL and longevity. Both types of analysis usually also report single-dimension measures of impacts, such as cases of illness or injury averted, or years of life extended. As typically implemented, both approaches focus primarily on economic efficiency and must be supplemented by other sources of information.

In particular, most policy makers are concerned with the distributional and ethical consequences of their choices. In the case of BCA, the Pareto Principle and the hypothetical compensation criterion take as given the distribution of resources at the regulatory baseline. Some argue that this presumption implicitly endorses that distribution as a just or fair starting point. Although CEA avoids this problem in part, it does not address the distributive implications of a regulatory action. The results of both BCA and CEA can be presented in disaggregate form to indicate the impact on different subgroups of concern. Ultimately, however, decision makers must engage in collective reasoning, consider additional information and the views of the public, and exercise judgment to determine whether the resulting distribution of costs and benefits argues in favor of an option that differs from the approach that provides the largest net benefits or appears most cost-effective across all groups. The incorporation of these sorts of deliberative processes is discussed in Chapter 4.

Furthermore, both BCA and CEA inevitably provide somewhat incomplete and imperfect estimates of regulatory impacts. Analysts may find it difficult to quantify all the major impacts of the regulatory options, and the results may be subject to significant uncertainty. Although these difficulties may reflect in part the limited time or resources available for a particular analysis, they often reflect more fundamental problems related to the status of the underlying scientific research base. For example, the relationship

TABLE 1-1 Comparison of Key Features of BCA and CEA

Approach for Valuing Benefits	Willingness to Pay	Health-Adjusted Life Year
Accounts for health-related impacts	Yes	Yes
Accounts for nonhealth impacts, such as ecological effects	Yes	Excluded from effect measure, may be included as an offset to costs
Accounts for altruistic values or concerns about impacts on others	Depends on study design	Depends on elicitation method and question
May be influenced by income or wealth	Yes	No
Consistent with utility theory	Yes	Only under restrictive assumptions
Summary Measure	**Net Benefits**	**Cost-Effectiveness Ratio**
Decision criteria	The option where benefits exceed costs by the largest amount is the most economically efficient; options with benefits less than costs should not be selected	Compare the incremental cost-effectiveness of different options to determine whether an increase in the effect measure is worth the increase in cost; options that are dominated (i.e., have higher costs and lower benefits than others) should not be selected
Incorporates assessment of uncertainty	Yes	Yes
Indicates the equity or fairness of the distribution of impacts	No, must be assessed separately	
Indicates the importance of impacts that cannot be measured in quantifiable terms	No, must be assessed separately	

between a specific hazard addressed by a regulation (e.g., air pollution, contaminants in food or water) and health risks may not be well understood by scientists. As a result, both BCA and CEA reports must discuss the uncertainty of the estimates and highlight important impacts that could not be quantified.

Table 1-1 summarizes the key similarities and differences between BCA and CEA based on the overview contained in this chapter. Other differences in the implementation of these approaches are discussed in Chapter 2. The table focuses on what is possible under each approach; in reality, deficiencies in the research base or other factors may limit the ability of a particular analysis to include all of the features noted in the table. The Committee encountered some of these challenges in conducting the three case studies, as discussed later in the report.

ORGANIZATION OF THE REPORT

This chapter introduced the charge of the Committee, provided an overview of the regulatory development process, identified key features of BCA and CEA, and noted their important differences. This last section outlines the organization of the remainder of the report.

Chapter 2 discusses current practices for the conduct of regulatory economic analyses and reviews the various approaches used by individual federal agencies.

Chapter 3 presents criteria for selecting integrated measures and survey instruments, reviews alternative HALY measures and HRQL survey instruments, and describes different strategies to obtain estimates for regulatory CEA.

Chapter 4 reviews the aspects of risk regulation that policy makers need to consider that are *not* reflected in the cost-effectiveness ratios, including ethical issues related generally to CEA as well as those related to the population and risk characteristics that are not fully captured in the effectiveness measures.

Chapter 5 concludes the report by presenting the Committee's recommendations for valuing health benefits in the economic analysis of regulations, including recommendations for additional research and data collection.

The appendixes to this report discuss three case studies of regulatory CEAs that the Committee conducted in collaboration with federal agency staff (Appendix A), include commonly used HRQL survey instruments (Appendix B), and provide the full text of OMB Circular A-4 (Appendix C). A glossary and list of acronyms are also included as Appendix D.

2

Characteristics of Major Regulations and Current Analytic Practices

The U.S. Congress has granted the executive branch broad authority to develop regulations addressing health and safety risks. At the federal level, the Office of Management and Budget (OMB) has primary responsibility for coordinating and reviewing the economic analyses that support these regulations, and has developed detailed guidelines for these analyses. This chapter builds on the information provided in Chapter 1 to discuss the general approaches to health and safety regulations authorized by Congress and summarizes current practices for analyzing their impacts. It provides background and context for the Committee's recommendations.

TYPES OF RISK REGULATIONS

The starting point for the issuance of federal regulations is authorizing legislation developed by Congress. This legislation generally establishes a legal basis or standard for the regulations and lays out the considerations to be taken into account by the agency in developing the regulations. Although the government issues thousands of different types of regulations each year, only a few are economically significant health and safety regulations subject to the OMB requirements for benefit–cost analysis (BCA) and cost-effectiveness analysis (CEA). If the relevant statute prohibits the consideration of costs or BCA, then the executive branch cannot countermand the statute in developing the regulation. (See *Whitman v. American trucking* (U.S. S. Ct. 2001).) The use of economic analysis in developing regulations has been subject to judicial challenge and may be upheld or rejected depending on the wording of the specific statute.

Statutory Standards

Under the U.S. Constitution, Congress has wide authority, upheld by the courts, to enact legislation to protect the public's health and safety. The U.S. Supreme Court has generally permitted Congress to delegate this discretion to the federal regulatory agencies. When Congress authorizes individual agencies to examine particular risk exposures, such as those associated with air or water pollution, it may establish an approach based on health alone (prohibiting consideration of cost); on the best available technology (including the consideration of cost); on feasibility (which depends on cost but not on BCA); on the least burdensome alternative to achieve a given goal (implying CEA); or on reasonableness (implying BCA). At times the legislation will be silent as to the type of standard or will take a mixed approach. Many of these authorizing statutes have both health- and non-health-related goals; for example, they may require that agencies address impacts on the natural environment as well as on human health. In addition, some statutes establish other factors that must be considered, such as the impact on sensitive populations.

The following discussion sketches the statutory and regulatory context for the economic analyses of regulations that are the subject of this report and of the Committee's recommendations. We consider legislative standards and procedural requirements for agency deliberations and policy determinations, supplementing the discussion of the regulatory development process in Chapter 1.

Health-Based Requirements

Health-based statutes establish a general goal of reducing the risks of death, illness, and injury. In Section 3(8) of the Occupational Safety and Health Act of 1970, for example, Congress gave the Secretary of Labor broad regulatory authority to adopt standards "reasonably necessary or appropriate to provide safe or healthful employment." Section 6(b)(5), for toxics, requires the Occupational Safety and Health Administration (OSHA) to "set the standard which most adequately assures, to the extent feasible, on the basis of the best available evidence, that no employee will suffer material impairment of health or functional capacity. . . ." Immediately following OSHA's benzene and cotton dust regulations, industry groups argued that the statutory language required OSHA to use BCA in promulgating regulations. However, after a series of cases, the Supreme Court concluded that the statute did not require OSHA to use BCA and that the agency could instead rely on epidemiological and other scientific findings to establish safe levels of exposure.

Even though nothing in a health-based statute may prohibit an agency from taking costs into account, the courts expect regulatory actions to be based on sound scientific evidence that establishes an appropriate level of public safety. Indeed, one concern about a health-based standard is whether it amounts to zero tolerance. Except for a now-repealed amendment that explicitly enacted a zero-tolerance standard for new food additives, courts have provided agencies with considerable discretion to issue regulations that focus on more significant risks to human health and safety.

On occasion, Congress has specified a threshold of risk exposure. For example, Section 112 of the Clean Air Act set a threshold that certain carcinogenic emissions must be controlled if they produce an incremental risk of cancer of 1 in 1 million over a lifetime. For the most part, the risk exposure thresholds are established by the agencies as part of the regulatory development process. For example, the Environmental Protection Agency (EPA) explicitly considers health risk in hazardous waste listing decisions under the Resource Conservation and Recovery Act. Where the individual incremental cancer risk exceeds 1 in 100,000 over a lifetime, a wastestream will be considered for listing, and if the cancer risk exceeds 1 in 10,000, there is a presumption that listing is required (Hazardous Waste Management System, 59 Fed. Reg. 66,072, 66,077 (1994)). OSHA uses a 1 in 1,000 threshold for occupational exposures that create fatality risks (Adler, 2003).

Section 112 of the Clean Air Act, which regulates hazardous air pollutants, directs the Administrator to set an emission standard "at the level which in his judgment provides an ample margin of safety to protect the public health." In *NRDC v. EPA*, 824 F.2d 1146, 1164 (D.C. Circuit 1987), the court interpreted what constitutes an ample margin of safety by noting that:

> This language permits the Administrator to take into account scientific uncertainty and to use expert discretion to determine what action should be taken in light of that uncertainty. . . . Once "safety" is assured, the Administrator should be free to diminish as much of the statistically determined risk as possible by setting the standard at the lowest feasible level.

Other statutes also focus on reducing unreasonable risks to health, such as the Federal Insecticide, Fungicide, and Rodenticide Act; and the Consumer Product Safety Act. In general, such statutes may also require agencies to take other factors into account, such as harm to natural resources or ecological risks.

Technology-Based Requirements

Statutes may require that agencies apply the "best available technology" (BAT) in setting regulatory standards. The BAT approach allows the regulatory agency to consider a range of factors, including costs, but it usually does not require industry to develop new technologies. Rather, it requires industry to adopt available technologies to reduce emissions or toxic exposures. But stating such requirements is much easier than implementing them. As noted in *NRDC v. EPA*, 863 F.2d 1420, 1427 (9th Cir. 1988):

> Technology-based limitations under BAT must be both technologically available and economically achievable. To be technologically available, it is sufficient that the best operating facilities can achieve the limitation. To demonstrate economic achievability, no formal balancing of costs and benefits is required; BAT should represent a commitment of the maximum resources economically possible. . . . EPA has considerable discretion in weighing the costs of BAT.

Hybrid Requirements

The above types of standard-setting requirements may be combined as well as supplemented with other factors for consideration by regulators. For example, Section 112 of the Clean Air Act first requires industries to use maximum achievable control technology standards to reduce toxic emissions, but then requires EPA to promulgate more stringent regulations if excess cancer risks exceed a threshold of 1 in 1 million. Thus, for example, the nonroad diesel rule (the subject of one of the Committee's case studies) was authorized by two separate provisions of the Clean Air Act, which differ in focus. Section 213 is BAT based, instructing EPA to set standards that achieve the largest emissions reduction achievable through the use of available technology and allowing the EPA Administrator to consider the cost, lead time, noise, energy, and safety factors associated with the application of such technology. In contrast, Section 211(c) requires EPA to regulate fuels as needed to reduce adverse effects on human health or welfare, as well as to prevent impairment of emissions control devices.

Another example of a hybrid approach is the Safe Drinking Water Act. This statute requires EPA to set standards that are as close as "feasible" to the level at which there are no known or anticipated adverse health effects associated with exposure to the contaminant, taking into account an adequate margin of safety and considering the effects on sensitive subpopulations. "Feasible" is defined as the use of the best technology and treatment techniques examined for efficacy under field conditions, taking cost into consideration (Section 1412(b)(4)(D)). However, EPA can, at its discretion, establish an alternative standard that "maximizes health risk reduction benefits at a cost that is justified by the benefits" (Section 1412(b)(6)(A)), with certain exceptions for small water systems.

This balancing of costs and benefits has been upheld by some courts, which have required agencies to consider the costs of a regulation as well as its benefits. For example, the Fifth Circuit has stated with respect to both the Occupational Safety and Health Act and the Toxic Substances Control Act (TSCA) that the government must show ". . . substantial evidence that the benefits to be achieved [by a regulation] . . . bear a reasonable relationship to the costs imposed by the reduction [before it can] . . . show that the standard is reasonably necessary to provide safe or healthful workplaces" (*American Petroleum Institute v. OSHA*, 581 F.2d 493, 504 (5th Cir. 1978); *Corrosion Proof Fittings v. EPA*, 947 F.2d 1201, 1223 (5th Cir. 1991)).

Several statutes identify other types of factors that an agency must take into account in developing regulations. Some require consideration of particular aspects of the health risks addressed. For example, the Food Quality Protection Act requires consideration of the susceptibility of infants and children to pesticide residues (Section 408(b)(2)(C)).

Others require certain types of analysis. In the case of SDWA, the 1996 amendments require the assessment of costs and benefits and identify factors that must be addressed. In particular, EPA must consider:

• the quantifiable and nonquantifiable health risk reductions associated with controlling the contaminant of concern and any co-occurring contaminants;

• the costs of compliance with the control requirements;

• the incremental costs and benefits associated with each alternative under consideration;

• the effects of the contaminant on the general population and on groups within the population that are likely to be at greater risk of adverse health effects from drinking water contaminants, "such as infants, children, pregnant women, the elderly, and individuals with a history of serious illness";

• the increased health risks, if any, that may result from compliance with the proposed standard, including risks associated with co-occurring contaminants; and

• other relevant factors, including the quality of the available information supporting the analysis, the uncertainties in the analysis, and factors relating to the degree and nature of the identified risks (Section 1412(b)(3)(C)(i)).

Thus it is important for regulatory agencies to generate scientific bases for rules and to consider the least restrictive alternatives (i.e., those least burdensome to industry), but to also balance costs and benefits, usually through BCA or CEA. In reviewing challenges to regulations, courts will not prescribe which general methodology an agency should use to estimate costs and benefits. As noted later, however, courts will not hesitate to question the particular methods and reasoning that agencies use in constructing their analyses.

Examples of Recent Regulations

As noted in Chapter 1, the federal requirements for CEA that are the subject of this report apply mainly to economically significant health and safety regulations. To identify the types of regulations that may be subject to these requirements, the Committee commissioned a review focusing on those agencies that recently issued economically significant regulations with quantified health and safety impacts, and/or that were in the process of doing so (Robinson, 2004). This review identified seven such agencies: EPA, the Food and Drug Administration (FDA), the Food Safety and Inspection Service (FSIS), OSHA, the National Highway Traffic Safety Administration (NHTSA), the Federal Motor Carrier Safety Administration, and the Consumer Product Safety Commission (CPSC).[1]

From January 2000 through June 2004, these agencies finalized 18 economically significant regulations with quantified health and safety impacts, listed in Table 2-1. Although they represent a relatively small proportion of all regulations issued each year, these regulations have substantial effects. For example, in fiscal 2003, an OMB summary indicates that only 3 of the 4,312 final rules published were economically significant rules with quantified health and safety benefits (OMB, 2003b, 2004). However, the 18 rules listed in Table 2-1 had estimated net benefits totaling close to $200 billion annually. If only costs are considered, six of these rules resulted in annual costs estimated to be greater than $1 billion. In terms of benefits, eight of the rules had estimated gross annual benefits exceeding $1 billion and, of these, three had estimated gross annual benefits exceeding $10 billion.

The majority of the quantified benefits addressed in these regulations were those attributable to EPA requirements for control of air pollution. Related benefits include increased life expectancy (the avoidance of premature mortality or preventable deaths), as well as reduced morbidity related to respiratory and cardiovascular effects. The other regulations addressed a wide variety of acute and chronic conditions as well as various types of injuries, which led to varying degrees to preventable mortality.

The Committee's review also identified several economically significant

---

[1]CPSC is an independent agency not subject to OMB review. It is included in this discussion because it is currently working on economically significant rules with safety impacts.

TABLE 2-1 Summary of Recent Major Health and Safety Rulemakings (January 1, 2000–June 30, 2004)

Agency	Authorizing Statute(s)	Rulemakings
EPA: Office of Air and Radiation	Clean Air Act	• New vehicle emissions • Heavy-duty diesel engines • Spark ignition engines • Reciprocating internal combustion engines • Nonroad diesel engines
EPA: Other offices	Toxic Substances Control Act; Safe Drinking Water Act	• Lead paint abatement • Arsenic in drinking water
FDA	Federal Food, Drug, and Cosmetic Act; Public Health Service Act	• Shell egg labeling and storage • Juice processing • *Trans* fat labeling • Dietary supplements containing ephedrine alkaloids • Bar codes for human drug products and blood
FSIS	Federal Meat Inspection Act; Poultry Product Inspection Act	• *Listeria* control in meat and poultry
OSHA	Occupational Safety and Health Act; Construction Safety Act	• Ergonomics program • Steel erection safety
NHTSA	Transportation Equity Act for the 21st Century; Transportation Recall Enhancement, Accountability, and Documentation Act	• Occupant crash protection (air bags) • Tire pressure monitoring
FMCSA	Interstate Commerce Commission Termination Act	• Truck driver hours of service

SOURCE: Robinson (2004).

regulations that the agencies were developing that were likely to include quantified health and safety impacts. The types of health impacts that the agencies expected to assess for these rules are listed in Table 2-2. No other agencies appear to be planning to develop such regulations in the near term.

Judicial Review of Regulatory Analyses[2]

The use of CEA and BCA to assess the impacts of these types of regulations has been subject to judicial scrutiny. In general, the courts defer to

___

[2]Based on Jacobson and Kanna (2001).

TABLE 2-2 Health Effects Likely to Be Quantified in Forthcoming Major Health and Safety Rulemakings

Agency	Potential Quantified Health Impacts
EPA	• Numerous cardiovascular and respiratory conditions • Lung, stomach, bladder, and other cancers • Pathogen-related illnesses
FDA	• Pathogen-related illness • Hepatitis C-related liver disease and other effects • Numerous conditions associated with dietary supplements
FSIS	• Pathogen-related illness • Cancers and coronary heart disease
OSHA	• Chronic obstructive pulmonary disease and other respiratory conditions • Lung and other cancers • Hearing loss • Suffocation and explosion-related injuries
NHTSA	• Vehicle crash-related injuries
CPSC	• Fire-related injuries

SOURCE: Robinson (2004).

regulatory agency expertise, but agency decisions must be well reasoned and not "arbitrary, capricious, an abuse of discretion, or otherwise not in accordance with a law" (Administrative Procedure Act, 5 U.S.C. 706(2)(A)). In addition, agency actions must be supported by substantial evidence when the record is viewed as a whole, and agencies must explain the rationale and factual basis underlying their decisions. Within this framework, agencies have a great amount of discretion when constructing economic analyses. The scope of judicial review over agency decisions is narrow, and courts must not substitute their own judgment for that of the agency, particularly in matters requiring technical expertise. Generally, courts defer to the agencies on issues related to the preparation of the regulatory analyses that support their rulemakings.

However, many courts have not hesitated to question the methods and the reasoning agencies used in constructing BCAs or CEAs. In *Corrosion Proof Fittings* v. *EPA*, 947 F.2d 1201 (5th Cir. 1991), the court was highly critical of the BCA methodology EPA used to justify a complete regulatory ban of asbestos. The court was "troubled" by EPA's strategy of discounting future calculated costs while failing to discount future calculated benefits, thus significantly "skewing" the analysis and calling its validity into question. The court also found that EPA violated TSCA by failing to consider less burdensome alternatives between a total ban and no action, and by failing to assess the risk of substitute products such as vinyl chloride in pipes and nonasbestos automobile brake linings.

Some courts have gone even further in arguing that regulatory activity must take into account the possibility that regulations may improve safety in one area, but reduce it in another. Known conceptually as "risk–risk" analysis, the notion is that regulations imposed to save lives can also have the effect of costing lives through the substitution of less safe products or other changes. A related argument, "health–health" analysis, is that by increasing the costs of production, regulation results in lost jobs and income, pricing some consumers out of the market for safer products ("richer is safer").[3]

Take, for example, challenges to fuel economy standards.[4] In *Competitive Enterprise Institute* v. *NHTSA*, 956 F.2d 321 (D.C. Cir. 1992), a group of national automobile lobbyists petitioned NHTSA to relax the fuel economy standards for model year 1990 cars. NHTSA had the authority to relax the standards but declined to do so, based in part on an agency BCA indicating that the more stringent fuel economy standards produced a total net benefit. The plaintiff filed suit, claiming the agency had failed to assess the impact of additional automobile accident fatalities that were being caused by downsizing cars in response to the stricter standards. The court was critical of NHTSA's reasoning throughout its rulemaking process, but was most concerned about the agency's failure to include the additional fatalities in its BCA, stating:

> Even if the 27.5 mpg standard for model year 1990 kills "only" several dozen people a year, NHTSA must exercise its discretion; that means conducting a serious analysis of the data and deciding whether the associated fuel savings are worth the lives lost. When the government regulates in a way that prices many of its citizens out of access to large-car safety, it owes them reasonable candor. If it provides that, the affected citizens at least know that the government has faced up to the meaning of its choice. The requirement of reasoned decision-making ensures this result and prevents officials from cowering behind bureaucratic mumbo-jumbo (at p. 27).

---

[3]See *International Union, United Auto Workers* v. *OSHA*, 938 F.2d 1310 (D.C. Cir. 1991), Judge Williams concurring at p. 1326: "And larger incomes enable people to lead safer lives." A range of views on "risk–risk" and "health–health" analysis can be found in the following sources: Wildavsky (1980), Viscusi (1994), Graham and Wiener (1995), and Sunstein (1996).

[4]This case is used to illustrate courts' consideration of risk–risk trade-offs; the discussion here should not be taken to imply any Committee judgment about the merits of the arguments.

Following remand to NHTSA, the agency considered the safety implications of more stringent fuel economy standards. A different three-judge
panel upheld NHTSA, ruling that the agency's action was adequately supported by the record (*Competitive Enterprise Institute* v. *National Highway Traffic Safety Administration*, 45 F.3d 481 (D.C. Cir. 1995)).

CURRENT PRACTICES FOR REGULATORY ANALYSIS

In recent years, OMB has issued a series of guidance documents to
improve the economic analysis of the types of regulations discussed above.
Initially, these documents focused on using BCA to estimate social costs
and benefits, noting that analysts should also report the distribution of
impacts across subgroups of concern. Until recently OMB paid relatively
little attention to CEA, indicating only that it can be useful in certain cases
where benefits are difficult to value in monetary terms.

These guidance documents are based on the requirements of Executive
Order 12866, as discussed in the first chapter. They provide requirements
that OMB expects agencies to follow as well as information on preferred or
"best" practices, recognizing that agencies' ability to implement the recommended approaches may be constrained, for example, by limitations in the
available research base. The most recent version of these guidelines was
published by the Bush Administration in September 2003 as OMB Circular
A-4, *Regulatory Analysis*, after extensive public comment, interagency review, and independent peer review. The new guidelines became effective in
January 2004 for proposed rules and January 2005 for final rules.

OMB Circular A-4 is intended to help analysts define good regulatory
analysis as well as to standardize the way benefits and costs are measured
and reported. Figure 2-1 illustrates in simplified form the process specified
in the Circular, which is included in full in Appendix C.

Although it is similar to earlier guidelines, the Circular provides substantially more detailed information on the criteria for high-quality analysis, imposes certain new requirements, and alters the details of some of the

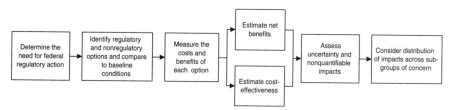

FIGURE 2-1 Key Components of OMB Circular A-4

previous guidance. Chief among the new requirements are those related to the use of CEA. The key analytic requirements of the Circular are summarized in Table 2-3.

These requirements are designed to support decisions regarding the appropriate approach for addressing a particular policy problem. OMB

TABLE 2-3 Key Analytic Requirements of 2003 Office of Management and Budget Guidelines

Requirement	Guidance
Type of analysis	Both BCA and CEA
Monetary valuation of morbidity	Prefer estimates of willingness to pay from stated or revealed preference studies plus any additional economic costs of illness, may use health utility studies
Monetary valuation of mortality	Agency discretion in selecting value of statistical life estimates, may adjust for income growth or time lag but not age, caution on use of value of statistical life year
Effectiveness measures for health and safety	Use integrated measures that combine consideration of morbidity and mortality where appropriate, report more than one measure as well as estimates of physical impacts
Effects on children and the elderly	Avoid measures that place lower values on benefits accruing to these subpopulations, apply CEA when children are affected
Cost estimates	Include costs and savings related to private-sector compliance, government administration, losses in consumers' or producers' surplus, discomfort or inconvenience, or loss of time in work, leisure, commuting, or travel
Discounting	Present costs and benefits undiscounted and discounted at both 3 and 7 percent; may consider other rates; intergenerational impacts require special consideration
Uncertainty analysis	Discuss qualitatively, present sensitivity analysis, and complete probabilistic analysis as appropriate; probabilistic analysis required if impact is greater than $1 billion annually
Nonquantified or nonmonetized effects	Highlight in presentation of impacts
Distributional impacts	Quantify impact on different segments of the population when important, including both transfers and total social costs and benefits

SOURCE: OMB (2003a).

encourages agencies to consider a wide range of regulatory and nonregulatory options that vary, for example, in terms of stringency or the nature of the requirements (e.g., providing information, creating market-based approaches, or establishing performance standards). In assessing these options, OMB instructs agencies to compare the options to a baseline (sometimes referred to as the "no action" alternative) that represents current and potential future conditions in the absence of the regulation.[5] When statutory language limits the consideration of desirable alternatives, OMB requires the agency to discuss these constraints and estimate their impacts.

The following briefly summarizes those aspects of the 2003 guidance that are most relevant to the discussion in this report, and then provides examples of current valuation practices. This section concludes with a summary of cross-cutting OMB requirements that affect both CEA and BCA.

Benefits Analysis Guidelines

OMB devotes a significant portion of the contents of Circular A-4 to the valuation of benefits. It discusses the monetary valuation of morbidity, mortality, and other impacts (e.g., ecological effects) in BCA, as well as approaches for constructing effectiveness measures in CEA. It also provides guidance related to judging the quality of the studies used for valuation.

This guidance on measuring effectiveness in CEA has implications for BCA as well. OMB supports the use of monetized health-adjusted life year (HALY) measures in BCA when suitable willingness-to-pay estimates are not available, and many agencies follow this practice, as discussed in Box 2-1.

OMB highlights three areas of concern related to the application of integrated HALY measures (OMB, 2003a):

- HALY measures may lead to CEA results that differ from the results of BCA because HALYs must meet certain restrictive assumptions to be a valid representation of individual preferences.
- HALY measures may affect the perceived fairness of the analytic approach, for example, if lower values are used for life-extending interventions affecting persons with disabilities. Rather than using different estimates of life expectancy or health-related quality of life (HRQL) for different subgroups, OMB recommends that analysts use general population averages.

---

[5]OMB recognizes that in some cases, it will be desirable to present multiple baselines that differ, for example, in terms of assumptions regarding the future impact of other regulations or compliance with existing regulations.

BOX 2-1
Monetized Health-Adjusted Life Years in Benefit–Cost Analysis

In discussing approaches for assigning dollar values to morbidity impacts in BCA, the OMB notes that if suitable willingness-to-pay studies are not available, agencies may combine HALY studies "typically . . . based on the standard gamble, the time tradeoff or the rating scale methods . . . with known monetary values for well-defined health states . . . to estimate monetary values" (OMB, 2003a, p. 29). The Committee's review of current practices found that several agencies, most notably the FDA and the NHTSA, use monetized HRQL indexes in some form when valuing nonfatal illnesses and injuries (Robinson, 2004). Although the details of the approaches vary, each agency monetizes the HRQL values based on annualized estimates of the value of statistical life.* In addition, each agency adds the economic costs of illness to these monetized HRQL measures when estimating total benefits, although the types of costs included vary across agencies. This reliance on monetized HRQL estimates appears to stem largely from the shortage of stated or revealed preference studies of willingness to pay that address the health effects of concern to these agencies.

---

*The value of a statistical life refers to the value of small reductions in risk spread throughout a large population; it is not the value of saving the life of an identifiable individual.

•   Different HALY measures may yield varying results and provide different perspectives; hence OMB recommends that agencies apply more than one such measure in their analyses. OMB instructs agencies to disclose the underlying data used in their calculations so that OMB and the public can, if desired, recalculate the results using alternate measures and compare the findings across different rulemakings.

Circular A-4 also provides detailed information on the use of stated preference and other methods for valuing benefits, and notes that the criteria for evaluating stated preference studies for use in BCA also apply to the HALY studies used in CEA. Although some of these criteria (listed in Box 2-2) refer specifically to monetization, most are relevant to both types of research.

OMB also discusses the use of benefit transfer; that is, the practice of taking estimates from a prior study and applying them to a rulemaking. While noting that use of such transfers can be expedient, Circular A-4 advises that they should be considered a last-resort option and not used

BOX 2-2
Office of Management and Budget Criteria
for Evaluating Stated Preference Studies

When you are designing or evaluating a stated-preference study, the following principles should be considered:

- the good or service being evaluated should be explained to the respondent in a clear, complete and objective fashion, and the survey instrument should be pre-tested;
- willingness-to-pay questions should be designed to focus the respondent on the reality of budgetary limitations and alerted to the availability of substitute goods and alternative expenditure options;
- the survey instrument should be designed to probe beyond general attitudes . . . and focus on the magnitude of the respondent's economic valuation;
- the analytic results should be consistent with economic theory using both "internal" (within respondent) and "external" (between respondents) scope tests such as the willingness to pay is larger (smaller) when more (less) of a good is provided;
- the subjects being interviewed should be selected/sampled in a statistically appropriate manner. . . . The sample should be drawn using probability methods in order to generalize the results to the target population;
- response rates should be as high as reasonably possible. Best survey practices should be followed to achieve high response rates. Low response rates increase the potential for bias and raise concerns about the generalizability of the results. If response rates are not adequate, you should conduct an analysis of non-response bias or further study. . . . Statistical adjustments to reduce non-response bias should be undertaken whenever feasible and appropriate;
- the mode of administration of surveys (in-person, phone, mail, computer, Internet or multiple modes) should be appropriate in light of the nature of the questions being posed to respondents and the length and complexity of the instrument;
- documentation should be provided about the target population, the sampling frame used . . . the design of the sample including any stratification or clustering, the cumulative response rate . . . the item non-response rate for critical questions; the exact wording and sequence of questions and other information provided to respondents; and the training of interviewers and techniques they employed (as appropriate);
- the statistical and econometric methods used to analyze the collected data should be transparent, well suited for the analysis, and applied with rigor and care.

SOURCE: OMB (2003a, p. 23).

without explicit justification if the scenario considered in the study differs in significant ways from the regulatory scenario. The Circular describes the steps analysts should follow in conducting such transfers as well as the criteria for selecting studies, and indicates that the biases and uncertainties that result from the transfer should be acknowledged.

Current Valuation Practices

The Committee's commissioned review of federal agency practices revealed diverse approaches to the valuation of health and safety improvements (Robinson, 2004). While the OMB guidance provides a general framework for assessing the impacts of regulations, it allows the agencies substantial leeway in determining the details of the approach to valuation for both BCA and CEA.

The Committee's review suggests that regulatory analyses are usually completed under tight time frames with limited staff and budgetary resources. Analysts often must make many decisions about the analytic approach early in the rule development process, when they face substantial uncertainty regarding the regulatory requirements to be assessed, the overall schedule for the rulemaking, and the resources available for completing the analyses. The rulemaking schedule is usually too tight to allow time for new primary research on benefit values; analysts generally rely on preexisting studies, analytic methods, and quantitative models, as exemplified in the rules that were the basis of the Committee's case studies (see Appendix A).

These available analytic resources in some cases resulted from longer term efforts to develop valuation methods for overall program evaluation, separate from particular rulemaking efforts. For example, NHTSA's approach is based on its periodic studies of the national costs of motor vehicle accidents (NHTSA, 1996, 2002a), and EPA's approach has evolved as a result of its prospective and retrospective studies of the Clean Air Act (EPA, 1997, 1999).

Most of the analyses reviewed by the Committee provided a range of measures of regulatory impact, including estimates of the numbers of cases of preventable mortality and nonfatal illness and injuries averted as well as information on uncertainty and nonquantified impacts. All of the analyses included estimates of the costs of regulatory compliance, focusing on those costs expected to be most significant in the context of individual rulemakings. These costs often consisted primarily of direct compliance costs (e.g., the costs associated with implementing pollution controls or administering a new program) and any resulting savings. In some cases, the agencies also assessed the market impacts of price changes associated with the rulemaking; such impacts were generally small.

TABLE 2-4 Quantified Benefits of EPA's Nonroad Diesel Rule
(primary estimate for the year 2030)

Endpoint	Avoided Incidence (cases/year)
Human Health Impacts	
Premature mortality: Long-term exposure (adults, 30 and over)	12,000
Infant mortality (infants, under one year)	22
Chronic bronchitis (adults, 26 and over)	5,600
Nonfatal myocardial infarctions (adults, 18 and older)	15,000
Hospital admissions—respiratory (adults, 20 and older)	5,100
Hospital admissions—cardiovascular (adults, 20 and older)	3,800
Emergency room visits for asthma (18 and younger)	6,000
Acute bronchitis (children, 8–12)	13,000
Asthma exacerbations (asthmatic children, 6–18)	200,000
Lower respiratory symptoms (children, 7–14)	160,000
Upper respiratory symptoms (asthmatic children, 9–11)	120,000
Work loss days (adults, 18–65)	1,000,000
Minor restricted activity days (adults, 18–65)	5,900,000
Other Impacts	
Recreational visibility impairment (86 areas)	N/A

NOTE: Excludes a number of benefits that EPA was unable to quantify as well as EPA's analysis of uncertainty.

SOURCE: EPA (2004b).

Agency analyses of distributional issues tended to focus on the impacts of compliance costs, particularly on small businesses, reflecting the need to comply with related statutory requirements. However, some analyses provided information on the distribution of health impacts, for example, by reporting separate estimates of impacts on children or on individuals with preexisting health conditions.

Examples of the types of health effects examined are provided in Tables 2-4, 2-5, and 2-6. We present these tables to illustrate the ranges of benefits assessed; the source documents cited provide detailed information on the derivation of the estimates and the uncertainty surrounding them, as well as on the importance of nonquantified effects. Additional information on these estimates is available in the Committee's case studies and review of current practices (Robinson, 2004).

All of these agencies are in the process of developing methods for CEA to implement the new guidelines in Circular A-4. Adapting to the new guidance is relatively straightforward for several agencies; five of the seven agencies studied already use HALY-based measures in some form in their BCAs. In general, these approaches involve either transfers of estimates

TABLE 2-5 Quantified Benefits of Food and Drug Administration's Juice Processing Rule

Pathogen/Endpoint	Avoided Incidence (cases/year)
B. cereus	
Mild cases	340
Moderate cases	<0.1
Severe cases	0.3
Deaths	0
Subtotal	340
C. parvum	
Mild cases	2,890
Moderate cases	290
Severe cases	20
Deaths	1
Subtotal	3,200
E. coli O157:H7	
Mild cases	95
Moderate cases	60
Severe-acute cases	5
Severe-chronic cases	10
Deaths	<0.1
Subtotal	160
Salmonella (non typhi)	
Mild cases	1,590
Moderate cases	730
Severe cases	20
Reactive arthritis cases—short-term	50
Reactive arthritis cases—long-term	120
Deaths	1
Subtotal	2,340
Total	6,040

NOTE: Detailed estimates of incidence do not add to total cases in source document, due largely to double counting of cases that begin as acute and become chronic or long term.

SOURCE: FDA (2001).

from the available literature or the application of generic HRQL indexes using expert judgment.

For example, FDA has traditionally used monetized quality-of-life measures in its BCAs and now reports the results as both costs per quality-adjusted life year (QALY) and net benefits as discussed in Box 2-3. FDA's approach varies depending on the health effects assessed, and includes transferring QALY weights from an online, open-access database of health-related CEAs (see Box 3-6 for a description), using expert judgment to

TABLE 2-6 Maximum Abbreviated Injury Scale (MAIS) Categories Used in NHTSA Analyses

Injury Severity Category (based on risk to life)	Examples
MAIS 1: Minor Injury	Whiplash, bruise, broken tooth
MAIS 2: Moderate Injury	Closed leg fracture, finger crush
MAIS 3: Serious Injury	Open leg fracture, amputated arm, major nerve laceration
MAIS 4: Severe Injury	Partial spinal cord severance, concussion with neurological signs (unconscious less than 24 hours)
MAIS 5: Critical Injury	Complete spinal cord severance, concussion with neurological signs (unconscious more than 24 hours)
MAIS 6: Immediately Fatal	N/A

SOURCE: Examples provided in Miller et al. (1991); the Abbreviated Injury Scale was originally developed by the Association for the Advancement of Automotive Medicine.

apply existing indexes (e.g., the Quality of Well-Being Scale), and calculating condition-specific QALY weights based on an approach developed by Cutler and Richardson (1997; see also Scharff and Jessup, 2001). Within the Department of Agriculture, the FSIS reports that it is considering approaches similar to those used by FDA.

NHTSA has historically conducted CEA based on estimates of "equivalent lives saved," which represent the ratio of the dollar value of injuries (including monetized HRQL impacts and economic costs) to the dollar value of fatalities. For example, NHTSA estimates that the total value (economic and quality of life combined) of an injury in the least severe category is $10,396 (excluding noninjury costs). Because $10,396 is 0.31 percent of the per-fatality value ($3.4 million), NHTSA assumes that each injury in this category is equivalent to 0.31 percent of a life saved. NHTSA now uses the values that underlie this approach to calculate net benefits as well as cost-effectiveness ratios. This approach is summarized in Box 2-4.

EPA and OSHA are the two agencies that did not previously use HRQL measures in their BCAs. OSHA's plans are uncertain, but EPA recently completed a pilot CEA that transfers estimates of HRQL impacts from the existing literature for its Clean Air Interstate Rule (EPA, 2005a, Appendix G), as summarized in Box 2-5. EPA labeled its approach the Morbidity-

---

BOX 2-3
FDA's Benefit Valuation Approach

The FDA has used monetized QALYs in its BCAs for many years, and is now applying the same approaches to assess QALY gains in its CEAs. These approaches are evolving as a result of the agency's ongoing research and vary from rule to rule depending on the nature of the health impacts. FDA's juice processing rule, which was the subject of one of the Committee's case studies, illustrates one of the approaches used. (See Robinson, 2004, for others.)

The juice processing analysis is based on a 1998 assessment of the HRQL impacts of mild, moderate, and severe infections associated with exposure to four pathogens as well as resulting cases of reactive arthritis. To determine the per-case value of averting these health effects, FDA completed the following steps:

- FDA staff used the Quality of Well-Being Scale (QWB) to assess the utility losses associated with disease symptoms and related changes in functional status. For each health endpoint, the staff assigned the QWB codes that best described the expected average impacts of the illness (see Appendix B). The results were then weighted using the standard community values for this index, as discussed in Chapter 3. FDA then multiplied the weighted values by the duration of each health condition to determine the quality-adjusted life-day (QALD) gains associated with each averted case.

- The starting point for the dollar valuation of these gains was a value of statistical life (VSL) estimate of $5 million per premature fatality avoided. For non-fatal effects, FDA converted this estimate to a daily value by first annualizing it (at a 7 percent discount rate), which resulted in a value of a statistical life year (VSLY) of $230,000. FDA then divided the VSLY estimate by 365 days, resulting in an estimated value of $630 per day in perfect health. This estimate was then multiplied by the results of the QWB analysis to determine the dollar value of the utility losses. For example, if a day with illness resulted in a 60 percent loss in HRQL, then the value of that daily loss would be $378 ($630*60 percent).

- FDA then added the medical costs of illness to these monetized QALD estimates to determine the total value of the benefits associated with averting each case of illness.

SOURCES: FDA (1998, 2001).

Inclusive Life Year (MILY). This approach adds an estimate of the HRQL impacts of nonfatal cases of myocardial infarction and chronic bronchitis to an estimate of the number of life years lost to preventable mortality. These life years lost are not adjusted to reflect the HRQL expected in the absence of air pollution-related mortality.

BOX 2-4
NHTSA's Equivalent Lives Saved Approach

For many years, the NHTSA has reported the results of its regulatory analyses as costs per equivalent lives saved (ELS). This approach converts injuries to "equivalent lives" based on the relative monetary value of different injury categories. These values are calculated for a given year for different injury categories based on data from all motor vehicle crashes that occurred in that year. The fractional ELS values that result are then used in subsequent rulemakings. The most recent estimates were calculated as follows:

• NHTSA collected data on injuries for a national sample of motor vehicle crashes, then categorized each injured individual by Abbreviated Injury Scale (AIS) and body part affected. When multiple injuries occurred, the case was categorized according to its most life-threatening injury, that is, the Maximum AIS (MAIS) (see Table 2-6).
• NHTSA then estimated the economic costs of crashes for individuals in each of the MAIS categories. These costs were divided into two components: "non-injury-related" costs included those stemming from travel delays and property damage; "injury-related" costs included expenditures on medical treatment, emergency services, lost workplace and household productivity, employer replacement costs for workers with disabilities, legal and court fees stemming from litigation, and administration of insurance claims. These economic costs ranged from roughly $5,900 per MAIS 1 injury to $960,000 per fatality, if only the costs of injury are included.

BOX 2-5
EPA's Morbidity Inclusive Life Year Approach

The EPA's MILY approach sums unadjusted life years gained from averted premature mortality and QALY adjusted gains from averted morbidity. To implement this approach, EPA first searched the literature for estimates of the HRQL impacts of cardiac disease following nonfatal myocardial infarction and of chronic bronchitis. For each health state, EPA then developed a distribution of values that reflected the varying estimates found in the literature. These values were multiplied by a range of estimates of duration, taking life expectancy into account. The resulting range of QALY estimates were then combined with a range of estimates of life years gained to determine the total MILY gains attributable to the rule, using a probabilistic model.

To estimate net costs, EPA subtracted two items from the costs of regulatory compliance: the avoided costs of illness (including medical costs and lost earnings

- NHTSA next estimated HRQL impacts based on injury-related changes in functional status over time for individuals in each MAIS category. NHTSA used a functional capacity index applied by a panel of experts that considers the effects of injury on seven dimensions: mobility, cognitive/psychological, self-care, cosmetic, sensory, pain, and ability to work. In multiple-injury cases, the worst score (highest decrement in quality of life) in each category was used to characterize the case.
- The HRQL impacts were then multiplied by the value of a statistical life year (after first subtracting the value of after-tax wages and household production) to determine their dollar value. The resulting monetary value for the quality-of-life effects was then added to the economic costs discussed above to determine the total (or "comprehensive") average per-case costs of injuries in each MAIS category. These monetized quality-of-life costs ranged from roughly $4,500 per MAIS 1 injury to $2.4 million per fatality.
- Finally, NHTSA divided the comprehensive dollar values for each nonfatal MAIS category by the comprehensive value of fatalities ($3.4 million) to estimate the ELS ratio for injuries in that category.

The "injury only" values are designed for use in assessing interventions that avert injuries, but not the crash itself (e.g., by requiring protective measures such as air bags); the noninjury values are added to the injury values when the analysis addresses interventions that would avert the crash entirely (e.g., by reducing alcohol-related problems).

SOURCES: Miller et al. (1991); NHTSA (2002a).

for chronic bronchitis and myocardial infarction, but not for premature mortality), and the monetized value of those health and nonhealth impacts not captured in the MILY measure. These other benefits are valued based on willingness-to-pay (WTP) estimates to the extent possible; cost-of-illness estimates are used to value certain of the health endpoints for which suitable WTP estimates were not available. In addition to reporting the resulting range of costs per MILY, EPA separately reported each component used to construct the cost-effectiveness measure, including the estimates of life years gained from mortality risk reductions, the estimates of QALY gains for each of the morbidity endpoints, and the sum of these values (i.e., the total MILYs gained). Each of the estimates is presented using both 3 and 7 percent discount rates, and is accompanied by the estimates that bound the 95 confidence interval.

SOURCES: Hubbell (2004); EPA (2005a).

EPA's approach is equivalent to comparing HRQL with the pollution-related health conditions to perfect health for preventable mortality and to average health for the nonfatal endpoints. EPA notes that

> [t]his measure may be preferred to existing QALY aggregation approaches because it does not devalue life extensions in individuals with preexisting illnesses that reduce HRQL. However, the MILY measure is still based on life years and thus still inherently gives more weight to interventions that reduce mortality and morbidity impacts for younger populations with higher remaining life expectancy (EPA, 2005a, p. G-2).

EPA developed this approach in response to OMB Circular A-4 guidance, which suggests that life years lost to preventable mortality should be based on population averages and not adjusted for disabling or other conditions.

Other Guidelines Relevant to CEA

OMB's 2003 guidelines also discuss the estimation of costs in CEA, and include a number of general provisions that affect the analysis of costs and benefits in both BCA and CEA. Below, we summarize several key requirements that are most relevant to the Committee's deliberations.

Estimating Costs

In regulatory analysis, OMB notes that the valuation of both costs and benefits should be based on the concept of "opportunity cost," consistent with the general framework of welfare economics as introduced in Chapter 1. This concept recognizes that, because resources are limited, any decision to use them for one purpose means that they cannot be used for other purposes. Hence the value of a resource can be determined based on the value of its best alternative use.

OMB's discussion of the application of this concept to the analysis of regulatory costs is relatively brief, although this topic is addressed in detail elsewhere (see especially EPA, 2000a). Circular A-4 directs that the assessment of costs should generally follow the same guidance as the assessment of benefits, and notes that the analysis should address both costs and savings related to private-sector compliance and government administration, as well as changes in consumer or producer surpluses, discomfort or inconvenience, and time spent in work, leisure, commuting, or travel. Changes in technology or innovation that may affect the baseline and the impacts of the regulations over time should also be considered.

For BCA, OMB indicates that countervailing costs and benefits can be included in either the "cost" or "benefit" side of the analysis as long as they are not double counted, because the end result is the calculation of net benefits (benefits minus costs). For CEA, which involves the calculation of a ratio, the appropriate categorization of benefits and costs requires more attention. OMB advises that both public and private costs should be considered, and that

> [t]he numerator in the cost-effectiveness ratio should reflect net costs, defined as the gross cost incurred to comply with the requirements (sometimes called 'total' costs) minus any cost savings. You should be careful to avoid double-counting effects in both the numerator and the denominator of the cost-effectiveness ratios (OMB, 2003a, pp. 11–12).

Furthermore, OMB recommends that benefits not included in the effectiveness measure should be subtracted from the cost estimate before calculating the cost-effectiveness ratio if these excluded benefits can be measured in monetary terms. If the value of some of the ancillary benefits cannot be estimated, the analysis should note this so that the cost-effectiveness ratio can be properly interpreted as likely overstating costs relative to benefits.

Discounting Impacts over Time

The OMB guidance requires the use of discounting to reflect the timing of impacts that accrue during different periods or are distributed unevenly over time.[6] The Circular indicates that the same rate should be used to discount both costs and benefits, and that benefits should be discounted regardless of whether they are presented in monetary terms or as physical or HALY impacts. OMB requires that agencies present information on the time periods within which the undiscounted impacts are likely to occur.

OMB recommends that agencies estimate the net present value of benefits and costs using both 3 and 7 percent discount rates. These rates reflect the ongoing debate regarding the extent to which the economic impacts of regulations primarily affect investment or consumption. The 7 percent rate represents the opportunity cost of capital, that is, the real (net of inflation) before-tax rate of return on incremental private investment. The 3 percent rate represents the social rate of time preference, sometimes referred to as the consumption rate. The Circular also discusses cases where other discount rates may be considered, and considers several issues related to the appropriate treatment of intergenerational effects.[7]

---

[6]For example, most individuals generally would prefer to receive money today rather than at a later date because they can invest it and earn interest. Discounting involves adjusting numerical values to account for these types of time preferences.

[7]See Chapter 4 of this report for the Committee's discussion of accounting for intergenerational impacts.

Using Ratios

In addressing the interpretation of the results of economic analyses, OMB notes that ratios can be deceptive and that the net benefits (not the ratio of benefits to costs) is the correct BCA measure to consider in decision making. In CEA, OMB notes that ratios based on averages can be problematic, and instructs analysts to determine the cost-effectiveness of each option incrementally in comparison with the baseline and with each successively more stringent set of requirements.

Assessing Uncertainty and Nonquantified Effects

The OMB guidelines advise that, as appropriate, agencies should discuss qualitatively the main uncertainties in the calculations; use sensitivity analysis to assess the effects of changes in the approach on the resulting estimates; and develop formal probabilistic analyses of uncertainty using simulation models and/or expert judgment. Formal probabilistic analysis is required for all rules with impacts that exceed $1 billion annually.

Because a net benefit or cost-effectiveness estimate may be misleading if important impacts cannot be measured in monetary terms, OMB also emphasizes the importance of providing information on impacts that cannot be quantified or that can be quantified in physical terms but not assigned a monetary value (in BCA) or included in the effectiveness measure (in CEA). Hence analysts are required to clearly specify any nonquantified effects that should be considered in the regulatory decision.

Determining the Distribution of Impacts

In addition to estimating the total national impacts of the regulatory options, agencies are directed to describe distributional effects, that is, to report how benefits and costs affect subpopulations of particular concern. In this assessment, OMB indicates that analysts should consider the allocation both of total social costs and benefits (from the national BCA) and of impacts that represent transfers between different subgroups. The Circular defines distributional effects as the impact across gender, income and racial groups, industrial sectors, and geographic regions, as well as impacts that occur over time or across generations.

Communicating the Methods and Results

OMB emphasizes the need for clear communication of the regulatory options and analytic steps, including information on important assumptions and the sensitivity of the results to these assumptions. The Circular also discusses standards for information quality, instructing agencies to document that the analysis rests on the best obtainable scientific, technical, and economic information.

SUMMARY

The authorizing statutes for regulatory programs vary in the types of factors that they require agencies to consider. These may include the need to maximize risk reductions, avoid excessive costs, and/or apply the best available technologies. In addition, some statutes require agencies to consider impacts on particular groups of concern, such as children or sensitive populations, as well as to pursue goals other than improving health, such as reducing ecological effects.

The responsibility for implementing these programs is delegated largely to executive branch agencies, which develop many regulations each year. Economically significant health and safety regulations that are subject to OMB's requirements for economic analysis are a very small proportion of this total. However, these regulations have broad national impacts. For example, the 18 regulations included in the Committee's review produce roughly $200 billion in net benefits each year and include several individual regulations with national impacts well in excess of $1 billion annually.

The Circular A-4 guidance requiring agencies to begin conducting CEA in addition to BCA is now in force. Agencies have made significant progress in determining how to implement this guidance; however, the dollar resources available for related research are generally limited (Robinson, 2004). In addition, statutory and judicial deadlines, political pressures, and the desire to address health and safety risk in a timely manner often mean that these rules must be developed within a short time frame that does not allow for significant new primary research. As a result, the agencies frequently rely on valuation approaches that do not require a substantial investment of time or funding. These agencies generally transfer estimates from available studies or apply expert judgment rather than conduct new survey research. In some cases, the agency's approach has resulted from long-term projects that develop new methods or data for valuation.

Review of agency practices indicates that some agencies use monetized HALY measures for valuation in BCA, as permitted under current OMB guidance. Use of these measures in part reflects significant gaps in the WTP literature, which includes relatively few studies that address the health effects of concern in regulatory analysis. Although a detailed review of practices for monetizing HALY measures is outside the scope of the Committee's charge, it is clear that such approaches mix valuation measures from two differing, and not entirely compatible, frameworks. As discussed in Chapter 1, these approaches are based to varying degrees on the tenets of utility theory, and represent differing research practices and types of trade-offs.

The magnitude of the impacts of regulations for which economic analyses are required is great. The significance of these public interventions argues for careful attention to the development of high-quality, unbiased analyses that include thorough documentation of their limitations. Such analyses must be rigorous and conform to accepted professional standards for best practices. Data, methods, results, uncertainties, and limitations must be clearly communicated.

The rest of this report elaborates on these objectives for regulatory analysis and policy development. Subsequent chapters consider and make recommendations about the use of HALY measures in regulatory CEA, ethical and other nonquantified information to be considered in developing regulatory policies, and the construction and presentation of CEAs using health-related effectiveness measures. Importantly, the conclusions and recommendations presented throughout address the use of CEA *specifically for public policy analysis of interventions affecting the environment, public health, and safety*. Different characteristics of measures and criteria for use of a particular measure may be of greater relevance in other contexts than the criteria proposed here.

3

Measures and Strategies for Obtaining Health Benefit Values for Regulatory Analysis

As described in Chapter 2, federal agencies apply a variety of approaches to estimate and value the health-related benefits of regulatory interventions. Agencies are currently developing measures of health impacts for use in cost-effectiveness analysis (CEA) along with monetized estimates for use in benefit–cost analysis (BCA). These effectiveness measures include both single-dimension measures such as deaths or cases of illness averted and integrated measures of morbidity and mortality, that is, the health-adjusted life-year (HALY) measures that are a central focus of this report.

In this chapter the Committee describes different effectiveness metrics for health-related CEA and sources for estimates of health-related quality of life (HRQL) based on these metrics. We first introduce criteria for selecting among effectiveness measures for use in regulatory analysis, and then discuss various approaches in light of these criteria.

We cover much of the same ground as "Identifying and Valuing Outcomes," Chapter 4 of the report of the U.S. Panel on Cost-Effectiveness in Health and Medicine (PCEHM) (Gold et al., 1996b). The emphasis and detail of this report, however, are tailored for an audience of regulatory analysts and decision makers. We reiterate some of the material in the PCEHM report here so that this volume will be a largely self-contained reference. In many instances the Committee follows and endorses the PCEHM's interpretations and recommendations; in a few respects, our judgments differ, as summarized at the end of the chapter.

This chapter begins with a discussion of criteria for selecting among different HALY measures and for determining which approach to applying

67

these measures is most appropriate for regulatory analysis. We then describe and evaluate each approach in more detail. The subsequent sections of this chapter first briefly review the single-dimension measures common in statistical reporting systems and epidemiological studies, including case reporting of illness or injury, preventable deaths, and life years lost. This section also considers the contribution of mortality and longevity changes, relative to changes in HRQL, to overall estimates of effectiveness. Next we examine alternative HALY metrics, discuss their construction and theoretical roots, and methods for determining the relative values of specific health states. These metrics, survey instruments, and methods for eliciting preferences or values for particular health states are evaluated in terms of their practicality, reliability, and theoretical and empirical validity. In the following section we consider sources of health state values for regulatory analysis and review four commonly used generic HRQL survey instruments. The fifth section identifies data collection and research priorities as well as promising developments for improving the measurement of health effects for regulatory analysis. Last, we briefly summarize the Committee's findings and conclusions based on the material presented in the chapter.

CRITERIA FOR SELECTING HALY METRICS FOR REGULATORY CEA

As introduced in the preceding chapters, regulatory analysts face a series of choices in determining how to structure the effectiveness measure in their analyses. First, they may choose between a single-dimension or integrated measure. Although single-dimension measures, such as lives saved, life years extended, or cases of illness or injury avoided provide important information of interest to decision makers, analyses of major regulations generally include more than one health effect of concern. Thus our focus is on developing criteria for selecting among the integrated measures that are the main focus of the report.

The first choice that analysts face in selecting an integrated measure is whether to rely on the most commonly used approach—the quality-adjusted life year (QALY)—or one of the other HALY approaches. HALY approaches, which rest on how length of life is combined with a value or preference for a given state of health, are discussed in detail later in this chapter. They vary primarily in the extent to which they are widely accepted, available, and used. Because the requirements for regulatory CEA are already in effect and analysts need tools that are ready for use, the Committee's criteria for selecting among these HALY measures are largely practical ones. (The development and pursuit of a longer term research agenda are discussed separately at the end of this chapter.)

At this broadest conceptual level, the relevant performance characteristics of a HALY effectiveness measure for regulatory CEA conform to some straightforward criteria.

- First, the HALY metric should have a "track record," that is, it should be in relatively widespread use and methods for estimating index values, as well as estimates themselves, should be available in the literature.
- Second, the metric should be easy to understand and interpret. To some extent, the comprehensibility of a metric is a function of the extent to which it has been used, and thus depends on the first criterion.
- Third, the metric should be relatively inexpensive to use, both in terms of the availability of methods and values for immediate application and in terms of the development and collection of new values.

Of course, in addition to these practical considerations, measures must also provide valid and reliable estimates of the relative value of different health states. Assessing reliability and validity is, however, largely a function of the extent of the research base; the measures that do not meet the first criteria above are less likely to have been subject to extensive tests of validity and reliability.

As discussed in more detail in the following sections of this chapter, the Committee believes that the QALY best meets these criteria. Once an analyst makes the decision to use the QALY metric, the next set of choices involves determining how to apply this measure in the context of a particular regulatory analysis. As already discussed, analysts face the choice in BCA and CEA alike of conducting new research on benefit values or transferring estimates from existing studies. In CEA analysts have a third option: they can use generic indexes. The use of these indexes can be based on existing studies or new research; i.e., the analyst may transfer estimates from an existing study that used a generic index, or may use the index to generate new valuation estimates. As illustrated by the Committee's case studies, these indexes have the advantage of allowing the analyst to value new health states without the substantial investment of time and resources required for new primary valuation research. Each of these approaches is discussed in detail in the later sections of this chapter.

Because several generic indexes are well established and easy to use, the Committee expects that they will often be applied in regulatory analysis in the near term. As already discussed, regulatory analysts lack the time or resources to engage in the development of instruments for health status valuation in the context of individual regulatory analysis. Thus we focused our criteria for implementing the QALY measure on the choice among available generic instruments.

Several authorities have offered criteria for assessing the construction and performance of HRQL measures, primarily with respect to their use in

CEAs of health care services and in clinical outcomes studies. Box 3-1 presents standard performance criteria for preference-based HRQL survey instruments. While each of these features of an HRQL instrument may be

---

BOX 3-1
Standard Performance Criteria for HRQL Instruments

The PCEHM proposed that valuation approaches should have a *theoretical foundation* and be *empirically derived*. Economists and decision theorists tend to favor choice-based valuation such as standard gamble and time trade-off methods because they are more closely connected to utility theory. Some psychologists have also used techniques such as rating scales and magnitude estimation.

An ideal measurement method would satisfy a long list of criteria. While any given list is probably incomplete, some criteria deserve particular attention. For example, the ultimate standard of *validity* is *construct validity*, the extent to which an instrument accurately measures or identifies the thing it is intended to measure. Because HRQL is an unobservable construct with alternative theoretical foundations, there is some ambiguity and tension as to how to demonstrate an instrument's validity. Three subsidiary or partial aspects of validity that are more readily demonstrated are *content validity* (adequate or appropriate scope to the measure); *criterion validity* (the degree of correspondence of the instrument to an agreed-on measure of the construct); and *predictive validity* (ability to predict future behaviors and outcomes).

An instrument's valuation survey sample should be adequate in size and response rate, and the population from which the sample was drawn should be *representative* of the population of interest in the CEA. In the case of regulatory CEA, this would be the population affected by costs and/or benefits of the regulatory intervention.

A measure should be *reliable*, that is, exhibit consistency in repeated measurements by the same individual over time or across different groups drawn from the same population.

A measure should be *widely applicable* to a range of health states and conditions. It should be *sensitive*, that is, responsive to change, and not exhibit floor or ceiling effects in the range of anticipated effects. An HRQL instrument should be *flexible* and *universal*, as demonstrated by applications to and adaptations for cultural and language subpopulations and alternative administration formats.

An HRQL measure should be *well documented*, *transparent*, and *interpretable*. An instrument should be *feasible to administer*, *not burdensome for respondents*, and *acceptable* to users and the public. This may be judged by administration format, completion times, and rates of missing responses. Preference elicitation surveys should have satisfactory completion rates; if respondents consistently decline to make choices within an elicitation exercise, the measure or method may not be appropriate or adequately informative.

SOURCES: Gold et al. (1996b); Lohr et al. (1996); IOM (1998); Brazier et al. (1999b).

desirable, some are particularly important and take a specific form in the context of informing regulatory decision making.

As discussed later in this chapter, in applying these criteria the Committee found that no one HRQL index is obviously superior to the others in all respects for all applications. Thus, to designate any single instrument as a standard for all regulatory analyses would be arbitrary. Judging the appropriateness of a given instrument for a particular regulatory application depends not only on the features of the HRQL instrument, but also the characteristics of the affected population, the intervention, and the health research that underlies the risk assessment.

The Committee emphasizes the following criteria for choice of an HRQL instrument in a regulatory analysis.

First, *an HRQL instrument must be applicable to the range of health-related effects being evaluated.* Generic HRQL instruments are designed for application to a wide range of health states that can result from a variety of health-related risks or interventions. Still, as described below, each generic instrument has distinctive features absent from the others. For example, the Quality of Well-Being Scale (QWB) includes symptoms and problems in its valuation formula, along with functional attributes; the Health Utilities Index (HUI) instruments specify sensory and cognitive functions, which make them relatively sensitive instruments for conditions with these manifestations; and the SF-6D allows the use of widely collected SF-36 and SF-12 data sets.

Second, *the instrument should be sensitive enough to distinguish among health endpoints.* This criterion addresses the "fit" between the HRQL instrument, the health condition(s) of interest, and the risk assessment data used to estimate and characterize the health impacts. For example, a highly differentiated HRQL instrument may not be readily "mappable" onto epidemiological data about respiratory symptoms related to air quality if the later dataset is based on very general symptom-based categories. Conversely, if the regulatory health impacts of interest are very specific, such as functional limitations resulting from long-term effects of traumatic injury, and the domains of an HRQL instrument do not reflect those effects, that instrument might not be sufficiently sensitive. In the Committee's case study of child seat restraint anchoring systems, in which head injuries were a prominent risk, some but not all indexes included a cognitive function domain. In this case study, however, the similarity of estimates of QALY effects (as assigned by experts) across different instruments does not demonstrate that the more specific attributes are critical to the sensitivity of the instrument (see Appendix A, Tables A-11 and A-12).

Third, *a generic instrument should reflect the values or preferences for health of the population(s) of interest.* In most cases, for major regulations, those who will bear the costs and/or receive the benefits can be represented by the U.S. population as a whole. Hence it is the preferences of this population that will matter most for valuation. Of the generic instruments reviewed, only the QWB and the EuroQol Group's EQ-5D have preferences derived from the U.S. population. Whereas the U.S. EQ-5D valuation survey is recent and based on a nationally representative sample, the QWB valuation survey is about 30 years old and was conducted in a single community (San Diego, CA). The HUI-3 valuation survey was conducted with a representative sample from Hamilton, Ontario, Canada, and the SF-6D values are derived from a U.K. general population survey.

Fourth, as in the case of the HALY measure, *the HRQL instrument also must be acceptable to and understandable by survey respondents, policy makers, and the general public.* One indication of a measure's acceptability is the extent to which valuation survey respondents comprehend, and are willing to engage in, the preference elicitation exercise. In a broader sense, the ethical commitments and implications of the HRQL instrument and the health state values it generates must be viewed as legitimate by the ultimate users of the analytic results. Transparency, in the sense of relying on data that is publicly available (not proprietary), may also contribute to a measure's acceptability.

Finally, as in the case of the HALY measure, *the HRQL instrument should be as inexpensive to use as is compatible with the other objectives.* This criterion applies to considerations such as mode of administration (e.g., mail surveys are less costly than personal interviews) and also to the proprietary status of the instrument and related analytic tools.

SINGLE-DIMENSION MEASURES OF HEALTH-RELATED OUTCOMES

Cases of illness or injuries, deaths, hospitalizations, and days of work or school lost are commonly reported outcomes based on routine health information collection activities. These measures are familiar, easily comprehended, generally stable, and can be obtained or calculated from standard statistical sources. Tables 2-2, 2-4, and 2-5 in the previous chapter provide examples of specific single-dimension outcome measures used in regulatory analyses. The drawback of relying on these types of measures alone, without benefit of more comprehensive measures, is that they are not readily aggregated.

Mortality-based indicators have long dominated population-based health status measurement. They are also prominent in risk assessments and economic analyses for health and safety regulations. Life expectancy and age-specific death rates are familiar and straightforward health outcomes measures. Early analyses counted *preventable* or *premature deaths averted.*[1] With the advent of CEA in health care settings, analysts turned to counting *years of life saved*, thus reflecting differences in remaining life expectancies.

Much of the information needed to calculate integrated measures of morbidity and mortality relates to the determination of the relative values attached to different health states, yet changes in survival tend to swamp the impact of changes in HRQL in HALY calculations for health care programs. In a review of 63 studies that included 173 cost-effectiveness-ratio pairs that reported both cost per life year ($/LY) and cost per quality-adjusted life year ($/QALY), Chapman and colleagues (2004) found that quality-adjusting life years resulted in a median difference between LY and QALY ratios for the 173 ratio pairs of just $1,300. (The median ratios were $24,600/LY and $20,400/QALY.) In a separate review of 110 cancer prevention, early detection, and treatment interventions, Tengs (2004) also compared $/LY and $/QALY ratios. Consistent with the findings of Chapman et al., she reported a very high rank-order correlation between LY and QALY ratios. Both studies concluded that the difference in quality-adjusting life years would have affected decisions about cost-effectiveness in just a small proportion of cases (8 and 5 percent in the Chapman and Tengs studies, respectively, at a $50,000 decision threshold in each case).

The results of these two review studies suggest that accounting for mortality impacts may be more important than adjusting for the HRQL impacts associated with diseases for which the intervention saves many lives. In these cases, calculation of life years gained may capture the majority of the impact of the intervention on health. However, this will not be the case for programs or regulations that improve health and functioning but do not significantly change life expectancy, such as one might expect with mitigation of environmental exposures to lead or mercury. In the juice processing case study (summarized in Appendix A), for example, chronic illness impacts accounted for the majority of QALY gains.

HEALTH-ADJUSTED LIFE YEARS

HALY measures were designed to address the limitations of single-dimension measures. HALYs capture information about both length of life and the states of health experienced during those years. The virtue of such an index of health—that it combines information about diverse health-related conditions as well as mortality—also poses challenges. A HALY is a

---

[1]Throughout this report, we use the term "preventable" rather than "premature" deaths. These terms refer to decreases in the risk of death attributable to a regulation, in other words, expected gains in life expectancy.

relatively abstract concept, and some users of health statistics may find it harder to understand than more concrete and simpler health indicators, such as a change over time in the incidence of lung cancer or life expectancy in a population. Hence reporting the constituents of HALY measures and presenting cost-effectiveness ratios using specific outcomes such as preventable deaths remain important.

HALYs not only meld descriptive information about health states and longevity, they also incorporate judgments about the relative value of different states of health, taking into account their impact on functioning and subjective experience. Such judgments about HRQL may be individual, aggregated and averaged for a population, or reached collectively by individuals participating in an interactive or consensus process.

HALY measures are constructed in three steps. First, a description of a health state or disease condition is needed. Second, that state or condition must be given a value or weight, relative to other states and conditions. By convention, HRQL scales are anchored by values of 0 and 1, where 0 corresponds with death and 1 with the state of full, optimal, or "perfect" health. (States of health considered worse than death can be accommodated by negative values.) Third, the values for different health states or conditions must be combined with estimates of the duration in each health state over the predicted remaining life span. Figure 3-1 represents an illustrative health-adjusted life expectancy (for either an individual or a population, on average) as the shaded area on a two-dimensional graph where the vertical axis represents HRQL and the horizontal axis represents duration of life. When interpreted as an individual life, the figure suggests how one moves through different states of health, implying different levels of HRQL, over the course of a lifetime.

Several approaches to estimating HALYs are discussed later in this section and many are illustrated in the Committee's case studies. The most familiar and widely used measure is the QALY, and that is the metric given fullest consideration here. Before discussing the QALY and alternative metrics, we describe some general features of HALY measurement, using the QALY as the case in point.

Describing Health States

HRQL measurement relies on concepts such as "health status," "functional status," "well-being," and "quality of life." Although these terms, along with "health-related quality of life," are often applied interchangeably, in fact they encompass narrower or broader arrays of domains, with "health status" denoting a more restrictive concept and "quality of life" a more extensive one. Table 3-1 presents concepts and domains that fall within these broader rubrics.

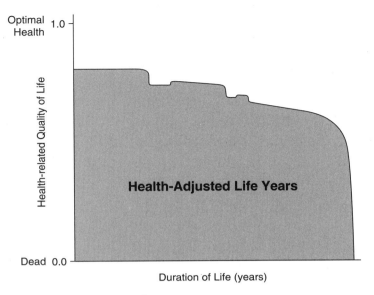

FIGURE 3-1 Health-Adjusted Life Years

At a minimum, the measurement of HRQL incorporates both the description of health status (which may include observable and unobservable symptoms, functional capabilities, and health perceptions) *and* the importance or value that people, individually and/or collectively, attach to these aspects of health. Health states may be described (and valued) either as related to or representing specific disease conditions or in generic terms. Valuations of generically described health states, using multiattribute health state classification systems, are reviewed in some detail later in this chapter.

HALY metrics such as QALYs have been constructed with tools from both psychometrics (the theory and techniques of measuring psychological phenomena such as attitudes) and utility theory (defined in Chapter 1). They are developed most often from some combination of psychological survey and decision-theoretical techniques. All generically described health states used in HRQL indexes depend on psychometric scaling and concepts to some degree. Such generic indexes thus share common features with health profiling instruments, such as the SF-36. Like other health status profiling instruments, the SF-6D was not designed to produce a preference-based index value.[2]

---

[2]The SF-36 is described later in the Chapter, when its derivative preference-based index, the SF-6D, is discussed.

TABLE 3-1 Concepts and Domains Used in Defining Self-Reported Health Status, Quality of Life, and Health-Related Quality of Life

Concepts	Domains	Attributes
Symptoms	Reports of physical and psychological symptoms or sensations not directly observable, such as energy and fatigue, nausea, and irritability	Frequency, severity, bothersomeness
Functional status		Frequency, difficulty, severity, ability, with help
Physical	Functional limitations and activity restrictions, such as self-care, walking, mobility, sleep, sexual	
Psychological	Positive or negative affect and cognitive, such as anger, alertness, self-esteem, sense of well-being, distress	
Social	Limitations in work or school, participation in community	
Health perceptions		Frequency, severity/intensity, satisfaction
Global	General ratings of health and quality of life, such as satisfaction or overall well-being	
Worries and concerns	About health, finances, the future	
Spiritual	Meaning and purpose of life or relationship to the universe	
Disadvantage/opportunity	Perceptions of stigma or reports of discrimination because of health condition	Frequency, impact
Resiliency	Reports of ability to cope or withstand stress and illness	Frequency, satisfaction, ability
Environmental	Evaluations of personal safety, adequacy of housing, respect, freedom, and so on	Satisfaction, importance

SOURCE: Reprinted from Patrick and Chiang (2000, Table 1).

Valuing Health States and Preference Elicitation Methods

The scaling of values associated with particular health states reflects the relative strength of preference for one state as compared with another. Health states must be located on an interval scale (and not simply ranked) in order to be incorporated in a HALY measure. This section reviews four methods for eliciting preferences for health states:

- Standard gamble (SG),
- Time trade-off (TTO),
- Category rating (CR) or visual analogue scale (VAS), and
- Person trade-off (PTO).

These preference elicitation techniques pose different questions and emphasize different facets of the relative value of various health states. Most analysts who use these valuation techniques recommend that results from two or more approaches not be combined within a single analysis, and that their interpretation and the discussion of results consider the elicitation method (Lenert and Kaplan, 2000).

Each of the four methods has particular strengths. Economists generally prefer metrics or instruments that use SG or TTO. These elicitation techniques produce relative preference weights using methods consistent with neoclassical economic utility theory, which requires choices reflecting an opportunity cost—the sacrifice of one valuable good for another. Preference or value elicitation methods grounded in utility theory correspond more closely than do psychometric approaches to the model of consumer choice.

Rating scale approaches such as CR or VAS are considered the least burdensome for respondents, although some studies have reported that respondents found the task more challenging than TTO or SG. CR or VAS are understood to reflect respondents' internal representations of health states in a comparative sense, and may be anchored or influenced by the actual health of the respondent (Krabbe et al., 1997).

PTO valuation methods have been designed to introduce other-directed interests and considerations into societal resource allocation and priority-setting contexts. In contrast with other techniques, the PTO approach does not purport to represent primarily self-interested or consumer preferences for health states. PTO has not been as widely applied as the other techniques.

Unless new surveys are conducted to elicit values for specific health states, the elicitation technique is part and parcel of the choice of a generic, multiattribute HRQL index. Thus, although the following discussion addresses elicitation methods in isolation from other features of valuation surveys, in practice these methods are not readily mixed and matched with the descriptive systems of different indexes. Nonetheless, considering the performance of different elicitation methods as such is helpful because the valuation (as compared with the characterization or description) of health states is what distinguishes QALYs from other HALY metrics.

Standard Gamble

Expected utility theory provides a normative model for individual decision making under conditions of risk or uncertainty. The SG is the only preference elicitation method directly linked to the axioms of expected utility theory. In order to establish the relative values of various health states on an interval scale, respondents must determine the conditions of indifference or equivalence between two outcomes. One of the alternatives, representing the health state (less than full health) of interest, is a certain outcome. The other alternative has two possible outcomes, one being full health and the other being immediate death. The respondent is asked to specify the risk of immediate death (with probability p) and the complementary probability of survival in perfect health $(1 - p)$ that would make this uncertain alternative just as attractive as the certain alternative of the impaired health state. On a 0-to-1 scale for health state values arrayed from death to full or perfect health, the value of the health state in question is then $(1 - p)$.

The relative values of different states of health elicited with the SG technique will reflect, to some degree, individuals' attitudes about taking risks. If the respondent in an SG is averse to taking risks, the value assigned to the certain, impaired state of health will be closer to 1.0 (optimal health) than if the respondent is not risk averse (Kahneman and Tversky, 1979; Loomes and McKenzie, 1989). The standard gamble is a cognitively demanding technique. Because SG explicitly uses probabilities of events to determine relative values, and probability information often is not well understood, empirical results do not confirm the prediction from expected utility theory that the relative values of different health states maintain a constant proportional relationship to risk. For example, when presented with probabilities that differ by an order of magnitude (a 1-in-100 risk versus a 1-in-1,000 risk), respondents do not treat them as representing a fully tenfold difference in likelihood. A method for adjusting SG responses to account for biases in probability weighting has been proposed by Bleichrodt et al. (2001), but this method has not been widely adopted.

Time Trade-Off

The TTO elicitation method is also considered consistent with utility theory because respondents must sacrifice one valuable good for another.

The TTO method was developed as an alternative to the standard gamble to avoid the cognitive challenges associated with choosing probabilistic outcomes. In a TTO elicitation, the respondent is asked to choose between two certain prospects, for example, to experience remaining life expectancy in a given health state (less than full health) or to live for a fixed number of years in full health, followed by immediate death. The number of years in full health is varied until the respondent is indifferent between the two prospects. The value of the health state is then given by the ratio of the number of years in full health to the remaining life expectancy.

The TTO method has proved practical and acceptable to survey respondents (Brazier et al., 1999a). It may be more comprehensible than an SG. Furthermore, the TTO method has intuitive appeal, as it involves the direct exchange of the two components of health, morbidity and longevity. The method has been shown to confound preferences for health states with time preference (the extent to which one discounts the value of states in the future). The TTO method relies on the fundamental assumption of QALYs that the weight assigned to a health state is independent of its duration, and so one will trade off a constant proportion of remaining years of life for a given improvement in health status, regardless of how many years remain. However, empirical work has demonstrated that the value of a health state may depend on its duration (Sackett and Torrance, 1978; McNeil et al., 1981). Other experimental results suggest that TTO may be better suited to valuing chronic conditions than temporary conditions (Dolan and Gudex, 1995). The TTO method nonetheless offers a useful and intuitively plausible first approximation of relative values for different states of health.

Direct Rating: Category Rating and Visual Analogue Scales

Direct rating approaches to preference elicitation ask respondents to assign a single number to a health state, usually on a scale of 0 to 100, with these anchors being the worst and best imaginable health states, or death and perfect health. Visual aids, such as the "feeling thermometer" in the EuroQol Group's generic HRQL survey instrument, the EuroQoL-5D (EQ-5D), are often used in this approach. (See Kind et al., 1998, for a reproduction of the "feeling thermometer.") If the direct rating scale is divided into discrete points of equal intervals that the respondent must select, the approach is called CR. If there are no constraints on the location of assignments between the anchor points, the approach is referred to as a VAS.

Direct rating approaches apply psychometrically based attitudinal scaling methods to questions related to health. Rating scale methods are familiar to many and have been used extensively in survey research. They are generally thought to impose the least cognitive burden among value elicitation methods. CR and VAS values have been treated as having interval properties as measures of strength of preference by their proponents (Revicki, 1992; Kaplan et al., 1993). Health state values generated by VAS tend to correlate more closely with health status indicators such as pain, functioning, and clinical symptoms, and with health status profile scores, than do values generated by SG and TTO methods (Brazier et al., 1999a).

Direct rating, however, lacks the theoretical support of the trade-off-based methods (Bleichrodt and Johannesson, 1997). Respondents to rating scale surveys are not told that, in calculating QALYs, rating an impaired state of health at 50 on a scale of 0 to 100 will be interpreted as considering 1 year of life in perfect health equivalent to 2 years of life in the impaired health state. Empirical findings of both clustering of responses away from the extremes of the scale and response spreading have raised concerns that CR and VAS do not reflect the interval-scale properties that are required for QALY valuation.

Person Trade-Off

The PTO represents a fundamentally different approach to establishing relative values for health states. This method was designed to inform societal decision making about investments in and priorities for health care interventions, and most notably was used in setting the original disability-adjusted life-year (DALY) weights (Murray and Lopez, 1996; Murray and Acharya, 1997). In a PTO exercise, respondents are asked to make choices about health interventions and health states for groups of people other than themselves. For example, a respondent may be presented with a situation in which a given number of people (x) have a particular health-related impairment A and another group of y members have a different health impairment B (the time in health states A and B are the same). The respondent is asked to choose which group to help if she could help only one group because of limited resources. By varying the number of persons in one or the other group (x') until the respondent concludes that helping x' persons with condition A is equivalent to helping y persons with condition B, the societal value of health condition A relative to health condition B is determined: $(1 - x')/(1 - y)$.

PTO choices incorporate concerns about relative health status and the distribution of benefits in the particular choice scenario. Specifically, PTO choices are more responsive to the relative severity of conditions involved and to life-saving interventions than are individual preference-based valuation techniques, reflecting an interest in benefiting the worst off (Nord, 1999). Yet, at the same time, participants in PTO exercises appear to take into account the total gains in health across all participants, even if those who are initially worst off are not necessarily helped (Dolan and Green,

1998). Several reviews of the PTO methodology applied in different contexts, including the World Health Organization's (WHO's) Global Burden of Disease DALY measure, have called for more research to refine and improve the reliability of the technique and specifically for further development of its theoretical rationale (Brazier et al., 1999a; Dolan, 2000; Green, 2001; Walker and Siegel, 2002).

The PTO technique is cognitively demanding and it requires posing a large number of choices to construct a robust set of relative values for different diseases (Green, 2001). It has also performed poorly, relative to other approaches, in tests of reliability and internal consistency (Patrick et al., 1973; Ubel et al., 1996).

Comparisons Among Elicitation Methods

This review reinforces the caveat stated at the beginning of the section: Each approach elicits relative health state values that incorporate different characteristics of the health states or aspects of the choices posed. For example, SG results incorporate attitudes about risk, most often risk aversion, so that SG-based values tend to be higher than values estimated with other approaches. Similarly, TTO elicitations capture time preferences and direct rating methods reflect elements of current health status.

In a study in which 69 public health professionals valued 12 health states according to each of the four previously described elicitation methods, Salomon and Murray (2004) explored the hypothesis that a consistent set of core valuations of health states underlies the preference estimates produced via each elicitation technique. In their modeling of responses, the authors estimated the contributions of various factors (e.g., risk attitudes, discounting, distributional concerns, and scale distortion effects) in explaining the differences among the valuation techniques, in order to isolate an underlying strength of preference. This study is encouraging with respect to the possibility of ascertaining consistent and stable preferences for health. At the same time, it suggests that comparing the results of studies using different valuation techniques should be approached with caution and that mixing valuation approaches within one study may be unwise.

In the following discussion, the Committee considers the relative performance of the three predominant elicitation techniques in terms of feasibility, reliability, and theoretical and empirical validity. Because the PTO approach differs from the other elicitation techniques in what it intends to measure, it is not included in this comparison. Furthermore, there is little evaluative research on the performance of the PTO.

Feasibility Of the three main elicitation methods, rating scale approaches like CR or VAS are the most feasible and least expensive, and are acceptable to respondents, with a high completion rate (95 percent and above). Some researchers have reported completion problems and difficulty in understanding the probabilistic choices with the SG (Froberg and Kane, 1989). In their more recent review of the literature, Brazier and colleagues (1999a) concluded that the SG methodology was comparable to TTO in terms of completion rates. Both the SG and the TTO may require an interview-based approach because of the complexity of the valuation exercises, in contrast with VAS, which is more amenable to a mail survey format.

Reliability Table 3-2 presents intrarater test–retest reliability results for the SG, TTO, and VAS methods from studies that resurveyed respondents at different time intervals, ranging from less than one week to a year. None

TABLE 3-2 Intrarater Test–Retest Reliability of the Standard Gamble, Time Trade-Off, and Visual Analogue Scale Techniques

Test–Retest Reliability	Standard Gamble	Time Trade-Off	Visual Analogue Scale
1 week or less	0.80[a] 0.77–0.79[b]	0.87[a]	0.77[a] 0.70–0.95[b]
4 weeks or less	0.82[c]	0.81[d] 0.63[e]	0.62[c] 0.89[e]
6 weeks		0.63–0.80[d] 0.85[f]	
10 weeks		0.73[g]	0.78[h]
6–16 weeks	0.63 (props)[i] 0.74 (no props)[i]	0.83 (props)[i] 0.55 (no props)[i]	
1 year	0.53[j]	0.62[j]	0.49[j]

NOTE: Correlation as specified; intraclass correlation coefficient: b, c, g, h; Pearson correlation coefficient: e, i; others unspecified. "Props" and "no props" referred to mode of administration, with or without specially designed aids in decision making (boards or cards).

[a]O'Connor and Pennie (1995).
[b]Bakker et al. (1994).
[c]O'Brien and Viramontes (1994).
[d]Churchill et al. (1987).
[e]Gabriel et al. (1993).
[f]Molzahn et al. (1996).
[g]Dolan et al. (1996a).
[h]Gudex et al. (1996).
[i]Dolan et al. (1996b).
[j]Torrance (1976).

SOURCE: As reported in Brazier et al. (1999a, Table 1).

of the three elicitation methods has been shown to perform consistently better than the others.

Theoretical validity   Several economists and QALY valuation researchers engaged in health-related CEA have noted that the ultimate test of validity should be the extent to which a technique or measure predicts the preference revealed in actual decisions (Brazier et al., 1999a; Dolan, 2000), consistent with the theoretic basis of welfare economics. In research on willingness to pay for risk reductions, the results from a stated preference survey (e.g., for safety interventions that reduce the risk of accidental death) can be compared with revealed preference studies (e.g., based on labor market studies of wage-rate differentials for risky jobs). It is more difficult to use revealed preference methods in studying choices in health and health care because the relative prices paid for treating different conditions cannot be assumed to reflect consumers' relative preferences. Thus the "gold standard" of validity testing is not available for HRQL stated preference results. Instead, validity testing has been conducted primarily within the psychometric tradition, and has focused on construct validity, that is, the extent to which measures discriminate among unlike health states and converge on like ones (Dolan, 2000).

Empirical validity   The SG and TTO methods have been compared in terms of producing logically consistent orderings of health states. In one study in which about 150 participants each compared 12 pairs of health states ordered in terms of level of impairment, TTO elicitations resulted in somewhat higher rates of logically consistent rankings (92 percent) compared with SG elicitations (84–88 percent), but this difference between methods was not statistically significant (Dolan et al., 1996a).

Internal inconsistencies in valuation have been found in some TTO studies as well. A recent study by Bleichrodt and colleagues (2003) concludes that these inconsistencies occur for short but not longer duration health states. They suggest that this phenomenon explains why TTO valuations sometimes exceed SG values, even though values elicited with SG approaches generally tend to be higher than those elicited by TTO. For example, the EQ-5D uses a relatively short-gauge duration of 10 years for comparison with remaining life expectancy; the authors argue that this leads to valuations that are too high.

Dolan (2000) argues that, although the SG and TTO methods are preferable in the abstract to rating scale approaches, both of these methods incorporate features that influence valuation. Because many people are averse to risk, they may assign a higher value to the intermediate health state that is certain. Because people generally have positive time preferences and value years in the near future more highly than those more distant, they will more readily trade off years of life closer to death. (Box 3-2 addresses the question of how this phenomenon relates to discounting QALYs.) Taken together, these measurement biases lead to higher SG values than TTO values for the same health states. Furthermore, many respondents are unwilling to accept any risk of death, or trade off any longevity, for a health improvement, leading to relatively high values for impaired health states (Reed et al., 1993). These results also suggest that individuals' preferences are not fully consistent with QALYs.

Although SG and TTO values are ordinally correlated with VAS values, their relationship is not proportionate. The practice of mapping from VAS to SG or TTO valuations has been reviewed by Brazier and colleagues (1999a,b) and directly evaluated in an original study by Krabbe and col-

---

BOX 3-2
The Time Trade-Off Method and Discounting

It has been argued that, because the TTO preference elicitation method incorporates respondents' time preferences, discounting QALYs elicited by TTO results in double discounting. The following demonstrates why this is not the case.

Time preferences in health are usually modeled with a constant discount rate, r, over time. Assume that a respondent has a positive time preference (r), meaning that she prefers that good things happen sooner and bad things happen later. In a TTO choice, then, the longer lasting health state alternative would diminish in value proportionately more than the shorter term alternative. Thus, to equilibrate the two options, the respondent would decrease the value assigned to the shorter term, better health state option, resulting in a lower TTO score for the health state of interest. TTO scores are negatively related to the respondent's positive time preference; however, they are not proportionally related.

If the individual's utility function can be represented by the discounting factor r, then QALY values could be adjusted by calculating the TTO score by dividing the discounted (at rate r) years in full health by the discounted years in the health state of interest. However, this works only at the individual, not aggregate, level (Johannesson et al., 1994). In societal evaluation, the discount rate reflects the time preferences assigned by the decision makers.

Although TTO preference scores are affected by the respondent's time preference, this effect is neither uniform nor proportionate. Individual time preferences for health have been found to be highly variable and range from positive to negative rates of discount (Dolan and Gudex, 1995). Conventional social rates of discount do not necessarily reflect individual time preferences. Because no method of accounting for time preferences exists at the aggregate or societal level, Drummond and colleagues (1997) recommend that, regardless of the elicitation method, QALYs should be discounted at the recommended social rate.

SOURCE: Drummond et al. (1997, pp. 184–185).

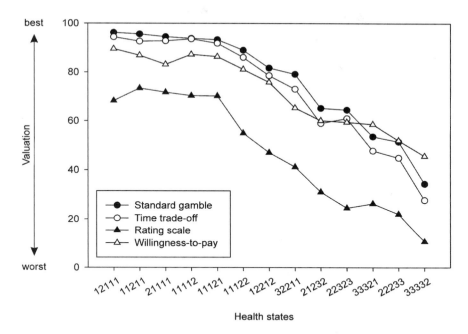

FIGURE 3-2 Mean Valuations for 13 EQ-5D Health States with Four Estimation Methods
NOTE: Each set of health state numbers refers to a specific combination of attribute levels for the EQ-5D survey instrument. See Appendix B for the corresponding descriptions.
SOURCE: Reprinted from Krabbe et al. (1997, Figure 1), with permission from Elsevier.

leagues (1997). Brazier and colleagues report that the seven studies they examined had inconsistent results with respect to the relationships between VAS and either SG or TTO.[3] Krabbe and colleagues' study comparing SG, TTO, rating scale (RS), and willingness-to-pay values for 13 generically described health states (taken from the EuroQol Group's EQ-5D classification system) did, however, find a consistent relationship between RS and TTO mean values, as shown in Figure 3-2. They estimated an algebraic power function for the relationship between the 13 mean RSs and TTO values with an R-squared of 0.96 (RS = 1 − (1 − TTO)$^\alpha$; α = 0.42).

---

[3]Krabbe et al. (1997) was published too late to be included in the Brazier et al. (1999a) review, which was completed in early 1997.

Conclusion This section has considered the performance of different elicitation techniques and the distinctive aspects of value implicitly conveyed by each one. Comparing methods for eliciting health state preferences directly may be less relevant for guiding CEA in regulatory analysis, however, than is comparing the specific HRQL instruments, or generic indexes, presented later in this chapter. The choice among alternative preference elicitation techniques is embedded in the choice of generic index, because each index relies on a valuation survey that employed a particular elicitation method. If health state values are elicited directly in new surveys, however, the researcher must choose a preference elicitation method.

Alternative HALY Metrics for Regulatory CEA

In the previous section we relied on the QALY as the construct for which different preference elicitation methods are applied. This section further considers the QALY and several other HALY constructs, in light of their suitability for regulatory CEA.

Quality-Adjusted Life Years

As noted in Chapter 1, the QALY was the first HALY metric, developed about 30 years ago as an outcome measure for CEA. It was designed to facilitate the maximization, in accordance with individual preferences for health, of aggregate health benefits for a given level of resources invested.

QALYs can be interpreted in different ways. When initially developed, the QALY was simply an index with an intuitive meaning, corresponding to the equivalent number of years in full health. More formally, QALYs can be thought of as an index for which relative values are calculated using utility theory or as a measure of economic utility (Gafni, 2004).

Pliskin and colleagues (1980) first proposed an underlying utility model for QALYs. This model applies to individual decision makers who are presumed to maximize expected utility when outcomes are uncertain. The authors derived the behavioral assumptions about preferences for health states and longevity that would be consistent with QALYs as a utility function, in situations where health status is constant over the life span. As described in the previous section, the SG and TTO are commonly used to determine the value of a particular health state that will last the rest of one's life in terms of the risk of death or the loss of life expectancy that the individual is willing to accept in order to achieve optimal health.

The behavioral assumptions of the utility-theoretical model are as follows:

• Individual decision makers follow the axioms of expected utility theory, which is based on preferences for outcomes that are uncertain. These are that (1) preferences for outcomes exist and are transitive; (2) preferences for an uncertain prospect do not depend on whether the prospect has one stage or two; and (3) preferences are continuous (von Neumann and Morgenstern, 1947; see Patrick and Erickson, 1993, for an exposition in terms of HRQL valuation).

• The proportion of remaining life that the individual decision maker would trade off for a given quality improvement is independent of the length of life remaining. That is, if someone with severe osteoarthritis would trade off 10 years of a remaining life expectancy (LE) of 40 years for 30 years free of disease followed by immediate death, then that person would be willing to trade off 5 years of a remaining 20-year LE to live free of disease.

• The utility for a health state is independent of its duration.

• An individual's health utilities are independent of nonhealth factors in her overall utility function. This means that preferences for income, leisure time, and other features of life do not affect her preferences for different states of health.

• Individuals are risk neutral with respect to gambles over life years (Dolan, 2000). Risk neutrality implies indifference among lotteries on future longevity that have the same life expectancy (and that are the same in terms of health).

An additional assumption that is required when health states vary over the life span is that preferences for health in different time periods are additive, in accordance with individual preferences for health.

Miyamoto and Eraker (1985) have investigated the behavioral content of the theoretical assumptions and concluded that:

> the QALY model deserves consideration as a description of patient preferences. . . because it concisely formulates two aspects of utility that are crucial to any viable medical utility model. . . . By summarizing risk attitude toward survival and the effect of health quality in a few easily assessed parameters, the QALY model provides a powerful and general instrument for describing patient values (p. 205).

As a measure of the production of health, QALYs are relatively simple and "modular," allowing longevity and HRQL to be equated, combined, and traded off at both the individual and population levels. Thus, despite some evidence that the independence and risk neutrality assumptions of the QALY model are violated in empirical studies, the model remains useful for decision making because its parameters can be readily estimated and it reflects trade-offs between survival and quality of life (Miyamoto and Eraker, 1985, 1988).

QALYs are by far the most commonly used metric in CEA. A literature survey of cost-effectiveness studies published over 20 years (1981–2000) in the medical and health services research literature identified 328 original CEAs that used a HALY outcome measure. All but one study, which used the healthy year equivalent (HYE) metric, used QALYs (Greenberg and Pliskin, 2002).

Healthy Year Equivalents

The HYE is an economic concept used to determine the number of years in optimal health that would produce the same level of utility for an individual as produced by a lifetime health *profile* (i.e., a particular succession of health states).

In a critique of the QALY model, Mehrez and Gafni (1990, 1991) proposed alternative approaches for estimating the relative values of alternative health states that do not rely on the strong independence assumptions posited by Pliskin et al. (1980) and the assumption of additivity over time. First, individuals may value two different sequences of health states that result in the same number of QALYs differently. Second, quality and length of life are *not* valued independently of each other, in contrast to a fundamental assumption of QALYs. Mehrez and Gafni addressed these empirical results by constructing dynamic health profiles extending over the course of life and then eliciting the relative values for these profiles in their entirety with a TTO elicitation technique.

The HYE approach requires comparing a large number of alternative health profiles. Although the HYE has an advantage in that some of the restrictive assumptions associated with QALYs do not apply, preferences must be elicited for specific health profiles, or sequences of health states, rather than for individual health states as with QALYs. Although proponents of the HYE metric contend that the greater methodological demands of the approach are justified in terms of its closer adherence to the theoretical conditions of utility theory, critics counter that developing an empirical base of HYE values for widespread use is not practical. The debate between proponents of QALYs and HYEs boils down to a choice between a simpler model that imposes a smaller information collection burden and a more complex but better fitting model that has demanding and costly data collection requirements.

Disability-Adjusted Life Years

The DALY is a measure of potential years of life lost to premature death, adjusted to include the equivalent years of healthy life lost through poor health or disability. Box 3-3 provides some background on the origin

---

BOX 3-3
The World Health Organization's Disability-Adjusted Life Year

DALYs were developed as a summary measure of population health for the WHO Global Burden of Disease study (Murray and Acharya, 1997). Three objectives motivated this project. First, international health policy debates previously had depended primarily on mortality statistics, and policy makers and researchers wanted to include the impact of nonfatal health outcomes in their assessments and deliberations. Second, to allocate resources across a spectrum of health interventions more effectively, a common measure was needed to estimate the relative magnitude of particular diseases in terms of their impact on longevity and disability. Last, such information could reduce existing allocative inefficiencies by comparing investments in different kinds of interventions for particular populations and societies.

The valuation of various health states using a variant of the PTO elicitation method was undertaken with WHO's concerns and objectives in mind. In 1995, health experts were brought together by WHO and first asked to determine the numbers of persons in full health and those with a particular condition that they would consider equivalent in terms of a given life extension (say, of one year). Next they were asked to determine the number of persons in the health-impaired group who would have to experience an improvement in HRQL to full health to be equivalent to gaining a life extension of one year for the fully healthy group. These PTO values were then compared and reconciled in a final weighting. The official DALY weights are available in Mathers et al. (2003), which can be downloaded from the WHO website (http://www3.who.int/whosis/discussion_papers/pdf/paper54.pdf).

---

of the DALY measure. DALYs are calculated by summing the life years lost from an optimal life expectancy, adjusted downward by any mental or physical disability caused by disease or injury. Like QALYs, DALYs can be discounted to present value. The DALY index scale is an inversion of the QALY scale: for DALYs, 0 corresponds to perfect health and 1 to death. DALY index values correspond to specific health conditions rather than to generically characterized health states.

The initial characterization of nonfatal health outcomes in DALYs was based on the International Classification of Impairments, Disabilities, and Handicap. DALYs focus on functional disability from diseases and other health-related conditions. In the WHO DALY study, health professionals constructed the descriptions of disabilities, and other groups of health experts valued the disabilities using the PTO method in a deliberative, iterative process (Murray and Lopez, 1996; Gold et al., 2002). These DALY condition weights do not purport to reflect individual utilities. Rather, they represent the relative social value of different states of health as judged by experts, ". . . a variant of QALYs which have been standardized for comparative [international] use" (Murray and Acharya, 1997, p. 704).

The DALY construct reflected two much-criticized analytical choices that are no longer considered essential for the measure. First, decrements in longevity were calculated from a worldwide optimum life expectancy, represented by that of Japanese women (82.5 years). The second distinctive feature was age weighting. Years lived in young adulthood were given a greater value in comparison to years lived earliest and at the end of the life span. Age weighting gives priority to the potential for improving health outcomes among the members of society most critical to the well-being of society as a whole, those in their productive years of life.

Age weighting and the use of optimum life expectancy are not, however, in principle necessary to the DALY construct. DALY weights may be determined based on any of the methods described earlier in this chapter, including PTO, SG, TTO, or RS. Some more recent applications of DALYs are not age weighted, use life tables for the actual target population, and apply DALY weights derived from sources based on different methods (see, e.g., de Hollander et al., 1999; Fox-Rushby and Hanson, 2001, for applications and discussion of analytic options using DALYs).

Saved-Young-Life Equivalents

QALYs and other individually based preference or utility measures are deemed by some to be inappropriate for societal resource allocation decisions. These measures do not adequately account for the value attached to saving lives relative to improving health or to the priority that may be given to improving outcomes for the most severely impaired, regardless of the size of the improvement. QALYs measure only the size of an improvement in health and disregard health state starting and endpoints. This reflects the irrelevance, in the calculation of QALY gains or losses, of all personal attributes except the quality adjustment to a life year and the number of aggregate QALYs. However, in surveys of people's preferences for public investments in health, their "health-related social welfare function" is rarely consistent with QALY maximization (Ubel et al., 1996; Menzel, 1999).

Nord (1992, 1999) has proposed several strategies to incorporate this concern for severity and life saving in HALY measurement. One of these approaches, related to the PTO valuation method described earlier, selects a single health care outcome as the common unit of measurement for all health-related outcomes. The common unit Nord proposes is the SAVE, the value of saving the life of a young person and restoring him to full health. To determine the relative societal value of a given health outcome, two equally expensive programs are compared. One program saves a young life each year and the other produces n health outcomes of type x each year.

Respondents are asked how many outcomes of type *x* would be considered as valuable as saving the life of one young person. This direct elicitation allows all aspects of the given health outcome to be taken into account, including the initial health states as well as the extent of potential gains in health and the characteristics of the persons who would benefit. Nord proposes this unit of measure as a common denominator for all societal investments in health and longevity improvements.

The SAVE measure, like the HYE, requires direct elicitation for many specific health profiles, and thus faces the same implementation difficulties. Index values for SAVEs are not available in the research literature and, as with PTO values more generally, the reliability of the technique has not been determined.

We take up the issue of societal values and QALYs again in Chapter 4, where we examine the ethical assumptions embedded in the QALY metric and strategies for addressing distributive and other ethical issues that arise in regulatory CEAs that employ QALYs.

Choosing a HALY Measure for Regulatory Analysis

The QALY is the obvious choice at this time for standardizing regulatory analysis on a single HALY metric. Researchers have completed only limited work using the HYE and the SAVE, and health state values using these metrics are not readily available. Furthermore, values for the wide range of health conditions considered in regulatory analysis are not likely to be developed in the near term using these approaches, given the complexities of establishing values (such as conditioning health state values on duration or transitions from prior health states) and the expense of related research. The HYE, while in theory superior to the QALY as a measure of preferences for health, would require a significantly more complex elicitation process, as would the SAVE, which is valued using variants of the PTO method. The DALY can be valued using a variety of methods consistent with QALY measurement. However, the inversion of the calculations, as *losses* averted from some normative life expectancy, introduces opportunities for confusion in interpretation if other results are presented as QALY *gains*.

Alternatives to the QALY have not undergone extensive reliability evaluation. Although the QALY can be criticized for not adhering to expected utility theory or for ignoring certain dimensions of societal values for health-related improvements such as severity or threat to life, it is feasible and widely used. In addition, the QALY is supported by a number of generic, multiattribute HRQL survey instruments and can be estimated for health endpoints in regulatory analysis using a variety of approaches.

SOURCES OF HEALTH STATE VALUES
FOR REGULATORY ANALYSIS

Relative values or preference weights for health states that represent endpoints in regulatory analyses can be obtained using a variety of sources. As already noted, the field of HRQL measurement was initially developed to inform medical technology assessment and resource allocation decisions. The data sets, information needs, and analytic priorities for these policy contexts tend, not surprisingly, to differ from those of regulatory analysts and policy makers. Consequently, the measurement tools that have been designed to answer questions of clinical effectiveness and efficiency in improving health outcomes are unlikely to be perfectly matched to the demands of regulatory analysis. The following discussion reviews various ways of obtaining preference-based HRQL values, focusing on the information needs and constraints of those involved with risk regulation. This section reviews:

- Primary elicitation of health state index values for specific conditions,
- Four commonly used generic HRQL survey instruments or indexes,
- Use of condition-specific indexes,
- Use of experts to assign health states,
- Use of data from routine population surveys,
- Use of health state index values from prior studies and benefit transfer practices, and
- Assessing uncertainty in the estimation of health-related effects from regulatory interventions.

The section concludes with a brief review of innovations in survey instruments and measurement techniques and key areas for further research and development of HRQL metrics and methods for regulatory CEA.

Primary Elicitation of Condition-Specific Index Values

One way to obtain index values for particular states of health is to elicit preferences for those states directly from the population whose interests are at stake, or from proxies for that population. For example, to value a reduction in a particular type of cardiac disease in the U.S. population, researchers might conduct a survey that described the effects of the disease and ask a representative sample of the U.S. population to value these effects. When QALY-based CEA was first introduced, direct elicitation of preferences for specific health states, conditions, or treatment outcomes was the only available approach (Bush et al., 1973; Torrance et al., 1973;

McNeil et al., 1978; Pliskin et al., 1980). Every CEA had to estimate values for the outcomes of interest. Generic HRQL indexes had not been developed, and a research literature reporting values that could be used "off the shelf" had not yet accumulated.

By the time the PCEHM issued its report in 1996, several generic HRQL survey instruments were available. The panel recommended generic health state classification systems as the preferred measurement approach in CEA because these systems offer the best opportunity to achieve consistency in the valuation of health states across studies and across different health interventions and diseases (Gold et al., 1996b).[4]

In some cases, existing studies may provide suitable, high-quality estimates for valuing the health states of interest in regulatory analysis. In the absence of such studies, new, primary research to value the health conditions targeted by a regulatory intervention might appear to be the most desirable course. However, it is unlikely to be a realistic option in the near term for the vast majority of regulatory analyses. Both the time available to conduct analysis of proposed regulations and the resource demands of survey research militate against undertaking original studies, except as part of a separate project without the constraints of regulatory analysis. In addition, federally sponsored survey research is subject to Office of Management and Budget review and approval under the Paperwork Reduction Act, which creates additional time and resource burdens and uncertainty. As a result, the sources of health state index values discussed in the remainder of this section are likely to be the more feasible options for regulatory CEA in the near term.

Generic HRQL Indexes

An alternative to directly eliciting preferences for specific conditions is to use a multiattribute health state classification system with predetermined index values for generically described health states. These indexes are widely used and accepted in medical CEA as a way to assign general population or "community" index values to highly disparate conditions and diseases, with minimal burden on respondents. Characterizing particular health conditions in terms of the conditions' generic features or attributes can be done in a number of ways: by patients with the condition, by members of the general public based on a detailed description of the condition or scenario, or by clinical experts familiar with the condition. These characteristics are

---

[4]In the context of regulatory CEA, directly eliciting preferences for health states is analogous to conducting an original willingness-to-pay survey to value health effects for BCA. Although some researchers have proposed standardizing valuation approaches for BCA, established generic methods like the indexes used in CEA do not exist.

then valued using the preexisting health state values developed for that particular index.

The case studies conducted by the Committee to inform and illustrate the discussion and recommendations in this report employed four generic indexes:

- The Quality of Well-Being Scale,
- The Health Utilities Index (in two versions, Mark 2 and Mark 3),
- The EuroQol-5D, and
- The SF-6D.

These instruments were chosen for in-depth examination from a much larger field of such instruments based on their widespread use in U.S. and Canadian health care outcomes and cost-effectiveness research (in the case of the first three instruments listed) or because the index values could be calculated from health profile data that are collected extensively in the United States (in the case of the SF-6D).

After briefly reviewing the structure of such instruments and the theories on which they are based, we describe each of them in turn. Tables 3-3 and 3-4 present the basic features of each of the four instruments in summary and comparative form. The instruments themselves and sources for their valuation or scoring algorithms are presented in Appendix B.

The use of generic health indexes to estimate preference-based HRQL values involves two steps. First, the health state of interest must be described in terms of the several domains of HRQL. (See Table 3-1 for a conceptual overview of these domains.) A given respondent characterizes or describes the health state according to the generic set of attributes offered by the index's standardized questionnaire. For example, under the EQ-5D, the respondent may indicate that the health state leads to "no" problems with walking about, "some" problems washing or dressing, and so forth. Once a health state has been characterized in terms of the domains of the generic instrument, a single index value for the overall health state can be calculated on a 0-to-1 scale.

These index values for health states are based on a separate valuation exercise (typically conducted with respondents drawn from a local community's residents or a nationally representative sample) that elicits preferences for health states (described generically, not as particular diseases or conditions) in terms of the survey instrument's HRQL domains. The relationship between general population *valuation* of health states and the *characterization* of health states using a generic HRQL index is depicted in Figure 3-3, for the case in which patients with a health condition describe the condition.

Index values for health states using multiattribute generic instruments

TABLE 3-3 Domains and Number of Attribute Levels for Generic HRQL Indexes

QWB	[QWB-SA]	HUI-2	HUI-3	EQ-5D	SF-6D-36	[-12]
Mobility (3)	[3]	Sensation (4)	Vision (6)	Mobility (3)	Physical functioning (6)	[3]
Physical activities (3)	[3]	Mobility (5)	Hearing (6)	Self-care (3)	Role limitation (4)	[4]
Social activities (5)	[5]	Emotion (5)	Speech (5)	Usual activities (3)	Social functioning (5)	[5]
Symptom/problem complexes (26)[a]	[58][a]	Cognition (4)	Ambulation (6)	Pain (3)	Mental health (5)	[5]
		Self-care (4)	Dexterity (6)	Anxiety/depression (3)	Bodily pain (6)	[6]
		Pain (5)	Emotion (5)		Vitality (5)	[5]
		Fertility (3)	Cognition (6)			
			Pain (5)			

NOTES: HRQL = health-related quality of life; HUI = Health Utilities Index; QWB = Quality of Well-Being; QWB-SA = self-administered format QWB.

[a]Each of the symptoms/problem complexes is measured as present or absent.

SOURCES: Feeny et al. (1996); Torrance et al. (1996); Kaplan et al. (1997); Kopec and Willison (2003); Brazier and Roberts (2004). See Appendix B for complete descriptions and sources for these generic indexes.

TABLE 3-4 Valuation Surveys for Generic HRQL Instruments

Index	Sampling Frame	Sample Size/Year/ Response Rate	Valuation Technique	Number of Health States Measured/Measured by Each Respondent	Number of Possible Health States
QWB	San Diego community residents	866 adults/ 1974–1975/NA	VAS	42/42	945
HUI-2	Ontario, Canada	293 parents, for children/NA/NA	VAS transformed into SG	21 with VAS; 4 with SG	24,000
HUI-3	Ontario, Canada community residents age 16+	504 adults/ 1994/65%	VAS transformed into SG	Modeling sample: 22–24 with VAS; 5 with SG Direct valuation: 73/16 with VAS; 9 with SG	972,000
EQ-5D					
U.K.	U.K. community residents age 18+	2,997 with complete data/1993/56%	TTO; VAS	42/13	243
U.S.	U.S. community residents age 18+	3,773 with complete data/2002/59%	TTO; VAS for own health state only	45/15	243
SF-6D	U.K. community residents age 16+	611 with usable data/ 1998/65%	SG	249/6 (for SF-36 version) 241/6 (for SF-12 version)	18,000 7,500

SOURCES: Kaplan and Anderson (1988); Feeny et al. (1995, 2002); Torrance et al. (1995); Dolan (1997); Brazier et al. (1999a, 2002); Fryback (2003); Kopec and Willison (2003); Brazier and Roberts (2004); Shaw et al. (2005).

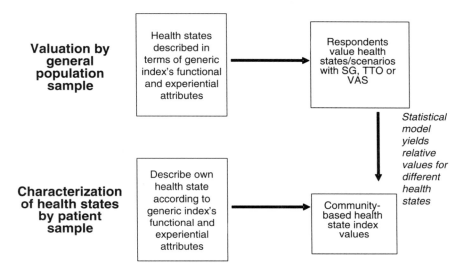

FIGURE 3-3 Measuring HRQL with Generic Instruments: Community Valuations, Patient Characterizations

can be estimated holistically or in decomposed form. In the holistic approach, respondents are asked to value a composite scenario reflecting a particular combination of functional and other characteristics represented by particular domain levels, using any of the elicitation techniques described above. In the decomposed valuation approach, respondents determine the relative value of each possible health-related attribute for each domain (e.g., pain, mobility, self-care) independently. When multiattribute systems are valued holistically, the weights for individual attributes and attribute levels are estimated through statistical modeling. The decomposed approach employs an algebraic approach to combining the single-attribute estimates. Weighting formulas can be additive or multiplicative under either approach.

Each of the generic indexes used in the case studies and described below has at least one set of values for all possible health states that is based on a general population or community valuation survey, presented in Table 3-4. The features of each instrument's standard or reference valuation survey are described below.

Quality of Well-Being Scale

History The QWB was developed from the first generic HRQL index, the Index of Well-Being, which was envisioned as part of a general health policy model to guide health services and health program investments (Fanshel and Bush, 1970; Kaplan et al., 1976; Kaplan and Anderson, 1988, 1996). Its early introduction and comprehensiveness made it a point of departure for the design of subsequent instruments (McDowell and Newell, 1996; Drummond et al., 1997). Until 1997, when a self-administered version of the QWB was released, the QWB had been available only in an interviewer-administered format. The interviewer-administered questionnaire takes about 15 minutes to complete and the self-administered version 14 minutes (Andresen et al., 1998).

Domains The QWB includes four dimensions: physical function, mobility, social function, and immediate symptoms or problems. The first 3 dimensions produce a total of 46 function levels, including death. In the interviewer-administered version, there are 27 symptom or problem complexes (including no symptom or problem), while there are 58 symptom or problem complexes in the self-administered version. The symptom/problem complex domain and related weights are unique to the QWB among the four indexes considered here.

Valuation The original community-based valuation survey for the QWB included 856 adults from a probability sample of households in San Diego conducted in 1974–75. This survey has been the basis for scoring all versions of the QWB since then. Each respondent in the valuation survey rated 42 descriptive health profiles using a CR procedure, with zero corresponding to death (Fryback, 2003). The survey asked respondents to consider the relative value of being in the health state in question for a single day. This short-term valuation period is unique to the QWB among the indexes considered here. The statistically modeled weighting formula is additive (i.e., it reflects no interactions between attributes) and yields summary index values between 0 and 1.

Availability Age- and sex-specific QWB norms for the U.S. noninstitutionalized population have been estimated from National Health Interview Survey (NHIS) data for 1986–88 and 1994 through a process of mapping NHIS responses to the QWB instrument (Anderson et al., 2004). The QWB questionnaires and weights are available to the public without charge.

Health Utilities Index

History The HUI family of HRQL measures (the HUI Mark 1, Mark 2, and Mark 3) is the second-oldest set of HRQL instruments. The earliest version of the HUI was developed in the late 1970s and early 1980s by Torrance and colleagues at McMaster University, Ontario, Canada, and incorporated in a CEA of neonatal intensive care (Boyle et al., 1983). The later versions of the instrument, the HUI-2 and HUI-3 (both of which are current, having succeeded the original index), were developed from the HUI-1. The HUI-2 was initially applied in studies of childhood cancer and was later modified for adult applications. The HUI-3 was developed for general application (Drummond et al., 1997). HUI questionnaires can be either self- or interviewer-administered, and proxy assessment versions (for completion by parents or caretakers rather than the subject) are also available.

Domains   The HUI-2 consists of seven domains: sensory, mobility, emotion, cognitive, self-care, pain, and fertility. The eight-domain HUI-3 is closely related to the HUI-2, with the sensory domain split into vision, hearing, and speech; a new attribute for dexterity; and the self-care and fertility categories eliminated. Some of these changes in domains (see Table 3-3) were made to reduce overlap in the constructs measured.

Valuation   The values for the HUI-2 were elicited from a random sample of 293 parents of schoolchildren in Hamilton, Ontario, and environs (Torrance et al., 1996). The valuation survey for the HUI-3 included a probability sample of the general adult population ($n = 504$) in Hamilton, Ontario (Feeny et al., 2002). For both valuation surveys, the VAS was used to elicit values within each domain while SG was used to assess utilities for the "corner states" (where one domain is at its worst level and all other domains are at their best levels). Respondents were asked to consider being in the health state they were valuing for the rest of their life.

The HUI instruments represent a direct application of multiattribute utility theory, which describes how different mathematical functions can be used to represent different types of interdependence among attribute values (Keeney and Raiffa, 1976; Torrance et al., 1982, 1995; Feeny et al., 2002). The HUI-2 and -3 scoring formulas are multiplicative, allowing for a limited form of interaction among domains. Each of the 8 HUI-3 domains has 5 or 6 levels, resulting in 972,000 possible health states and making it in this sense the most detailed of the four instruments with respect to the measurement of generic health-related characteristics.

Availability   Since 1990, the HUI-3 has been included in every major Canadian population health survey, and more recently in three major U.S. surveys: the Health and Retirement Survey 2000, the joint U.S.–Canada Health Survey (2002–03), and as part of the U.S. EQ-5D valuation survey. The latter two surveys allow for the calculation of U.S. population norms for the HUI-2 and -3. The HUI-2 and -3 questionnaires are available from their developers for a survey administration licensing fee.

The EuroQoL-5D

History   The EQ-5D instrument has been developed by the EuroQoL Group, a multidisciplinary network of researchers based largely in Europe. This research consortium was set up in 1987 and formally established under Dutch law in 1995, with the shared interest in creating a standard, simple, self-administered, generic HRQL index for use in economic evaluation and clinical outcomes studies. The EQ-5D is the simplest of the generic HRQL indexes. Initially, it was envisioned as an abstracting device that could be used in tandem with more specific HRQL measures, and serve as a bridge among particular studies and surveys (Williams, 1995).

The EQ-5D can be used as a self-administered mail survey or through phone or in-person interviews. It takes about a minute to complete, and data are less often missing than with longer, more complex HRQL surveys. The brevity that is the source of the EQ-5D's advantages is also, however, a limitation on sensitivity. In a side-by-side comparison to the HUI-3, little difference was found between the EQ-5D and the HUI-3 with respect to their ability to discriminate between respondents with and without a variety of self-reported health conditions. Those who are assigned to the best EQ-5D health state are, however, somewhat more differentiated by the HUI-3 (Houle and Berthelot, 2000). To address this limitation of the current EQ-5D, its sponsors have been developing a five-level version of the instrument, which would improve its ability to discriminate among health states (Kind, 2004).

Domains   The EQ-5D descriptive system has five domains: mobility, self-care, usual activity, pain/discomfort, and anxiety/depression. Each domain has the same three levels, designated as no, some, or extreme problems in the particular domain. The total number of health states is 243.

Valuation   One standard valuation method for the EQ-5D uses VAS rating. In addition, researchers in a number of European countries (including the United Kingdom) and in the United States have elicited weights for the EQ-5D using TTO methods (Dolan, 1997; Shaw et al., 2005). In the TTO valuation exercises, respondents were asked to regard the health state of interest as lasting for 10 years without change, followed by death. The U.K. TTO index values are the most widely used EQ-5D valuations in the English-language health outcomes literature. The TTO values have been analyzed in two different ways, by applying them directly to the health states for which they were elicited, and by constructing a statistical model in which the added impact is estimated for each attribute. In the statistical model, two interaction terms are included to allow for additional value or greater decrement in value if one or more attributes are at their best or worst levels (Dolan, 1997; Dolan and Roberts, 2002). More recently, Shaw and colleagues (2005) elicited EQ-5D values in a nationally representative U.S. sample using TTO methods.

Availability In 2000 through 2002, the EQ-5D was included in the Medical Expenditure Panel Survey (MEPS), a routinely conducted panel survey with roughly 24,000 to 37,000 U.S. noninstitutionalized adult respondents (depending on the year). MEPS is administered by the Agency for Healthcare Research and Quality. This survey provides U.S. national norms for the EQ-5D. Estimates of chronic condition index values have been developed from it as well (Sullivan et al., 2005). These condition-specific values were used in the Committee's Environmental Protection Agency (EPA) case study and are described later in this chapter. The EuroQoL Group has put the EQ-5D survey instrument in the public domain and thus users do not have to pay licensing fees to administer the survey or analyze data.

The SF-6D

History The SF-6D is the most recently developed generic, preference-based HRQL index (Brazier et al., 1998, 2002). It was designed to take advantage of the most widely used health status profiles in the world, the short-form health survey (SF-36) and its subset profile instrument, the SF-12. Two versions of the SF-6D are available, based on the 36-item and 12-item profiles, respectively. As discussed earlier, health profiling instruments produce quantified measures of health status but do not yield a single, preference-based value for HRQL as do index measures.

The SF-36 originated in research tools designed for the RAND Health Insurance Experiment, and was refined and applied in a series of medical outcomes studies that investigated specific conditions (Patrick and Erickson, 1993; Ware, 2000). Both the 36- and 12-item instruments measure general health in 8 dimensions, and yield 2 summary scores, 1 for physical health and the other for mental health, and 8 single-dimension scores. In the late 1990s, a British research group developed a simplified six-dimension health state classification system derived from the data collected in the SF-36. The SF-6D instruments use 11 items from the SF-36 (Brazier et al., 2002) and 7 items from the SF-12 (Brazier and Roberts, 2004). Their limitations include a floor effect (i.e., relatively high scores for physical function and role performance, at the lowest levels of these domains, compared with other indexes) and the fact that weights are available only from a U.K. valuation study.

Domains This index has six domains: physical functioning, role limitation, social functioning, pain, mental health, and vitality. The number of levels per domain depends on the profile questionnaire (either version 1 or

2) from which it was derived. For SF-6D states taken from the SF-36 version 2, each domain has from 4 to 6 levels, defining a possible total of 18,000 health states.

Valuation A representative sample of 836 residents of the United Kingdom participated in interviews and ranked and then valued a total of 249 SF-6D health states from the SF-36 version 2 (each participant rated 6 health states) using a SG technique. A scoring algorithm for the six-dimension model was developed using multivariate statistical methods. The same valuation survey was used to develop the scoring algorithm for the SF-12 version of the SF-6D as for the SF-36 version. There are also algorithms available to score responses to SF-12 and SF-36 version 1, which have fewer response categories than version 2.

Availability The attractiveness of the SF-6D instruments lies in their derivation from widely collected health profile data sets. However, scoring these instruments requires access to item-level data rather than the more widely reported physical and mental health summary scores. Item-level data are available for the SF-12 version 1 in MEPS for years 2000 to 2002. These data make it possible to calculate national age-specific population norms for the SF-6D as well as condition-specific norms.

The SF data sets and the latest versions of the SF-36 and SF-12 (version 2) questionnaires (from which the SF-6D questions were chosen) are proprietary, and must be licensed for use from the Medical Outcomes Trust. The SF-6D scoring algorithms are available free from their authors. Version 1 of each instrument is available free, and the algorithms to compute SF-6D scores from these versions are available from the authors (Brazier and Roberts, 2004).

Condition-Specific Indexes and Applications to Special Populations

Many HRQL instruments have been developed for specific diseases or conditions, such as asthma, cancer, depression, diabetes, and rheumatoid arthritis. Others have been developed for specific populations, such as children or nursing home residents.[5] These "targeted" instruments have been used in many health outcomes studies and CEAs of medical interventions or

---

[5]See the web-based Quality of Life Instruments Database, developed and maintained by the Mapi Research Institute and Mapi Research Trust, Lyon, France. It contains approximately 500 HRQL instruments, including generic instruments, condition-specific instruments, and population-specific instruments and is located online at http://www.qolid.org/ind_home2004.html.

prevention programs. More specialized classification systems can often provide greater sensitivity to changes in HRQL relevant to a particular condition or patient population than can generic instruments.

Condition-Specific Instruments

Evaluations to support the marketing of pharmaceutical therapies and to assess the effectiveness of other therapeutic and diagnostic interventions have led to the development of disease-specific health profiling instruments and preference-based indexes. Not all disease-specific instruments yield summary index values for calculating QALYs, however. Such profiling instruments may be used in conjunction with direct valuation of specific health states by patients.

Cost-effectiveness analysis, as compared with clinical outcomes research, depends on a measure of effectiveness that captures all aspects of health-related functioning and quality of life, and cannot rely on those that exclusively measure changes relative to a particular organ system or disease. The wider compass of the domains and attribute levels of a generic HRQL instrument, which make it less attuned to any particular health condition and its impacts on symptoms and function, also ensures that it can be applied broadly and provide comparability of results across health conditions. Although the PCEHM recommended that analysts use generic indexes, it concluded that, if disease-specific classification systems *are* used, health states still should be framed in terms of overall health. If necessary, default values should be assigned for domains found in generic indexes (e.g., social or role function) so that results from targeted instruments can be mapped onto a generic measure for comparability (Gold et al., 1996b).

In our case study analysis of the National Highway Traffic Safety Administration (NHTSA) rule establishing installation standards for child restraint anchoring systems, the Committee included a specialized instrument developed to assess the impact of traumatic injury on long-term functioning, the Functional Capacity Index (FCI), to value health effects (MacKenzie et al., 1996). Although the FCI is not a preference-based index, it does produce health state values, similar to those of the generic indexes, that reflect the relative impact of different traumatic injuries on long-term functioning (MacKenzie et al., 1996, 2004).

In this case study, both the health effects being measured (traumatic injuries and their long-term functional impacts) and the population affected by the regulation (children under 6 years of age) presented particular challenges. Although the FCI has been designed for application to adults, and in that respect offers no advantage over the generic indexes, it is designed for use 12 months after a traumatic injury. One version of the FCI predicts this long-term functional capacity from the categorical injury severity data that

NHTSA routinely collects. Appendix A describes the information available for estimating the kinds of injuries prevented by the child restraint rule and the Committee's approach to estimating long-term HRQL impacts for injuries to infants and young children. A fuller description of the FCI is included at Appendix B.

Special Populations

Applications of HRQL instruments to special populations raise several issues. One is the adaptation of generic instruments for use with language, ethnic and racial, and socioeconomic subgroups. A basic premise that underlies the use of an HRQL measure cross-culturally is that there is a universal or general quality-of-life concept that can be measured by a common set of indicators (Anderson et al., 1996). We have not attempted to determine the validity or consistency of specific generic instruments across population subgroups or cross-culturally; these sorts of evaluations have not been conducted in any systematic fashion. However, several generic instruments have been tested in subpopulations and/or are available in several languages. The EQ-5D is available in more than 80 languages, with all versions conforming to guidelines established for the instrument by the EuroQol Group. The recent U.S. EQ-5D valuation survey oversampled non-Hispanic black and Hispanic respondents to provide reliable subgroup estimates for these populations. The HUI questionnaires are available in 15 languages, and additional versions are under development.

Another important issue for HRQL measurement is the application of generic instruments, and their underlying valuations, to children. Children's HRQL measurement has been handled in several ways. First, parents and clinicians have served as proxy respondents, both in characterizing children's HRQL and in valuing children's health states and outcomes. Second, specialized instruments—frequently condition-specific instruments such as those for asthma or childhood cancer—have been developed for use with children or their proxies. Third, generic instruments have been designed or adapted for use specifically with children. For example, the HUI-2 was developed for use with children and was valued by parents (see Appendix B), and a "child-friendly" version of the EQ-5D with rephrased questions has been developed (Hennessy and Kind, 2002).

None of these strategies to address the special challenges of predicting and capturing changes in the HRQL consequences of illness and injury in childhood is entirely satisfactory. Although using standard generic indexes to value children's health outcomes allows for comparability with results for adults, these instruments do not capture many aspects of children's health-related well being. At the same time, while condition-specific HRQL instruments tailored for children may be more sensitive to changes in condition, they do not permit comparisons across different types of pediatric illnesses and impairments. Finally, both children and parents have important perspectives on children's HRQL, and instruments that focus on just one or the other offer only a partial view. Box 3-4 summarizes some of the considerations unique to valuing children's health outcomes and quality of life.

A recent literature review of QALY-based cost-effectiveness studies in pediatric populations found that the majority of such studies did not adhere to PCEHM recommendations to use generic indexes, SG or TTO valuation, and values elicited from the general population (Griebsch et al., 2005). The authors were unable to determine whether departures from these recommended practices were a result of ignorance or disregard of the recommended practices, or were instead a conscious choice to use an alternative approach that the researchers deemed more appropriate for children. For example, one concern with the use of parents as proxy respondents for their children is that parents may not be able to distinguish their own preferences from those of their child; this concern may lead researchers to use clinicians as proxy respondents instead (generally considered to be a less desirable approach because clinicians are less likely to be familiar with the ongoing HRQL impacts on their patients than are daily caregivers). Griebsch and colleagues argue that the evidence base for developing best practices, both in the characterization and description of health states and in valuing them for children, has yet to be established. Thus they conclude that the use of QALY-based CEA is not ready for standardization when used in pediatric populations.

Another challenge is that chronic illness or severe injuries that occur in childhood often have long-term impacts. Thus the requirements for appropriately assessing and valuing the impacts on HRQL change over time. Approaches that are appropriate for the childhood impacts may be less appropriate for impacts in the adult years and vice versa. However, if different instruments were developed and used for different ages, consistency could become a concern. This problem is compounded by the fact that the long-term impacts of childhood illness and injuries are often difficult to predict and can involve many aspects of well being, including social development and educational achievement.

The Committee's child restraints case study provides an example of these difficulties in prediction. The case study used generic HRQL instruments that included attribute descriptions that were inappropriately described or valued for young children, who cannot, for example, normally perform many self-care activities independently. The experts who applied these instruments noted that it was difficult to assess the long-term implications, and differed somewhat in their assessments of long-term effects.

BOX 3-4
HRQL Measurement for Children

Evaluating the HRQL of children poses particularly difficult choices and challenges about which there has been little consensus or resolution (Griebsch et al., 2005). These challenges relate to (1) the conceptualization of children's HRQL (do instruments developed for adults reflect the appropriate dimensions for children at particular developmental stages?); (2) the ability of children or their proxies to describe relevant aspects of children's health states adequately; and (3) the valuation of children's HRQL, including whose values should be reflected in the valuation and, to the extent that children's own valuations are desired, how these values might be elicited.

The construction and domains of HRQL instruments developed for adults may not be well suited to capture children's experience and functioning (Eiser and Morse, 2001a). Childhood is qualitatively different (culturally distinct) from adulthood, and ideally HRQL instruments for children should take account of particular developmental stages and thresholds (Landgraf and Abetz, 1996). This has implications both for the scope of the HRQL instrument and its format; it should measure developmentally important aspects of functioning, such as cognitive abilities, motor skills, social interactions, and body image, for example, and be calibrated for administration to children (or their proxies) at different developmental stages and ages. In addition, because children undergo relatively rapid changes in functional capacities, such as in self-care and mobility, at different rates, it is difficult to determine whether any observed changes are due to normal development or are the result of illness or intervention.

Generic HRQL survey instruments have been developed or modified for administration to children, and even more have been developed to assess HRQL in children with a specific disease. In a survey of the field of pediatric HRQL instru-

Assignment of Health States by Experts or Other Proxies

Proxies are used in HRQL assessments for a variety of reasons. As just discussed, parents may be asked to serve as proxies for children; caregivers, guardians, or family members for temporarily or permanently incapacitated adults (and children); and clinicians for patients. With the aging of the U.S. population and the growing incidence of conditions affecting cognitive functions, the use of proxy respondents for incapacitated adults can be expected to increase.

Proxies may be asked to (1) establish the relative values of different health states, or (2) describe or locate another person's HRQL using a multiattribute classification instrument. Pickard and Knight (2005) distinguish two proxy perspectives. The first is when a proxy describes another

ments, Eiser and Morse (2001b) identified 19 generic instruments developed or adapted for pediatric use and 24 condition-specific pediatric instruments. These pediatric instruments in some cases elicit responses from the child, in others from the parent, and in yet others from both parent and child. These authors argue that the perspectives of both parents and children are important for gaining a good understanding of children's HRQL. Although parent and child health state characterizations have shown good agreement in domains that reflect physical functioning, activity, and symptoms, characterizations in domains that reflect emotional or social health demonstrate less agreement (Eiser and Morse, 2001b). Clinicians tend to identify fewer deficits in HRQL domains when serving as child proxies than do parents and teachers (Eiser and Morse, 2001b). Most of the attention in developing these instruments has been on the characterization or description of health states in children, rather than on valuation. Where valuation is specifically addressed, as in the HUI-2, the values of parents have been elicited.

Likewise, the valuation of children's health states raises issues of whose preferences to take into account and how to measure preferences in children with limited but maturing cognitive and other capacities (Petrou, 2003; Matza et al., 2004). Many argue that children's valuation of their own health states should be included along with those of their parents in the societal value of these effects (Eiser and Morse, 2001a; Petrou, 2003). One study that evaluated the ability of children with asthma, ages 7 through 17, to comprehend and provide reliable responses to questions eliciting their preferences for different health states concluded that at least sixth-grade reading skills were necessary for SG exercises and that at least second-grade reading skills were necessary for using a VAS technique (Juniper et al., 1997). In addition to the challenges that valuation questions and elicitation techniques pose for children's and adolescents' valuation of their own health, a further valuation issue is how to include the effects of children's health on the well-being of parents and caretakers, as these effects are not captured by individual-level HRQL measures.

person's HRQL or assigns a relative value to HRQL as the person would rate himself. The second is when the proxy is asked to make those judgments about another's HRQL from the proxy's *own* perspective. In most cases the proxy perspective is understood in the sense first described; however, proxy surveys can be ambiguous and it is important to ascertain what proxy questionnaires and responses actually reflect.

This section does not discuss the important and well-documented issue of self-versus-proxy concordance and discordance in characterizing and valuing HRQL and functional capacities. Here we are considering experts as proxies in characterizing regulatory health endpoints in terms of the specific attributes of a multiattribute generic index. This exercise differs from individual self-descriptions on generic HRQL surveys or even experts' proxy descriptions for individual patients. Still, some of the findings from clinical and institutional settings, namely, that caregiver and professional proxies tend to rate quality of life as poorer within some domains and overestimate disabilities of patients, may carry over to expert elicitation exercises such as those described here (Magaziner et al., 1988; Rothman et al., 1991).

In the context of regulatory analysis, proxies may be most often used to describe the impacts of a health condition using the characterization scheme of a particular generic index. If it is not feasible to conduct a new survey of the population affected by the regulation to determine health state values, an alternative is to ask clinician experts (i.e., physicians and others involved in patient care) to characterize the health conditions of interest using a generic instrument. In these cases, index values for health states are obtained separately from community or general population valuation surveys. The Committee explored this approach in the three case studies conducted as part of its investigations. (See Appendix A for synopses of the case studies; and Robinson et al., 2005a,b,c, for complete reports.) Because of limited time and resources for preparing the case studies, we skipped or abbreviated several steps in eliciting expert judgments that are often recommended. Thus this discussion includes good practices in expert elicitation that we did not follow in the case studies. Box 3-5 summarizes the steps in using experts to assign the health endpoints specified in a regulatory analysis to a generic HRQL index to estimate the regulatory intervention's effectiveness.[6,7]

In regulatory analysis, health impacts are predicted based on one or more studies of the risks associated with a particular hazard. The descriptive information available for regulatory analysis may be developed from statistical reporting systems or epidemiological studies, and sometimes from animal studies and laboratory results developed for other purposes. These studies vary in the extent to which they provide detailed descriptions of the health impacts avoided or the characteristics of the affected population.

Assessing the health impacts associated with regulations differs from assessing individual patients' HRQL, because of both the limited risk information available and the lack of identifiable affected individuals. It is often

---

[6]For more information on expert elicitation practices, see Morgan and Henrion (1990), especially Chapters 6 and 7; Keeney and von Winterfeldt (1991); and Bedford and Cooke (2001), especially Chapter 10. Although these sources discuss practices developed in the context of risk assessment, they are generally applicable to a broad range of contexts involving expert judgment, including the estimation of HRQL.

[7]As already mentioned, federally funded survey research involving 10 or more respondents must be approved by the Office of Management and Budget under the Paperwork Reduction Act. This requirement makes a valuation strategy that employs experts more attractive relative to conducting population surveys, but can also limit the number of experts involved in any given survey.

necessary to supplement the information from these studies with information from other sources (as in all of the Committee's case studies), for example, to provide the data on symptoms, treatment, duration, affected population, and life expectancy needed for a QALY-based CEA. Depending on the available data, it may be necessary to characterize an average case, or a set of typical cases, that reflect the variation in health impacts. For example, the Committee's case study of nonroad diesel air emissions considered three severity levels for chronic bronchitis, and split the cases of cardiac disease into endpoints with and without angina and congestive heart failure. The results of the assessment suggested, however, that the HRQL instruments were not sensitive enough to distinguish between some of the endpoints. Pretesting these descriptions would have allowed us to determine the extent to which different scenarios are needed for the expert assessment process.

Regulatory analyses track the impacts of health effects such as cases of reactive arthritis, myocardial infarctions, or severe injuries over the full course of the disease or injury, which may include the predicted remaining life spans of the affected individuals. Asking clinical experts to estimate average HRQL impacts across time may be even more difficult and uncertain a task than is estimating HRQL for the typical or average patient with the condition.

Despite the difficulties and uncertainties engendered by an expert elicitation approach to applying generic indexes, as well as its cost, several features of regulatory analysis make such approaches potentially necessary. First, the health states of interest may differ from those measured in clinical outcomes studies (as discussed in a following section on use of index values from prior studies). For example, the characterization of health effects from environmental risks such as particulate matter in the air or carcinogens in drinking water may be more vague than the specific disease states described and assessed in clinical CEAs.

In addition, expert assignment allows one to focus on the HRQL impact of a single health effect in isolation from unrelated co-morbid conditions. This is important in regulatory analysis if the regulation does not avert the co-morbidities. For example, regulations that reduce diabetes incidence may also prevent the related heart disease, but will not prevent other types of illnesses. In the expert assignments conducted for each of the three case studies, nearly all the clinical experts reported that they considered the HRQL impacts of the condition of interest in isolation from potential co-morbidities. At the same time, this location of a single condition of interest on a health state classification instrument necessitates an additional step in calibrating the resulting values on a scale that reflects overall health, as described in Appendix A.

BOX 3-5
Expert Assignment of Health States
Using Generic HRQL Instruments

Several protocols for the formal elicitation of expert opinions regarding uncertain quantities are summarized in Morgan and Henrion (1990) and Bedford and Cooke (2001). These approaches vary in the details of their implementation; no generally agreed-on set of "best practices" has been developed specifically for use in HRQL assessment. However, these approaches generally consist of five basic steps:

• *Develop and pretest descriptions of the health endpoints.* Clear, unambiguous descriptions of the health states that will be the subject of the expert assignment process will help produce more reliable judgments. As illustrated in the Committee's case studies (see Appendix A), the basis for these descriptions should be the epidemiological literature and other materials used to estimate the types and numbers of cases of illness or injury averted by the regulation. A key issue is determining the extent to which these health states should be disaggregated for the assignment process to reflect different severity levels, disease phases, or other subcategories that may lead to variation in the attribute assignments. These descriptions should be reviewed and pretested (e.g., by asking a group of experts to complete the assignment process) to ensure that they provide the needed information and reflect the appropriate level of disaggregation of more globally described health conditions that persist and change over time.

• *Identify and recruit experts.* The second step involves identifying the experts (i.e., clinicians) who will be involved in the assignment process. The starting point for this step is the development of criteria for the selection process. These criteria may address the types of patients with whom each expert is familiar; taken together, the experts' range of experience should relate to the individuals whose health may be affected by the regulatory action in terms of age, health conditions, socioeconomic characteristics, and/or geographic distribution as relevant. In addi-

---

Approaches Based on Population Survey Data

The PCEHM urged the development of a standard catalogue of index values for "well-described health states" that would facilitate valid comparisons of CEA across conditions and illnesses and eliminate the need for collecting primary data for every analysis (Gold et al., 1996b). The PCEHM envisioned using generic indexes for which health states were *valued* by a general population or community sample, while people with particular conditions (rather than experts, as just described) *characterized* those health states according to the generic instrument's domains and attribute levels.

Researchers have responded to this call with different approaches. Table 3-5 presents an overview of efforts to develop sets of population-

tion, the criteria should identify the range of specialties needed to provide a complete perspective on different aspects of the HRQL impacts. For example, for traumatic injuries to children, relevant fields could include trauma surgery, orthopedics, general pediatrics, and rehabilitation medicine. Once the criteria are developed, relevant experts can be identified by querying professional contacts and through professional and scientific organizations.

• *Train experts in the assignment exercise.* The third step involves educating the experts in the assignment process so they have a common understanding of the health effects to be assessed, the attribute descriptions to be applied, and the overall task. An important component of this step is making the experts more aware of their own judgment processes and biases. This step is generally best accomplished by convening a workshop or training session.

• *Conduct expert assignments.* The fourth step involves asking the experts to assign the attribute levels to each endpoint. To the extent possible, experts should be asked to give a range of values rather than point estimates. For example, they could be asked to distribute a representative group of 100 patients across the different attribute levels to indicate the percentage they would expect to fall within each category. Ideally, this task should be completed in a structured one-on-one interview with each expert by a trained member of the project team. In-person interviews are generally desirable, but phone interviews or mail-in questionnaires may be used if necessary.

• *Assess results.* The final step involves analyzing the results of the assessment. This step should involve a feedback loop: asking each expert to verify the results and discuss the rationale for their assignments. The expert elicitation literature reflects some debate about whether, and how, to combine results across experts, including whether to allow interaction or to treat each set of results separately. Consequently, either of two approaches are reasonable. The group could be required to meet and discuss the attribute assignments until it reaches consensus; alternatively, the experts could exchange information anonymously, using processes generally referred to as "Delphi methods." In either case, the results should be reported as a range of values and not collapsed to a single point estimate.

based condition-specific index values during the past decade. The most recent versions of two of these conceptually distinct approaches are described below.

Catalogues of Chronic Condition HRQL Values

Sullivan and colleagues (2005) used the MEPS to develop EQ-5D index values for a number of chronic conditions, based on pooled MEPS data for the years 2000, 2001, and 2002 for respondents ages 18 or older. MEPS includes data on sociodemographic characteristics as well as responses to the EQ-5D health status questionnaire; valid responses were received for about 38,000 unique respondents. The researchers weighted respondents'

TABLE 3-5 Sources for Population-Based, Condition-Specific
HRQL Values

Source	Sampling Frame	Sample Size/Type/Year
Fryback et al. (1993)	Wisconsin township	N~1,400/Random sample adults ages 43–84 years/1991–1992
Gold et al. (1996a)	U.S. civilian, community-based population, ages 25–74	N~14,400/NHANES I probability sample/1971–1975; N~10,200/NHANES I Epidemiological Followup Study (NHEFS)/1982–1984; N~8,300 (reinterviewed in 1987)
Gold et al. (1998)	U.S. civilian community-based population, all ages	N~84,400/merged NHIS samples/ 1987–1992
Sullivan et al. (2005)	U.S. civilian community-based population, age 18+	N~28,800/MEPS nonduplicated sample/2000+2001
Cutler and Richardson (1999)	U.S. civilian community-based population	N~110,000/NHIS/1990
Stewart et al. (2005)	From Fryback et al. (1993)	N~1,400 respondents with complete QWB data/See Fryback et al.

NOTES: EVGGFP = Five-item global health status measure: excellent, very good, good, fair, poor
MEPS = Medical Expenditure Panel Survey
NHANES = National Health and Nutrition Examination Survey
NHIS = National Health Interview Survey
SEER = Surveillance, Epidemiology, and End Results Program

attribute scores using a model derived from a valuation survey of a representative sample of the U.S. adult population (Shaw et al., 2005; see Table 3-4 for a summary of the survey). They then calculated mean EQ-5D condition values for those respondents reporting each condition. These "with condition" values reflect both the condition itself and any co-morbidities, indicating the overall health of the individual. To separate out the effects of these co-morbidities, the researchers then used regression analysis to determine the marginal impact of the condition of interest alone, calculated as a decrement from median population health. These marginal decrements in EQ-5D values controlled for the effects of age, gender, race, ethnicity,

Survey Instrument(s)	Elicitation Method	Condition-Specific Index Values
SF-36; QWB; chronic medical condition; EVGGFP rating	TTO; rank ordering of health states	28 conditions
NHEFS mapped onto HUI	Constructed HUI based on responses to NHEFS questions	18 conditions
NHIS self-rated health (EVGGFP scale) activity limitations	Derived from HUI-2 weights	130 illnesses and conditions
EQ-5D	TTO	68 conditions
NHIS self-rated health status; chronic conditions from NHIS + SEER	Statistically inferred	21 conditions and 2 co-morbid health states
See Fryback et al.	Statistically inferred, based on Fryback et al.	33 chronic conditions

income, and education as well as co-morbidities. The marginal decrements can be added across conditions.

In their article, Sullivan et al. (2005) report the results for 74 clusters of chronic conditions (clinical classification categories) and for 10 priority conditions of particular interest to health care researchers. Estimates for individual conditions (by three-digit International Classification of Disease Version 9, or ICD-9, codes) are also available from the authors. The Committee used preliminary estimates of individual condition (ICD-9) marginal chronic condition decrements as one valuation approach in the air quality case study.

Statistically Inferred HRQL Values

Another approach to obtaining relative values for chronic conditions is statistical inference. Researchers have demonstrated that self-reported health status predicts changes in functional status and mortality and is correlated with specific aspects of health. Cutler and Richardson (1997) first proposed this approach using National Health Interview Survey data. The approach has been developed further in more recent work by Stewart and colleagues (2005) using a data set that included extensive health status information and HRQL valuations (see Fryback et al., 1993, described in Table 3-5).

Stewart et al. used ordered probit and ordinary least squares regression analyses to examine the effect of specific symptoms and impairments reported on the QWB survey on self-rated overall health status and, separately, on TTO valuations of current health. They estimated health effects as analogous in form to disutility weights (i.e., index-value decrements) for 30 chronic conditions, based on the likelihood of people with each chronic condition experiencing each symptom/impairment and on the regression coefficients for each symptom/impairment. The approach considers interaction effects between pairs of symptom/impairments.

The earlier model developed by Cutler and Richardson was adapted for regulatory analyses by the Food and Drug Administration (FDA) to estimate HRQL values for reactive arthritis and heart disease (Scharff and Jessup, 2001). Although this general approach must be used with caution because it does not directly value health states, it could stimulate the development of descriptive systems based on symptoms and conditions. Condition-specific values could be particularly useful in the context of regulatory analysis because the risk assessments underlying these analyses frequently report health-related impacts in terms of cases of particular diseases.

Incorporation of Health Profiles and HRQL Questions and Instruments in Routine Population Surveys

Routine and periodic national health surveys in the United States have included various health profiles, HRQL questions, and generic HRQL instruments over the past few decades. Table 3-6 lists the major surveys and the profiles, questions, and instruments they have included. Coordination among and long-term planning for these data collection activities have been minimal.

The apparently ad hoc and sporadic collection of HRQL data stems from several circumstances. First, multiple agencies with different if overlapping missions and interests have collected HRQL data. Second, every survey is constructed with both budgetary constraints and constraints related to response burden. Competition for time and space on questionnaires

TABLE 3-6 HRQL Measurement in National Health Surveys

Survey	Sample/Format/ Periodicity	HRQL Information Collected	Response Rate/ Other Comments
National Health Interview Survey	~94,000 persons of all ages in 37,000 households/personal interviews/annual	SRHS, health conditions, ADL, IADL, "Healthy Life Expectancy" calculation based on LE and SRHS	87%; includes ~12,000 < 18 years; proxy response for children < 12; excludes institutional residents, military
Medical Expenditure Panel Survey	15–19,000 adults 17+ years/personal interviews and phone/annual, in 2-year cohort panels	EQ-5D in 2000–03, SF-12 2000–present, ADL, IADL, functional disabilities, usual activities, chronic conditions	85–88% (2001) EQ-5D and SF-12 self-administered in mail survey
Behavioral Risk Factor Surveillance System	~300,000 adults 18+/telephone/ annual, continuous	SRHS, "Healthy Days" measure	53% (median); range: 32–66%; conducted within each state by health department
National Health and Nutrition Examination Survey	~5,000 adults and children/personal interview, physical exam, lab tests/annual	"Health Days" questions administered to all participants 12+ years	Each survey focused on particular health problem in addition to core data
Medicare Current Beneficiary Survey	~16,000 Medicare beneficiaries/personal interview/annual	SRHS, ADL, IADL, chronic conditions	
Medicare Health Outcomes Survey	~200,000 initially, 60,000 follow-up (longitudinal)/mail with phone follow-up/annual	SRHS, "Healthy Days," SF-36, ADL, chronic conditions	Survey of Medicare beneficiaries in managed care plans; 1,000 respondents/ plan
Medicare Fee-for-Service CAHPS	~200,000/mail with phone follow-up/ annual	SRHS, SF-12, ADL	600 Medicare beneficiaries in each geographic area
Medicare+ Choice CAHPS	~200,000/mail with phone follow-up/ annual	SRHS	600 managed care enrollees per plan area

NOTES: ADL = activities of daily living; IADL = immediate activities of daily living; LE = life expectancy; SRHS = self-reported health status; Healthy Days measure: core includes four questions encompassing SRHS, number of physically and/or mentally unhealthy days within the past month, and restricted activity days within the past month.

SOURCES: Fleishman and Lawrence (2004); Haffer (2004); Moriarty (2004); CDC (2005); NCHS (2005).

is keen for both reasons. Third, there has not been an ongoing focus or forum for coordination among agencies that design and field health surveys. Following the release in 1998 of the Institute of Medicine report, *Summarizing Population Health*, an Interagency Working Group on Summary Measures of Population Health was formed within the Department of Health and Human Services. The Working Group met for several years but is now inactive. Increased reliance on HRQL measurement for regulatory analysis will require more regular and coordinated surveys for valuation and establishment of population baselines.

Health State Index Values from Prior Studies and Benefits Transfer

When it is not practicable for analysts to conduct primary research on HRQL values for the specific health states and affected populations addressed by regulatory CEAs, another alternative is to use estimates from published research, commonly referred to as "off-the-shelf" values or preference weights.[8] This strategy, known as "benefits transfer" by welfare economists, refers specifically to using values estimated in one context (the "study scenario") in a new context (the "regulatory scenario"). Generally, these contexts differ in at least some respects, for example, in the specific details of the health state addressed or in some of the characteristics of the affected population. Because of these differences, a benefit transfer strategy is rarely the preferred approach; as noted in Chapter 2, the Office of Management and Budget (OMB) guidance describes it as a "last resort" because it may introduce uncertainties and biases of "unknown magnitude" (OMB, 2003a). However, the Committee's review of current practices (Robinson, 2004) suggests that regulatory agencies often rely on transfers because they lack the time and resources needed to conduct new primary research.

Guidance for transfer of benefit values has been relatively well developed in the context of regulatory analysis and natural resource economics (see, e.g., Desvousges et al., 1998). While the specific criteria for study selection are described in various ways in different sources, they generally involve consideration of both the quality and the applicability of the study. "Quality" refers to the extent to which the study adheres to generally accepted best practices for the particular type of study. It also relates to the accuracy, reliability, and completeness of the underlying data sources, and the appropriateness of the approaches used for sampling and survey administration, including sample size, response rate, and estimated standard er-

---

[8]We avoid the term "off-the-shelf" and instead refer to "health state index values from prior studies" and "benefits transfer" for consistency with the terminology used in guidance for regulatory analysis.

ror. The appropriateness of the techniques used for statistical or econometric analysis should also be considered.

"Applicability" includes the similarity between the health effect assessed in the study and the effect addressed in the regulatory analysis, and the similarity between the populations affected. For the health effect, similarities in factors such as symptoms, treatments, severity, and duration should be considered. For the population affected, factors such as age, gender, and/or baseline health may be of interest.

In addition, analysts should consider the extent to which there are opportunities to adjust the study data to better match the regulatory scenario. In some cases, the researchers may be willing to supply the original study data so that the results can be reestimated using different techniques or breakouts (to better match the characteristics of the affected population). Results can also be combined across studies using meta-analysis or other statistical methods. See, for example, Tengs et al. (2001) and Tengs and Lin (2003) for a meta-analytic approach to estimating index values for stroke.

The technique of benefits transfer relies heavily on the judgment of the analysts conducting the analysis. Thus, it is important that analysts be explicit about the studies reviewed, the criteria used to select particular studies and values from these studies, and the uncertainties involved. Where more than one study provides suitable values of reasonable quality and these values differ noticeably, the range of estimates should be used in a sensitivity analysis or in a probabilistic model (see Briggs, 2001; Briggs et al., 2002; Claxton et al., 2005).

These considerations and strategies are generally applicable when transferring health state values for QALY-based CEA. In recent years, researchers at the Center for Risk Analysis at the Harvard School of Public Health developed a comprehensive, open-access registry of CEAs. It contains detailed information on analyses published over a 25-year period in the health and medical literature that use HALYs as the effectiveness measure (Bell et al., 2001). It should be noted that many medical outcomes and effectiveness studies that do not include a CEA also estimate and report HRQL values and the CEA Registry does not include these sources of original HRQL values. Nevertheless, this registry is a convenient source of health state index values for regulatory CEA and has been used by agencies such as FDA and EPA for this purpose. Box 3-6 describes the registry in greater detail.

In work commissioned by the Committee to support its case study effort, Brauer and Neumann (2004, 2005) reviewed health state values in the CEA database with respect to their applicability to the EPA case study of air quality improvements. Informed by the development of the EPA case study analysis and Brauer and Neumann's work, we identified the follow-

---

BOX 3-6
The CEA Registry

The CEA Registry is a repository of information that currently includes more than 500 distinct health and medical CEAs published between 1976 and 2001. The database was developed through a computerized search of the English-language literature using the medical subject headings and/or text keywords "quality-adjusted," "QALY," and "cost-utility." Two trained readers independently abstracted data on the health state description, corresponding point estimates and ranges for health state index values, method of elicitation and the source of the estimates (e.g., general population or patient samples), cost-effectiveness ratios, and a wide variety of reporting practices. The readers met to reconcile their results, and a third reviewer adjudicated any discrepancies. Details of this work are described on the Registry website, along with selected data from each study (http://www.tufts-nemc.org/cearegistry).

SOURCES: Chapman et al. (2000); Neumann et al. (2000); Bell et al. (2001); Harvard Center for Risk Analysis (2003).

---

ing steps and questions that regulatory analysts should consider when reviewing available studies. These build on recommendations by the PCEHM as well as the benefits transfer guidance referenced earlier. There is some arbitrariness to the ordering of selection criteria used in this approach; selecting appropriate values for a particular set of health endpoints involves discretion and requires judgment on the part of the regulatory analyst. The format for reviewing potentially applicable index values is also useful for deriving possible ranges of values for uncertainty analysis.

The first step in applying index values from the research literature is to define the health endpoints in the regulatory analysis as precisely and accurately as possible. Because many disease and injury-related conditions are dynamic processes, regulatory health endpoints may be best represented by a series of health states, each with its own HRQL implications, which change over time. This could require either a relatively complex model of different health states that represent disease progression or, alternatively, simplifying assumptions about states of health and functioning on average over an extended time.[9] Box 3-7 and Appendix A describe how these chronic health states were defined for the Committee's air quality case study, including our review of health state values in the CEA Registry.

The next step is to assess the applicability of the health states available

---

[9]See Weinstein et al. (1987) and Sullivan et al. (2005) for examples of models of disease progression.

in the published literature, that is, the extent to which a particular study addresses the same health state as defined by the risk assessment that underlies the regulatory analysis. The applicability of a particular study's health state values depends most importantly on similarities in the clinical descriptions of the health states, such as the severity of disease and the timing and duration of any treatment, as well as characteristics of the study population, including age, sex, and co-morbidities.

The third step is to assess the appropriateness of the method used to elicit the health state values. Most importantly, analysts should consider the following features: type of population surveyed, elicitation technique, and sample size. As already noted, the PCEHM recommends using index values derived from a community valuation survey in CEAs intended to inform broad societal resource allocation decisions. Deriving health state index values from a sample that represents the population subject to the costs and benefits of the regulation to the maximum extent possible will enhance the credibility of the estimates. In Chapter 4 we consider the implications of the valuation perspective in greater depth.

Within the category of elicitation techniques, values from a generic instrument (such as the EQ-5D or the HUI) or those elicited directly with TTO or SG are preferred. Less desirable are values elicited by an RS technique or values from clinicians, other experts, or author judgment. Larger sample sizes are better than smaller ones, and more recent studies are preferred to older studies, if other characteristics of the studies are comparable.

This format for reviewing potentially applicable health state index values is also useful for deriving possible ranges of such values for sensitivity analysis.

The Committee's review of published studies for applicable health state values for the air quality case study revealed both the advantages and drawbacks of using index values from prior studies for regulatory analysis. On the positive side, it confirmed that the published literature can be a fruitful source of health state values for at least some regulatory health endpoints, and that using index values from the published literature is a relatively simple and inexpensive approach. On the other hand, the case study team found that the health state descriptions in published studies often did not match the description of health endpoints as described in the underlying health research used in regulatory risk assessments, and may not correspond on dimensions such as disease severity, patient age, or baseline risk factors. In addition, quality varies considerably across outcomes studies and CEAs in the literature, and published studies are not always clear about their methods.

Because published studies employ different populations and elicitation methods, the individually "best" estimates for particular health endpoints

BOX 3-7
An Example Using Health State Index Values
from Published Studies

The Committee's case study based on the EPA nonroad diesel engine rule (EPA, 2004a,b) provided an opportunity to investigate the use of published health state index values to develop estimates of the HRQL impacts of air quality improvements. The nonfatal health endpoints (disease conditions) assessed in the case study were "chronic bronchitis" and "myocardial infarction" (MI), that is, the course of cardiac disease following a nonfatal heart attack, based on the risk assessment studies used by EPA (Abbey et al., 1995; Peters et al., 2001).

As commissioned by the Committee, Carmen Brauer and Peter Neumann of the Harvard Center for Risk Analysis searched the CEA Registry's catalogue of preference weights, updated through 2001, to identify estimates related to these regulatory health endpoints. They found 127 health states and preference weights in the respiratory and cardiovascular disease categories published since 1994.

The Committee case study team reviewed the original studies that appeared to be most promising as a source of health state values in the case study. Two studies were selected as the basis of the chronic bronchitis and post-MI health endpoints. For chronic bronchitis, estimates came from a Canadian study of alternative treatments for patients with acute exacerbations (Torrance et al., 1999). Over a 1-year period, the researchers asked the patients to complete assessments (including the HUI-3 questionnaire) after each acute exacerbation as well as once every 3 months. During the study period, the health state index values for these patients averaged 0.79 or 0.76 (depending on the treatment), calculated with the standard community-based valuation formula for the HUI. The mean value for both groups combined was approximately 0.78, when weighted by the number of participants in each group. This estimate was used for all cases of chronic bronchitis.

within a regulatory analysis may not be derived from consistent methods. For example, the published index value estimates for cardiovascular and respiratory conditions used in the EPA case study were based on different generic instruments, the EQ-5D with U.K. population values and the HUI-3 with values from a single Canadian community, respectively. Because no tenable alternatives for HRQL values for the different conditions were available, in the case study we violated the *prima facie* rule of using values derived with consistent elicitation methods. Perhaps most important, different studies of similar endpoints reported significantly different estimates. As discussed in Box 3-7 and below, the uncertainty in both the estimation of health impacts and the estimation of preferences for the health states associated with those impacts underscores the importance of reporting key limitations and discussing their implications, as well as conducting quantitative analyses of uncertainty.

A study by Oostenbrink et al. (2001) provided estimates for the course of cardiac disease following nonfatal MI. This Dutch study followed patients after infrainguinal bypass surgery to compare the effects of different drug treatments. The researchers administered the EQ-5D survey instrument to study participants and used the standard U.K. population-based TTO valuation survey results to value the health states (Dolan, 1997). For those patients in the overall study sample who later experienced an MI, their subsequent index values averaged 0.58. The case study team used this estimate for all of the post-MI health states included in our assessment.

Other studies provide widely varying results. Although the values from these other studies appeared less suitable for transfer than the ones selected by the case study team, they show how different sources yield a wide range of HRQL estimates. Brauer and Neumann (2005) report index values for chronic bronchitis that range from 0.37 to 0.75, depending on the study approach, the disease severity, and the age of the patient.

Estimates for post-MI health states also varied, in part because of the different populations studied, the different approaches to HRQL measurement used, and the different severities of illness considered. For example, one study reports an index value of 0.33 for the hospitalization period, angina studies report a range of 0.67 to 0.95, studies of congestive heart failure yield values ranging from 0.46 to 0.70, and (paradoxically) a study of angina and congestive heart failure combined yields values ranging from 0.82 to 0.85 (higher than the value for heart failure alone from other studies). Although the team considered using different estimates for cases with and without congestive heart failure or angina, we were unable to find an internally consistent set of weights that addressed all of the combinations of these conditions of interest.

Uncertainty in Health Status and Preference Measurement

Uncertainty pervades all aspects of risk assessment and economic analysis of regulatory interventions to reduce health and safety risks. In its 2002 report, *Estimating the Public Health Benefits of Proposed Air Pollution Regulations*, a consensus committee of the Board on Environmental Studies and Toxicology of the National Research Council called for greater attention to the sources and analysis of uncertainty in developing and promulgating regulatory interventions. In particular, the committee recommended more extensive use of probabilistic uncertainty analysis.

OMB has also long encouraged the use of probabilistic analysis. Circular A-4 mandated that agencies conduct probabilistic uncertainty analyses as part of the economic analyses of regulations with a cost or benefit estimate exceeding $1 billion annually (OMB, 2003a). OMB also requires analysis of uncertainty for rules with less substantial impacts, but probabilistic methods need not be used.

In this section we consider sources of uncertainty and its treatment in the measurement of health effectiveness only. As outlined in the report of the PCEHM, the cost-effectiveness ratio is the end of a process of estimation, synthesis, and modeling. Uncertainty in cost-effectiveness analysis can stem from estimation of the numerical values of factors that are inputs of the analysis or from the analytic model or modeling process (Manning et al., 1996). One major source of uncertainty in HALY estimates for regulatory CEA is the estimation of the health impacts of the proposed intervention—the number of cases of each fatal and nonfatal health effect averted, the severity of disease or disability incurred, and so on.

Even taking the quantified estimates of cases averted as givens, however, uncertainty remains in the characterization and measurement of HRQL effects of those conditions. At least four aspects of HRQL measurement contribute to the uncertainty of the ultimate values assigned to the estimated health-related impact of a regulation:

• Variability in preferences across individuals, which contributes to uncertainty in estimating population means;
• Variability in the estimation of preferences for health states depending on the elicitation technique;
• Differences in the specificity and scope of attributes included by the generic HRQL instruments; and
• The statistical models that assign relative health state values for each of the generic instruments.

The case study results, in particular the case study of foodborne illness in which the same groups of experts assessed the regulatory health endpoints with four generic indexes, demonstrate that the instrument used to value health effects does indeed affect the results. The estimates of QALY losses averted with the juice processing rule ranged from 1,300 for the QWB and SF-6D, to 1,500 for the EQ-5D, to 1,900 for the HUI-3, using a 3 percent discount rate. This yielded cost-effectiveness ratios ranging from $13,000 to $18,000 per QALY. (See Tables A-5 through A-7.) Whether this range of estimates is significant enough to affect the regulatory decision is unclear, because this particular rulemaking did not include quantified information about other regulatory options.

In the case study of nonroad diesel emissions, which estimated QALY losses averted using the EQ-5D, but according to different approaches (expert assignment as compared with a catalogue of index values from a population survey), the variability in estimates was even less. The results ranged from 109,000 QALYs (based on the catalogue values) to 120,000

QALYs (based on expert assignment), using a 3 percent discount rate, which produced a small difference in the cost-effectiveness ratios (Tables A-16 and A-17).

The expert assignment of regulatory health endpoints using generic indexes, as described in the preceding section, also introduces additional uncertainty into the analysis. In debriefing interviews following the assignment exercise, experts raised concerns about several aspects of the task. First, characterizing a condition (the regulatory health endpoint) with a single multiattribute index response is difficult and imprecise, as the quality of life and functional impacts of chronic conditions change over time. Second, the disease descriptions were not always well distinguished from each other, or readily described by a generic index's attributes. Last, some experts expressed skepticism about the ability of clinicians to characterize the impact of a condition on patients' functioning and experience, despite having professional familiarity with the condition.

RESEARCH AND DEVELOPMENT OF METRICS AND VALUATION METHODOLOGIES

From the many fruitful avenues of research in the measurement and valuation of health-related quality of life, we focus on three issues with particular relevance to regulatory CEA:

- correlating and estimating conversion factors among generic indexes so that values based on different instruments can be compared;
- using information about ordinal rankings of health states to develop HRQL value scales with interval properties; and
- applying insights and best practices from willingness-to-pay survey research to HRQL valuation.

Correlations and Conversions Among HRQL Measures

CEA results based on different HRQL instruments are not readily comparable because the various instruments include different domains and rely on different value elicitation techniques. Furthermore, no one instrument has achieved preeminence in the field. These circumstances have stimulated interest in research that correlates and develops conversions or cross-walks among the various instruments so that estimates and analyses based on different measures might be compared and combined.

Using data from more than 11,000 respondents to the 2000 MEPS, Franks and colleagues (2006) have calculated the relative decrements in HRQL for 47 risk factors and health conditions based on several preference-based measures, including the U.S.-valued EQ-5D, the SF-6D (SF-12 version), and a statistically modeled HUI-3. Correlations between the estimates for these risk factors and health conditions using the three metrics were in all cases greater than 0.90.[10] The authors concluded that, although the particular HRQL instruments would yield different cost-effectiveness results in absolute terms, the different measures are unlikely to produce different orderings of incremental cost-effectiveness ratios because of their consistent rank ordering. Table 3-7 presents the summary results of studies that have examined correlations between and among HRQL instruments.

A set of ongoing studies sponsored by the National Institute on Aging promises to contribute substantially to our understanding of the relationships among different HRQL instruments.[11] First, a nationally representative telephone survey of U.S. adults over the age of 35 is co-administered the EQ-5D, the HUI Mark 2/3, the SF-36 version 2, and QWB instruments. This survey will be another source of national norms for each index and will provide algorithms to convert values derived from one instrument to each of the others. Second, to evaluate the responsiveness of each measure to different conditions and to check the cross-walk algorithms and the effects of the mode of survey administration, a related study will survey two groups of patients periodically over 6 months, one a group of patients undergoing cataract surgery and the other patients with congestive heart failure. In its entirety, this research effort (planned to be completed in 2008), should provide much better and more comparable information about the performance of different HRQL instruments than is now available.

Using Ordinal Data for HRQL Valuation

Ranking of health states is often used as a preliminary step in preference elicitation exercises involving TTOs or SGs. Recent studies have explored using aggregated ranking data to predict health state valuations that closely match interval-level values produced by TTO methods (Salomon, 2003; Salomon and Murray, 2004). These findings, along with the consistency of the ordinal rankings of health states that different generic instruments produce (as just discussed), suggest that ordinal preferences may have broader applications in health state valuation than are currently exploited.

---

[10]The estimated values were adjusted for sociodemographic factors that are distributed differently among persons with various risk factors and conditions.

[11]Information on the project is available at http://www.healthmeasurement.org/NHMS. html.

Best Practices in Stated Preference Surveys and Benefits Transfer

Much of the debate among experts on the relative merits of stated preference willingness-to-pay measures and QALY measures revolves around the protocols for and methodological rigor of surveys that elicit monetary "prices" or HRQL index values. The recommendations of an expert committee on contingent valuation convened by the National Oceanic and Atmospheric Administration in 1992 articulated such protocols for willingness-to-pay studies (Arrow et al., 1993).[12] The PCEHM (Gold et al., 1996b) serves a similar role in defining best practices in CEA, although this guidance is much less specific with respect to validity tests and methodologies for establishing the credibility of various preference elicitation techniques.

Researchers familiar with both willingness-to-pay and QALY measurement have called for cross-fertilization and even a synthesis of valuation practices across these fields (Johnson et al., 1997, 2000; Smith et al., 2003; Krupnick, 2004). For example, they have proposed that the choices underlying QALY valuations be interpreted using standard preference functions, making QALY results consistent with monetized health benefit measures. As another example, willingness-to-pay studies suggest that individual responses to risk and choices involving health depend on baseline conditions for other components of well-being (e.g., age, health status, and income), and that these factors should be taken into account in QALY measurement (Smith et al., 2003).

SUMMARY AND CONCLUSIONS

This chapter has reviewed a variety of health-related outcomes measures useful in CEA, focusing in particular on HALY measures and generic indexes for estimating QALYs. In particular, the Committee has formulated criteria for the selection of HRQL instruments and characterized alternative strategies for obtaining health state values for use in QALY-based CEA of regulatory interventions. In great measure, our recommendations conform to the guidelines and underlying rationales of the PCEHM, whose 1996 report constitutes the reference standard of best practices in CEA for clinical and public health interventions.

In two areas, however, our conclusions differ somewhat from those of the PCEHM, although the differences are more a matter of emphasis than of disagreement. These differences at least in part reflect the Committee's focus on effectiveness measurement for regulatory analysis, and the analytic

---

[12]See Mitchell and Carson (1989), Payne et al. (1999), Smith et al. (2002), Freeman (2003), and Krupnick (2004) for additional discussions of contingent valuation methodology.

TABLE 3-7 Correlations and Cross-Walks of HRQL Measures

Source	Sampling Frame	Sample Size/Type/Year
Gold et al. (1998)	U.S. civilian community-based population 0–85+	N~720,000/representative, random/ 1987–1992
Rizzo et al. (1998); Rizzo and Sindelar (1999)	U.S. civilian community-based population age 18+	N = 19,525/NMES, nationally representative (weighted) randomized sample/1987
Nichol et al. (2001)	Enrollees insured by Southern CA Kaiser Permanente	N = 6,921/longitudinal study; random and geographic subsamples stratified by Rx use/1992–1995
Franks et al. (2003)	NY community health center patients age 18+	N = 240/Convenience sample, predominantly Hispanic and black/NA
Franks et al. (2004)	U.S. civilian community-based population age 18+	N~13,000 complete responses to both EQ-5D and SF-12 questions/MEPS household sample/2000
Lawrence and Fleishman (2004)	See Franks et al. (2004)	See Franks et al. (2004); sample split in half for derivation and validation
Hawthorne et al. (2001)	Australian community population and hospital inpatients and outpatients age 16+	Community: N = 396 Inpatients: N = 266 Outpatients: N = 334/NA

NOTES: ADL = activities of daily living; AQoL = Assessment of Quality of Life instrument; EVGGFP = five-item global health status measure: excellent, very good, good, fair, poor; NHIS = National Health Interview Survey; NMES = National Medical Expenditure Survey; WHOQOL-Bref = World Health Organization Quality of Life abbreviated assessment instrument

Survey Instrument(s)	Condition-Specific Index Values (y/n; if so, list conditions)	Correlations with Other Indexes
NHIS: EVGGFP, ADL	130 illnesses and conditions	Yes: QWB (Beaver Dam) R2 = 0.78; HUI (NHEFS) R2 = 0.86 for conditions
Linking NMES responses to HUI-1 and EQ-5D questions	7 conditions: diabetes, atherosclerosis, cancer, myocardial infarct, heart disease, hypertension, stroke	Yes: EQ-5D and HUI-1 imputations had correlations ranging between 67% and 74%
SF-36; HUI-2; chronic disease score	No	SF-36 and HUI-2: 50% of variation in HUI-2 predicted by SF-36 scores
SF-12; EQ-5D; HUI-3	No	HUI-3 and EQ-5D: 0.69; predicted HUI/HUI: 0.71; predicted EQ w/EQ: 0.77
SF-12; EQ-5D	No	Regression of EQ-5D scores onto mental and physical component summary scores of SF-12; physical component R2 = 0.67; mental component R2 = 0.47
SF-12; EQ-5D	EQ-5D values reported for: asthma, diabetes, emphysema, high blood pressure, heart attack, stroke	Mean EQ-5D scores predicted from mean physical and mental component summary scores R2 = 0.61
AQoL; SF-6D (36); WHOQOL-Bref; EQ-5D; HUI-3; Finnish 15D	No	Spearman correlations of AQoL with EQ-5D: 0.73; HUI-3: 0.74; 15D: 0.80; SF-6D: 0.74

traditions and goals of regulatory decision making. First, we do not place the same emphasis on the theoretical grounding of QALY measurement in utility theory as did the PCEHM. Rather, we have taken an explicitly practical and instrumental approach to the measurement of health-related effects of regulatory interventions.

Second, the Committee in principle favors direct elicitation of preferences for the health states of interest over the use of generic indexes, whenever well-designed and executed preference elicitation studies for the appropriate health endpoints and the affected populations exist or are feasible. In practice, we recognize that such original research will often not be possible to support regulatory analysis. The use of generic indexes, possibly with expert characterization of the health states of interest, and the transfer of health state values from existing research databases are the more likely, and also acceptable, approaches.

Before turning to the ethical implications of QALY-based CEA and the larger context of regulatory policy determination, we reiterate the major conclusions and insights discussed throughout this chapter.

Single-dimension measures such as deaths averted and life years gained are informative measures of effectiveness in regulatory analysis.

For practical reasons, the QALY is currently the best among the family of HALY measures to use in regulatory CEAs. The QALY is in widespread use, it is flexible in application, and the construct has the advantage of simplicity and comparatively modest informational demands.

No single elicitation technique or common generic index for QALYs is superior in all respects to the alternatives. Given the current state of the art in HRQL measurement, however, the EQ-5D has several important advantages over other generic indexes. The EQ-5D:

- *Has been valued using a nationally representative U.S. sample.*
- *Uses a choice-based elicitation method (TTO).*
- *Is simple and inexpensive to administer.*
- *Can be used without charge (i.e., it is not a proprietary instrument).*

Several strategies for obtaining health state values for regulatory CEA are available. In the absence of new studies valuing the health impacts of interest, QALY estimates based on well-developed, generally accepted, and widely used generic HRQL indexes are desirable. These values may be derived from a number of sources, including population surveys, transfer of index values from prior studies, or by using experts to characterize health endpoints with generic indexes.

The measurement of HRQL in children poses special challenges in characterizing, reporting, and valuing health states, and is particularly in need of further research and development of approaches and instruments.

Nationally representative data that support HRQL measurement are essential for QALY-based CEA for regulations. To date, efforts to incorporate HRQL measures into national health surveys have been ad hoc and unsystematic.

HRQL measures and methods can be improved with further research. In particular, establishing the relationships among and conversion factors for estimates derived from the most commonly used generic HRQL instruments would make integration and synthesis of the results from different studies possible and thus expand the tools and data available for regulatory analysis. In addition, it would improve the reliability of cost-effectiveness comparisons among different analyses and regulations.

Standards of good research practice such as those that have been developed for stated preference valuation surveys for BCA offer a model for developing best practice standards for HRQL valuation instruments, surveys, and studies.

4

Beyond Ratios:
Ethical and Nonquantifiable Aspects
of Regulatory Decisions

Benefit–cost analysis (BCA) and cost-effectiveness analysis (CEA) provide summary measures of the economic efficiency of health and safety regulations—of the net benefits they deliver and of the cost per life year or quality-adjusted life year (QALY) saved. In measuring net impacts on social welfare, both BCA and CEA implicitly contain normative assumptions regarding the relative value of different contributors to well-being. It is important that we understand the ethical assumptions implicit in BCA and CEA and consider the implications of these assumptions when using the resulting information to make decisions about regulating risks. In this chapter the Committee discusses ethical and other unquantified considerations in regulatory analysis and decisions, particularly with respect to QALY-based CEA.

Normative assumptions are implicit in how the benefits measures are constructed in BCA and CEA. In CEA, for example, effectiveness measures such as life years or QALYs weight lives saved by considering remaining life expectancy. They thereby assign a greater weight to saving the life of a younger person than an older one, if other factors are equal. In BCA, willingness-to-pay measures in theory can be designed to address a wide range of factors, but in practice may not address important dimensions of the population affected or the nature of the risks.

Other normative issues arise due to factors that are excluded because of the focus on efficiency or because of data or methodological limitations. Such considerations relate to:

• The distribution of the effects across different population subgroups;
• Impacts that cannot be quantified easily; and
• Features of the risks that are not easily captured in the benefits measures.

Economic analysis is only one of many kinds of information that contribute to decisions related to regulation of health and safety risks. Regulatory decisions should and do reflect a number of considerations in addition to aggregate estimates of costs and benefits.[1] The goal of this chapter is to discuss the assumptions and methodological limitations inherent in such analysis that, from the Committee's perspective, are most important to consider in making decisions.

More specifically, the aggregate nature of net benefits or a cost-effectiveness ratio means that these measures by themselves cannot capture the distribution of benefits or of costs in a population. Aggregate estimates of QALY gains or cost-effectiveness ratios do not indicate the distribution of impacts over time or the magnitude of individual gains. Summed QALYs do not distinguish between health gains made within the course of a single life or across generations. Nor do they indicate whether the QALY gains represent small health improvements widely dispersed throughout a population or larger gains allocated among relatively few people.

Summary benefit–cost and cost-effectiveness measures also omit benefits that are difficult to quantify. Such benefits include health and nonhealth effects for which numerical estimates are not available, for example, because the scientific research base is inadequate to support quantified estimates of impacts or because relevant monetary values or effectiveness measures have not been developed. Policy makers and the general public may also care about characteristics that are not captured in QALYs nor by many of the other valuation measures used in CEA or BCA, such as the degree to which the risk is observable or controllable, and whether the risk is especially dreaded.

In this chapter, we first examine the ethical and normative[2] assumptions implicit in the calculation of the cost-effectiveness ratio, including the

---

[1]This position is reflected in the recommendations of previous expert panels and current Executive Office of the President guidance (U.S. Panel on Cost-Effectiveness in Health and Medicine, Gold et al., 1996b; Institute of Medicine Committee on Summary Measures of Population Health, IOM, 1998; Executive Order 12866, EOP, 1993; and Circular A-4, OMB, 2003a).

[2]In this chapter, "normative" refers to a variety of value-based judgments and beliefs, including some that are not ethical or moral in nature. For example, the fact that some people consider death from cancer worse than death from other causes is by itself not an ethical concern, though it involves a value-based judgment that guides their behavior.

construction of the metric most commonly used in CEA to value health outcomes, the QALY. In the second and third sections of the chapter, we identify important normative and distributional concerns that are not reflected in cost-effectiveness ratios and that should be taken into account in regulatory decisions. In the fourth section, we discuss the importance of an accountable, public deliberative process to bring together information from economic analyses with information about the ethical, qualitative, and distributive aspects to craft regulatory policies. The final section summarizes the Committee's conclusions.

ETHICAL ASSUMPTIONS IN QALY-BASED CEA

The QALY's strengths as the effectiveness metric in CEA are largely practical ones. The QALY is well established; it has been applied in hundreds of studies over several decades, is supported by generic health assessment survey instruments, and allows morbidity and mortality information to be readily combined. However, the QALY incorporates certain ethical commitments and ignores others. This section identifies some of the ethical implications of using the QALY as a unit of measurement for valuing health outcomes in CEA.

As discussed in Chapter 3, a QALY can be thought of in several different ways. Most simply, it is an index with an intuitive meaning, namely, an index that relates a particular state of impaired health (of a given duration) to some number of years in optimal health. More complex interpretations of the QALY, such as an index derived from utility theory or even as a direct measure of utility, are debatable, and are valid only under certain restrictive assumptions. When used in CEA for regulatory analysis, the QALY is probably best interpreted in its intuitive sense, as a *measure of health improvement or production* that facilitates comparisons with other opportunities for health gains. This pragmatic interpretation of the measure avoids the need to demonstrate that the QALY has particular properties consistent with the utility theory that underpins BCA and welfare economics.

Valuing Life Years Compared with Valuing Lives

Perhaps the most basic normative commitment entailed by using QALYs as an outcome measure in CEA is valuing some form of *life years*, rather than whole lives or preventable deaths. This move from treating all deaths equivalently to denominating losses and gains in terms of the extent of changes in longevity is illustrated by Table 4-1. Using lives as an impact measure assigns the same value to a preventable death regardless of whether the person is young, middle aged, or elderly, while the use of life years

TABLE 4-1 Lives, Life Years (LYs), and Quality-Adjusted Life Years (QALYs)

	Preventable Deaths	LYs[a]	LYs Discounted at 3%[a]	LYs Discounted at 7%[a]	QALYs[b]	QALYs Discounted at 3%[b]	QALYs Discounted at 7%[b]
Age (in years)							
5	1	73	29	14	65	27	13
35	1	44	24	14	37	21	12
75	1	12	10	7.9	9.1	7.6	6.1
Ratio of values by age							
5/35	1		1.7	1.2	1.0	1.8	1.3	1.1
5/75	1		6.1	2.9	1.8	7.1	3.6	2.1
35/75	1		3.7	2.4	1.8	4.1	2.7	2.0

[a]Based on age-specific life expectancy for 2002 (NCHS, 2005).

[b]Based on EQ-5D norms for the adult U.S. population (Hanmer et al., 2006); assumes HRQL is 1.0 for individuals through age 9, and midway between 1.0 and the value for persons age 20 for individuals ages 10 through 19.

shows the difference in impact of preventable mortality on younger and older individuals. Furthermore, adjusting life years for health-related quality of life (HRQL) in the QALY calculation increases the difference between the impact estimates for a younger as compared with older person.

Using QALYs gained, rather than deaths averted, as the measure of effectiveness in CEA has analogous implications in the BCA context. As discussed in Box 4-1, analyses in which monetized estimates of the value of preventable deaths vary by age have been highly controversial. Similarly, CEA using life years or QALYs gained as the effectiveness measure also appears to disadvantage older people, who have shorter average remaining life expectancies during which they can benefit from interventions. Some argue that shifting from valuing whole lives to any form of life years unfairly discriminates against older people, who may value the remainder of their lives as highly as do younger people. Similar arguments can be put forward for people with life expectancies shortened by their socioeconomic status or preexisting health conditions or disabilities.

A countering perspective is provided by those who hold that everyone should be given an equal chance to have a "normal" or full lifespan and that averting deaths among those who have achieved a normal lifespan should not count for as much as averting deaths among much younger persons. One implication of this view is that measuring life-preserving gains in terms of years of life does not *unfairly* disadvantage older people relative to younger people (Harris, 1987; Williams, 1997). In addition to this nor-

---

BOX 4-1
The "Senior Discount" Controversy

Analytic approaches that assign a lower value to premature mortality among the elderly have been the subject of heated debate in the context of BCA. In particular, the Environmental Protection Agency's use of estimates that reflected the value of remaining life years in a sensitivity analysis of air pollution-related policies led to a significant public outcry (Skrzycki, 2003). Based on a survey of older adults' willingness to pay for remaining life years, the analysis placed a lower value on premature mortality among the elderly (referred to as the "senior discount" in the subsequent policy debates). The controversy led the Office of Management and Budget (OMB) to issue a memorandum requiring agencies to avoid age adjustments (Graham, 2003a). OMB Circular A-4, which extends the guidance to CEA, amends the instructions regarding age adjustments (OMB, 2003a). The Circular notes that population averages, rather than values reflecting differences among subgroups, should be used in assessing both health-related quality of life and life expectancy to support the perceived fairness of the analytic approach.

---

mative argument, survey results suggest that, in the abstract, people judge saving the lives of younger as compared with older persons more important (Cropper et al., 1994).

Presenting the results of a CEA in several forms, using deaths averted, life years extended, and QALYs gained as alternatives, is one way to broaden perspectives on gains in life expectancy. In addition, reporting disaggregated estimates of regulatory impacts by key age and population characteristics—such as income, race, gender, or other factors relevant to the particular intervention—also increases the transparency of the justification for and implications of the regulatory action. Both strategies facilitate ethical deliberation.

A QALY Is a QALY Is a QALY

In contrast with the willingness-to-pay measures used in BCA, which may be affected by wealth and hence may vary depending on individual financial resources, by construction the value of a QALY is assumed not to vary with income. Although the relationship between willingness to pay and wealth is complex and depends on the characteristics of the good or service (see Freeman, 2003), the fact of this relationship can lead to concerns that the BCA results will be weighted toward the interests of wealthier members of society. In practice, regulatory analysts generally use willingness-to-pay values or ranges of values that reflect averages from the relevant research, rather than assigning different values to health risk reductions affecting richer and poorer people.

QALYs value an improvement in health of a given magnitude the same regardless of the characteristics of the person experiencing the improvement. They ignore the relative economic standing of affected populations in representing the value of health gains and reflect an ethical commitment to the income-independence of health as a societal value.

In addition, each QALY unit is of equal value in all contexts. Regardless of the individual to whom a QALY accrues, the states of health preceding or following the period in question, how widely health gains are distributed within a population, how impaired one beneficiary of a health gain is relative to another, or how a given impairment affects the lives of different persons, a QALY always carries the same value. Other health metrics, such as the healthy year equivalent, the saved young life equivalent, and the age-weighted disability-adjusted life year, each convey a different aspect of the distribution of health gains that the QALY omits.[3] However, none of these alternative HALY metrics are superior to the QALY in practice. No single metric can reflect all significant aspects of particular sorts of gains in health and longevity. The QALY, like any construct, imperfectly captures all aspects of what we value in good health. We know of no weighting scheme that is able to accurately reflect the full range of societal values relevant to regulatory decisions; in reality, these weights may vary depending on the particular decision-making context. Presenting supplementary information about the size and characteristics of the exposed population, the per capita magnitude of the risk, and the distribution of expected benefits will help respond to these concerns.

The Source of HRQL Values

The question of perspective in valuing HRQL has several dimensions. One has to do with the source of relative health state values, that is, whether they come from the general population, patients or persons experienced with the health state in question, or experts such as clinicians. The other dimension concerns the method for eliciting HRQL values and, more specifically, whether those values reflect individual preferences for one's own health or preferences for societal investments in health more broadly.

Whose Values Count?

The appropriate evaluative standpoint from which to determine the relative values of different health states, conditions, and disabilities in CEA

---

[3]These HALY measures are discussed in Chapter 3.

depends on the context of the decisions that the analysis is intended to inform. In clinical studies to compare the effectiveness of alternative treatments, for example, the values of patients may be most appropriate. In contrast, for societal decisions about resource allocation in health care settings, *community values* (i.e., the aggregated and averaged judgments of a representative sample of individuals in the general population) regarding the relative desirability of different states of health should be used (Gold et al., 1996b).

Because most economically significant regulations for which CEA is required affect all segments of society in terms of their costs and/or benefits, valuations (both for directly elicited values for specific health outcomes and valuation surveys underlying generic HRQL indexes) generally should be based on representative samples of the general U.S. population. Analysts will need to consider this issue in the context of individual regulations, however, because some rules disproportionately affect certain subgroups. For example, a regulation might impose costs and provide benefits primarily for elderly people or for residents of a single geographic area. In this case, values based on the affected subpopulation would be preferable.

If obtaining subpopulation values is not feasible, it would be important to conduct uncertainty analysis on the possible differences in valuation. Little is known about the differences in health state valuation across sociodemographic subpopulations in the United States with the notable exception of the recent U.S. EuroQoL-5D (EQ-5D) valuation survey (Shaw et al., 2005). This survey oversampled the two largest minority populations, Hispanics and non-Hispanic blacks, so that reliable subpopulation estimates could be calculated.

A related analysis that compared U.K. and U.S. results for these two large and methodologically consistent EQ-5D valuation surveys found significant differences in the values for particular health states (Johnson et al., 2005). These differences were not constant or systematic across health states; those characterized by severe problems had the largest discrepancies, with U.S. valuations exceeding the U.K. valuations. Although these findings suggest that it is important that the health state index values be derived from a population comparable to the one of interest, it may turn out to be less of an issue in practice than in the abstract. As illustrated by the case studies, regulatory analysis involves comparing health status with and without the condition of interest. More research would be needed to determine whether such estimates of *changes* in health status are as dependent on the population surveyed as are the estimates for particular conditions (Franks et al., 2006).

Some research shows that preferences for particular health states are quite similar for different groups of people, when patient valuations are compared with those of nonpatients, and when the valuations of different socioeconomic and ethnic groups are compared (Kaplan and Bush, 1982; Llewellyn-Thomas et al., 1982, 1993; Balaban et al., 1986). Other studies, however, suggest that people who have experienced a disease or disabling condition will tend to value that state more highly than those with no experience (Sackett and Torrance, 1978; Najman and Levine, 1981; Slevin et al., 1990).[4] One possible explanation for this latter finding is that those with the condition or impairment have made adjustments or adaptations that result in lesser losses in HRQL than are anticipated prior to any illness or disability.[5]

Discrepancies in valuations of impaired or disabled health states between a general population and those with experience of the condition have led some to challenge the validity of general population valuations, arguing that they are uninformed and potentially discriminatory. Recent research findings in psychology and behavioral economics suggest that people incorrectly predict the impact of changes in their circumstances on their sense of well-being (Kahneman et al., 1997; Wilson et al., 2001; Gilbert and Ebert, 2002; Riis et al., 2005). If health state index values are intended to represent the relative effects of different conditions on people's lives rather than reflecting apprehensions and prejudices about those conditions, then values elicited from people lacking knowledge about the conditions may be biased.

Furthermore, people with disabilities and disability advocacy groups have objected to being "assigned" lower HRQL values than are those without disability, on the grounds that the practice leads to the devaluation of persons living with disabilities and to perpetuation of stigma associated with particular conditions (Wang, 1992; Silvers, 1996). If a health condition or disability—human immunodeficiency virus disease or paraplegia, for example—is valued lower by the general public because it is stigmatizing, using this valuation in a public policy analysis may reinforce, and be taken as condoning, such prejudice.

Wasserman and Asch (2004) have suggested an alternative way to establish the relative values of preventing particular injuries and impairments. They propose that relative values should be based on the costs of restoring capacities and improving various aspects of quality of life for those who are impaired. For example, facilitative and adaptive technologies for persons with speech or writing disabilities can restore communications

---

[4]This *valuation* question must be distinguished from the task of *characterizing* the experience of a particular health condition or disability according to a multidimensional generic survey instrument. The descriptive task is always best carried out by those who are familiar with the condition, as discussed in Chapter 3.

[5]Such adaptation is not only psychological; it can involve substantial investments in rehabilitation, personal assistance, assistive technologies, and physical accommodations in the built environment (IOM, 1997).

abilities. The cost of providing someone who has lost capabilities through injury with the equipment and services that restore functioning could be used to establish an upper bound on the cost of that injury or impairment, relative to unimpaired health. Such investments could well exceed what is now spent on rehabilitative services for some conditions. Thus this approach to valuation is more demanding than a cost-of-illness estimate based on historical spending. Initial estimates (for the United Kingdom) of the costs of restoring capacities have been made for some conditions (Smith et al., 2004). We recognize that this strategy is not practicable in the near term, and would likely be feasible only for some kinds of disabling conditions. In concept, however, it offers an alternative to preference-based measures that avoids the apparent devaluing of lives spent with impairments.

The use of general population valuations does not necessarily result in material disadvantage for those with impairments or disabilities (Gold et al., 1996b). Because the perspective is ex ante in regulatory analysis and it cannot be known with certainty who ultimately *will* be affected, the values of those *potentially* affected (represented by the general population for most economically significant health and safety regulations) are appropriate in this context. This perspective takes account of the loss of capacities and opportunities that attend illness and injury. It reflects the societal value accorded having greater rather than lesser capacities and more rather than fewer opportunities.

If a subset of the general population receives the benefits and pays the costs of the regulation, then the values of this subpopulation should be used. In particular, there may be instances where the costs and benefits of a rule predominantly affect people with a preexisting illness or disability addressed by the regulation. In this case, the affected population is the same as the patient population, and patient values would be appropriate. Later in the chapter we consider the circumstances under which the lesser values placed on health improvements among those with impaired health or disabilities can be ethically problematic.

Individual Preferences and Societal Values

As noted in Chapter 3, empirical research suggests that each elicitation technique—standard gamble, time trade-off, category rating, and person trade-off (PTO)—produces somewhat different relative values for states of health. One distinction among these four elicitation methods is that the first three techniques query individual preferences, while the PTO method is socially oriented. PTO exercises ask for judgments about the equivalence of health improvements and life extensions for groups of people who differ in their states of health, age, and other relevant characteristics (Richardson and Nord, 1997; Nord, 1999). Respondents are asked "to compare the relative benefits of treating different conditions in a context of comparing equivalent numbers needing to be treated to produce equal social benefits" (Ubel et al., 1998, p. 43).

The results of PTO exercises suggest that values other than the maximization of potential aggregate health benefits, as measured by conventional QALYs, affect decisions to allocate health improvements among groups. Allocation choices using PTO tend to give greater weight to improving the health of more severely impaired groups relative to those with lesser problems (Nord, 1999). PTO elicitations also tend to distribute potential health gains more widely among groups able to benefit (Menzel et al., 1999).

Because of the broad and essentially social nature of health and safety regulation, the PTO method may be particularly appropriate for valuing health outcomes in this context. As noted in Chapter 3, much work remains to be done, however, to develop the PTO technique and the empirical base from which to estimate values. The Committee concludes that research to develop better approaches to societal valuation for regulatory CEA is warranted.

Combining Morbidity and Mortality in a Single Measure

As detailed in Chapter 3, QALYs combine information about changes in survival and morbidity in a way that reflects individuals' preferences for trade-offs between longevity and quality of life. This fundamental property of the QALY mirrors the actual situation of patients who face medical treatment choices that involve a risk of death. However, when QALYs are also used to compare very different health-related interventions, this framework may not mirror the actual choice as closely. Analyses of regulatory interventions are likely to encompass broader arrays of health-related effects for large population groups. CEA will at times involve the aggregation and synthesis of many health outcomes and of impacts across diverse groups of people, as illustrated in the examples in Chapter 2. In addition, evaluating the health impacts of regulatory interventions requires *combining* the benefits of increased length of life and improved quality of life for a population, rather than *trading off* longevity against improved quality of life for a given individual.

When health outcomes are aggregated and averaged across diverse conditions and populations, a single summary measure will mask disparities in impacts among age or other population groups. For example, in the Environmental Protection Agency (EPA) analysis that was the subject of the air quality case study, the summary measure masks the range of impacts on the very old, the very young, and those with preexisting conditions. Thus EPA presents disaggregated results for mortality and morbidity and for different age groups (see Table 2-4). The Committee's recommendations, presented in the final chapter, address the need for reporting disaggregated analytic results in regulatory analyses.

Summary

This section briefly reviewed the ethical assumptions embedded in QALY-based CEA. Using QALYs in regulatory analysis widens the application of this analytic tool and introduces a complex normative construct to a new audience. Understanding what the QALY does and does not reflect in the measurement of health effects should help regulatory analysts and policy makers interpret and communicate their analytic results. In particular, analysts should keep in mind the need to present information on the nature of the individual health effects and the characteristics of affected population groups because QALYs subsume these distinctions. The societal perspective of regulatory analysis is best reflected by valuation of health states and conditions by people affected by the regulation. At the same time, it is important to keep in mind the potential biases in the valuation of some health states due to unfamiliarity, lack of experience, or because the states carry stigma. The rationale for using health state values elicited from community-based sample surveys in regulatory analysis is to reflect the preferences and values of the population likely to receive the benefits and/or bear the costs of the intervention.

ETHICAL AND OTHER IMPLICATIONS OF RISKS AND OF INTERVENTIONS TO ADDRESS RISKS

In this section we consider the ethical, distributional, and other factors relevant to decisions about regulating health and safety risks that are not captured in CEA.

Dimensions of Value Affecting the Acceptability of Risks

Not all kinds of risks are the same. Risks may differ in ways that can affect their acceptability for individuals and for society as a whole, as well as their assessment from an ethical point of view. How government agencies should address risks that differ in kind and in acceptability (both to individuals and the larger community) is a question that can be addressed only as part of broad, public, and deliberative discussions.

Regardless of whether the value of risk reductions is measured by cases averted, willingness to pay for health improvements, or QALY gains, the measure is likely to exclude some aspects of the risk reductions that are valued by society. For example, a 1-in-100,000 reduction in the risk of death may be valued differently depending on the source of the risk; society may place a higher value on reducing risks associated with unpleasant sources (e.g., hazardous waste sites) than on risks associated with enjoyable activities (e.g., riding a motorcycle). This difference in valuation will not be reflected in single-dimension measures of benefit, such as cases avoided or years of life extension, nor will it be reflected in QALY measures focused on health-related impacts on quality of life.[6]

Because QALY-based CEA does not and cannot account for the nature of the risk itself and societal perceptions and values related to it, some features of risks must be considered explicitly by decision makers alongside the summary results of economic analyses. The psychological aspects of risk perception and risk assessment have been well studied (Slovic et al., 2000, 2004). At the same time, the normative significance of the public's perceptions of risks has been challenged (Margolis, 1996). Without joining this debate, the Committee proposes that the following characteristics be considered in regulatory impact analyses along with the presentation of quantified results:

- Knowledge about or understanding of risks,
- Degree of personal control, and
- Source or nature of risks.

These dimensions may affect the justification for regulatory action as well as the value placed on the resulting risk reductions. For example, as discussed in Chapter 1, regulation may be justified in cases where there is an externality, such as in the case of pollution that imposes health risks that are not controllable by the individual affected. Regulation may also be justified where information is lacking; for example, certain pathogens in food may not be easily detectable by consumers. However, this section focuses more specifically on the need to incorporate the value placed on these risk dimensions in the regulatory decision-making process, rather than on the initial justification for considering regulatory action.

Three aspects of risks bear on our *knowledge or comprehension* of them: To what extent are they easily detectable by the senses? Are their effects delayed or more immediate? Are they relatively well understood? Although these features of risks do not have direct ethical implications, they can affect the personal, social, or moral acceptability of certain risks or at least raise issues that should be discussed concerning the value placed on reducing them (Cranor, 1995).

If risks can be avoided because they are *easily detectable*, as in some traffic-related situations, we can use our basic human sensory capabilities

---

[6]Although willingness-to-pay estimates could, in theory, incorporate the values associated with features of particular risks, in reality such estimates rarely address all aspects of the risks.

to provide some protection against possible harm. At the very least, we may believe that we will have some opportunities for self-protection. These kinds of risk exposures may be more acceptable to us than risks for which we cannot provide any degree of self-protection by exercising normal human capacities, such as in the case of an undetectable toxicant in the air. As a result, we may value reduction in undetectable risks more than detectable risks.

Risks with *delayed effects* often lack an immediate feedback mechanism that would allow individuals or a community to implement timely protections. A pesticide released into the environment that immediately killed all exposed frogs would alert us to a problem meriting attention. By contrast, release of a pesticide with long-delayed but potentially devastating effects may receive less attention, and could lead a community to value precautionary measures more highly. Although the timing and duration of the risks, including related latency periods, are captured to some extent in the QALY measure, such measures may not fully incorporate the different values placed on reducing immediate versus delayed risks.

Some risks allow us a *degree of personal control*; for example, the care one takes in operating chainsaws or other kinds of equipment will obviously affect the likely degree of harm. Other risks are not subject to significant personal control by those facing the risk, such as toxic air pollutants. The degree to which one can control exposure to a hazard, and whether or not the hazard results in harm, can affect acceptability of the hazard and the value placed on risk reductions. Many risks are regulated because they are not subject to significant personal control and individuals can do little or nothing to protect themselves.

A third aspect of risks that bears on their acceptability includes intrinsic or contextual features of special concern, such as risks that are particularly *dreaded* (Slovic, 2000). Dreaded risks may reflect concerns about particularly unpleasant diseases or ways of dying (e.g., from cancer) or risks that could materialize as especially catastrophic harms, such as failure of nuclear power plant containment measures. Certain risks or outcomes may be dreaded because of stigma attached to them, such as HIV-positive status or paraplegia, as mentioned earlier.

These features point to important aspects of risks that could affect people's assessment of their acceptability and the degree of care with which they are approached. The above list is not exhaustive; rather, it is designed to suggest a variety of considerations that are likely to affect personal, social, or moral judgments regarding the value of risk reductions. Individuals' judgments about the acceptability of risks may also be affected by considerations such as whether the risk activity provides significant benefits; the degree, if any, of participation in decisions that have created the risk or the exposure; and how reliable a governmental agency is in providing protections from risks (Cranor, 1995; HM Treasury, 2005). Such dimensions of risk merit public deliberation and input.

Nonquantifiable Impacts

The economically significant health and safety regulations subject to OMB's requirements for CEA will have some risks that can be quantified (e.g., in terms of cases averted) and valued (e.g., in terms of QALY gains or willingness to pay for risk reductions). In addition, some of these regulations will have quantified nonhealth benefits. When these regulations provide additional health and/or nonhealth benefits that cannot be measured in numerical terms, care should be taken to ensure that these impacts are considered in the decision-making process. As discussed in Chapter 1, the existing guidance for regulatory decision making emphasizes the need to consider these nonquantifiable impacts.

In some cases, these nonquantifiable effects result from the limitations of the underlying health research. For some risks, a link to clinical disease has not been established definitively. For example, research shows that ozone changes the structure of lung tissue, but the implications of these changes for long-term health are not yet well described (Gilliland et al., 1999; Hubbell et al., 2005). Such "precursor" or intermediate biological conditions that might lead to adverse clinical effects in the future are not included in the quantitative measures used in CEA or BCA.

There are other risks, unrelated to human health, that may be reduced or prevented by regulations. Because they are not related, CEA based on single-dimension health measures or on QALYs will not capture them. For example, not only may dioxins released into surface water threaten the public's health, they may also have substantial environmental effects because they accumulate in many organisms, are persistent, and disrupt endocrine systems. The visibility improvements associated with the air pollution rule considered in the Committee's EPA case study are another example. Such consequences will not be captured in the effectiveness measure of a CEA that focuses only on human health protection. If quantified, however, such impacts could be included as an offset to costs.

Summary

This brief discussion provides some background on the particular features of risks that may affect the value placed on regulations designed to reduce or eliminate them. Three points emerge from this discussion. First, insofar as CEA aims to provide objective assessments of population health as measured by clinical disease, it may miss or undervalue other considerations, including nonquantified and nonhealth impacts, that should enter into public decisions concerning risk regulation. If such considerations cannot be incorporated into the cost-effectiveness calculus, they must be reintroduced into the decision-making process as an adjunct to summary economic information.

Second, the failure to account for the distinctive features of risks may in some circumstances lead to misinterpretation when cost-effectiveness ratios for different regulations are compared. Because CEA is a tool for comparing different interventions aimed at the same end, ignoring the different value dimensions of the risks involved or the contexts of the risks may well result in misleading comparisons and ultimately to poor regulatory decisions.

Last and most importantly, the multiple value dimensions of risks deserve public and deliberative consideration as regulatory options are devised and considered; these aspects of risk are as relevant for the decision as the results of economic analyses. Although in theory monetized estimates of the benefits of regulations could capture some of these characteristics, in practice they may not be fully captured by either BCA or CEA. The information conveyed by a cost-effectiveness ratio may be of interest because it presents costs and health-related effects in isolation from other pieces of information about the risk and the intervention. However, the cost-effectiveness ratio is, by itself, not an adequate basis for decision making and must be supplemented by other information. Even if not all stakeholders agree on the normative implications of a particular risk or intervention (and it seems unlikely that there will be unanimity), invoking these implications and discussing them ensures that qualitative information is not ignored in the decision. Disagreements about the relevance and importance of the different aspects of risks create an even greater need for public debate, both in preregulatory priority setting and in the development of and public comment on the regulation itself. Box 4-2 illustrates how these concerns might be summarized in the presentation of the results of economic analysis.

DISTRIBUTIONAL CONCERNS ABOUT RISKS AND REGULATORY INTERVENTIONS

By itself, a QALY-based CEA cannot address an important and difficult set of distributional questions and choices, including how much priority we should give to the sickest or the worst off in valuing health effects; when we should allow modest benefits to many people to outweigh significant benefits to fewer; when we should allocate resources to produce "best outcomes" as compared with giving more people fair chances at some benefit; and how the costs and benefits of regulatory interventions are distributed within the overall population. Both CEA and BCA can provide

---

BOX 4-2
Risk-Related Considerations for Regulatory Decisions

Characteristics of Risks: Do the risks averted by the rule have characteristics that affect the value society places on reducing them but that are not reflected in the quantified effectiveness measures used to assess the policy? For example:

- Are the risks not subject to significant personal control?
- Are the risks particularly dreaded?
- Are the risks undetectable by the senses?
- Are the effects of the risks delayed, rather than immediate?
- Are the risks not well understood?

We use the three case studies—on food safety, air quality, and child restraints anchoring—to provide examples of how risk-related concerns might be summarized in a regulatory impact analysis.

Food safety. *Personal control and detection:* In the absence of regulation, consumers generally lack the ability to determine whether a particular batch of juice contains pathogens. *Understanding:* Information about these risks emerges gradually as outbreaks occur, and the probability of individual exposure is relatively slight. Thus consumers may not fully understand the potential consequences.

Air quality. *Personal control and detection:* Air emissions from nonroad engines and sulfur in diesel fuel can severely affect many individuals whose ability to detect and avoid exposures in the course of daily life may be very limited. *Dread:* The associated risks include a relatively high rate of premature death and may include forms of cardiac and respiratory illness (e.g., congestive heart failure, emphysema) that are particularly dreaded.

Child restraints anchoring. *Dread:* Not only are children's lives and well-being highly valued in general, but severe injuries from motor vehicle crashes, such as traumatic brain injury, are particularly dreaded by parents and others. *Understanding:* The high rate of improper installation of child restraints in the absence of the rule suggests that attachment requirements were not well understood.

---

disaggregate information on impacts, if the underlying research on risks and effects supports separate estimates. However, standard analytic practices in BCA and CEA generally do not weight the results to reflect societal values across these dimensions. For example, a QALY decrement of 0.2 is not adjusted to reflect a preference for averting illnesses among particularly vulnerable groups. Similarly, values assigned to risk reductions of a given magnitude in a BCA generally do not depend on the distribution of impacts.

Although for both CEA and BCA values could, in theory, be adjusted to reflect distributive concerns, a consensus on how to weight across such dimensions does not exist. Thus distributive considerations must be explicitly discussed as part of the process of developing and issuing regulations along with the summary analytic results.

As noted in Chapters 1 and 2, regulatory agencies are required to conduct analyses of the distributional impacts of regulations. As discussed below, society may particularly value regulations that address subpopulations that are vulnerable or already disadvantaged, such as those who are physically susceptible to environmental or other health risks, are less than fully capable of representing their own interests, or are economically disadvantaged or vulnerable. Children, elderly people, those who are chronically ill or especially susceptible to a particular risk, low-income or minority communities, and local populations affected by a geographically concentrated risk or intervention are relevant subpopulations that may merit special consideration. Box 4-3 refers to the case studies to illustrate how information about populations disproportionately affected by a risk or an intervention might be presented in a regulatory analysis.

Children

Current Presidential guidance to federal agencies directs that particular consideration be given to the assessment of health and safety risks that disproportionately affect children. Each agency must, with respect to its rules, "to the extent permitted by law and appropriate, and consistent with the agency's mission . . . address disproportionate risks to children that result from environmental health risks or safety risks" (EOP, 1997, Section 1). OMB Circular A-4 further instructs that, for any rulemaking action expected to result in an economically significant health or safety rule that may disproportionately affect children, the agency must evaluate the health or safety effects on children. This account should address why the proposed regulatory intervention was selected over other potential and reasonably feasible alternatives that the agency considered. The focus of these instructions, however, is more on avoiding disproportionate harms than on providing a greater degree of protection.

Circular A-4 also directs that agencies use CEA as the *primary* analytic framework when children are the predominantly affected group. Secondarily, a BCA may be conducted. However, whenever a BCA is conducted and benefits accrue to both children and adults, "the monetary values for children should be at least as large as the values for adults (for the same probabilities and outcomes) unless there is specific and compelling evidence to suggest otherwise" (OMB, 2003a, p. 31).

BOX 4-3
Distributional Considerations in Regulatory Decisions

Distribution of Impacts: Do the baseline (preregulatory) or postregulatory costs or risks disproportionately affect certain segments of the population?

- The unborn or future generations
- Infants and young children
- Elderly people
- Persons with disabilities or preexisting health conditions
- Those particularly vulnerable to the risks of concern
- Members of minority groups
- Members of low-income groups
- Those residing in particular geographic locations

Below are some brief examples of distributional considerations in the cases of food safety, air quality, and child restraints anchoring, based on information provided in the agencies' regulatory analyses.

Food Safety: The juice processing regulation prevents foodborne illnesses, which can be especially severe for persons with poor immune system function, including people with human immunodeficiency virus, people receiving chemotherapy, and organ transplant recipients. Young children and elderly people are also likely to be more susceptible to more severe forms of these illnesses. Compliance costs are likely to be passed on to consumers of fresh juices, through very small but widely distributed increases in prices to cover production cost increases. Elderly people and young children consume somewhat more juice than the overall population on average.

Air Quality: Reductions in particulate matter due to cleaner exhaust from non-road diesel engines and reduced sulfur in diesel fuel will disproportionately benefit elderly people, young children, and individuals with preexisting conditions. Reductions in premature mortality will accrue largely among elderly persons; infant deaths also will decrease. Cardiovascular disease will be reduced among older adults, as will acute episodes among those with preexisting cardiac disease. Acute respiratory episodes and hospitalizations will be reduced among persons with chronic respiratory conditions, such as asthma. Individuals who work in industries that rely on nonroad engines (e.g., construction, agriculture, industry, mining, and airports) may be disproportionately affected. Compliance costs are likely to be passed on to consumers of products in related markets. The EPA estimates that related price increases are likely to be less than 0.1 percent, however.

Child Restraints Anchoring: This regulation provides additional protection from the risk of injury or death for young children restrained in car seats. Compliance costs are likely to be passed on to consumers in the form of higher prices. The National Highway Traffic Safety Administration estimates that these costs will average $6 per vehicle and $17 per child restraint.

These guidance documents reflect the exceptional value society places on children's lives and well-being, as well as recognizing their particular susceptibility to serious and long-lasting harm from health and safety risks. Table 4-1 illustrates how the use of life years or QALYs, instead of preventable deaths, weights the health impacts for children more heavily, relative to impacts on older persons. As discussed in Chapter 3, the difficulties of valuing children's health outcomes are both empirical and conceptual. Setting aside the practical problems of measuring HRQL for children, the concern remains that an individually based HRQL metric does not fully capture the high value placed on children's well-being and health by parents and society. Although some have suggested that HRQL measurement should encompass the effects of an illness, injury, or disability on the entire family in which it occurs, this demanding approach has not been implemented.

Population Health Data and Subgroups

Another potential problem for valuation is that the major population health surveys exclude some subpopulations of concern. As discussed in Chapter 3, the National Health Interview Survey and the Medical Expenditure Panel Survey are household surveys, limited to noninstitutionalized, civilian populations. By design, excluded populations are homeless people; those who are migrant or have no fixed residence; and persons in prisons, group homes, nursing homes, and other institutions (Meyers and Andresen, 2000). Undocumented aliens, migrant farm workers, and others with reasons to avoid contact with government officials or data collection activities are unlikely to be represented in survey samples. In addition, members of these groups may be particularly susceptible to certain kinds of risks targeted by regulations, such as pesticide controls and workplace safety practices.

The exclusion of the groups just mentioned from routine population health surveys is also a problem for the valuation surveys underlying generic HRQL indexes, and calls into question the extent to which they can be assumed to represent accurately the values of the general population. The significance of this omission depends on whether the excluded groups represent a large enough percentage of the population to affect the survey results, and whether the values of excluded groups differ to a significant degree from the values held by those included in the survey. Although the recently conducted U.S. valuation survey for the EQ-5D used a stratified sample designed to include the three largest racial/ethnic groups in sufficient numbers to provide disaggregate results for whites, Hispanics, and non-Hispanic blacks, disaggregated results were not presented in the initial publications from this survey (Luo et al., 2005; Shaw et al., 2005).

Another issue with respect to low-income populations and some minority populations, such as blacks and Native Americans, is that their life expectancy is lower and their HRQL worse than that of others in the population (NCHS, 2004). If health gains are calculated for such subgroups based on subgroup population health status and longevity norms, then the potential to benefit from life extensions will be proportionately lower for these subgroups.

Calculation of Health Gains

Some health risks subject to regulation disproportionately affect those whose health is impaired already. In the case of air quality interventions, for example, the elderly and those with preexisting cardiac or pulmonary conditions are more likely to suffer adverse health effects. One of the most difficult issues to address is whether and how to disaggregate the general population in calculating gains in health due to a regulatory intervention. Both OMB guidance and the PCEHM's recommendations for the reference case CEA direct the use of general population averages rather than health state index value estimates for subpopulations. (These requirements are discussed in more detail in Chapters 1 and 2; see Appendix C for the relevant text of Circular A-4.) The implications of these requirements for regulatory analysis depend on whether the general population is in fact representative of the population that achieves the health gains. For the types of economically significant health and safety regulations addressed by this report, the population affected will often reflect the same distribution of preexisting disabilities or health impairments as the general population. In such cases, using general population averages is analytically correct and will not disadvantage those who are disabled or in impaired health.

The OMB and PCEHM requirements are more problematic in a case where the affected population does not reflect the same distribution of preexisting disabilities or health impairments as the general population. For example, if individuals with heart disease represent 10 percent of the general population but 50 percent of the population affected by the regulation, using population averages may not accurately capture the QALY gains attributable to the rule.

In the air pollution example, reductions in preventable mortality may predominantly affect individuals with preexisting heart or respiratory conditions. Such deaths occur primarily among elderly people, and population averages for the affected age groups include a relatively high rate of heart and respiratory disease. EPA concluded that, because both the general population and the affected population in these age groups have comparably high rates of these preexisting conditions, the use of population averages may provide a reasonable best estimate of the impacts of its rule. However, this conclusion is the subject of debate and scientific uncertainty.

It is also important to remember that the population affected undergoes changes in health status over time. Rules tend to remain in place for extended periods, however. Thus people who are not affected at the outset may develop conditions later such that a regulatory intervention is especially beneficial.

In cases where the health impairment or disability *is* related to the risk or intervention of interest, QALYs could unfairly value life-extending interventions for people with chronic illness or disability. For example, suppose decision makers are comparing two regulations that are equally costly, one of which affects only individuals with preexisting disabilities and another that affects individuals in better health. Also assume that the first intervention, which extends for 10 years the lives of 100 people with a chronic condition or disability valued at 0.75 (on a scale where 1.0 corresponds to optimal health and 0 corresponds to death), would produce 750 QALYs. If the second intervention extends for 10 years the lives of 100 people in near optimal health—0.95, for example—the gain would be 950 QALYs. In this case, focusing solely on the QALY gains would lead decision makers to select the second intervention, even though it extends the same number of lives as the first. Hence the use of QALYs for evaluating and prioritizing life-saving interventions appears to discriminate against people with impaired health or disabilities by assigning less value to extending their lives simply because of their disability. The reduction of average HRQL that occurs with increasing age produces the same general effect in comparisons between life extensions among 20-year-olds and 70-year-olds.

An alternative to assessing QALY gains based on comparison to actual health status is an approach that assumes that affected individuals would be in optimal health as a result of the intervention. As discussed in Chapter 2 (see Box 2-5), EPA recently presented QALY-based results that do *not* adjust life years gained to reflect the less-than-optimal HRQL that would be expected during those additional years of life (EPA, 2005a, Appendix G). Instead, EPA calculated health gains due to averted mortality as life years spent in optimal health.

In our case study of air quality improvements, we followed a different practice. We estimated the gain in QALYs due to increased life expectancy based on average health state values for the general population in each age group assessed. This approach assumes that, in the absence of the regulation-related risks, individuals would face the same degree of impairment as the average member of the U.S. population of the same age. The Committee concludes that EPA's practice—which essentially gives greater weight to QALY gains from life extensions than from HRQL improvements—was less transparent than the alternative, namely to calculate all

QALY gains the same way regardless of whether morbidity or mortality is affected *and* to present those gains in disaggregated form so that the differences in the types of impacts are apparent. Appendix A provides additional discussion and presents the results of the Committee's case study analysis.

The Treatment of Future Generations in CEA

Although many regulations have the potential to affect future generations, those where the costs are incurred primarily in the near term but the benefits occur largely in the future (or vice versa) pose particular ethical issues, especially if the effects of the policy are not easily reversible. Such is the case, for example, with regulations governing the construction of nuclear waste repositories. Construction may impose costs on the current generation, whereas future generations may be affected by the release of radiation if safeguards fail. Contaminants with reproductive or developmental effects provide other examples; controlling exposures among members of the current generation will benefit the subsequent generation. Assessing the impacts of these types of regulations poses analytic as well as ethical challenges regardless of whether BCA or CEA is used to estimate costs and benefits.

Future Effects

Perhaps the biggest issue associated with rulemakings relates to the ability to predict future conditions with and without the regulation. This problem pervades all aspects of the analysis. For example, Harrington et al. (2000) compared the predicted and actual costs of several regulations, and found that one of the key factors leading to overestimates of future costs was the difficulty inherent in predicting technological innovation. Such innovations may affect the benefits of a rule as well as its costs.

The regulatory analyses reviewed by the Committee applied varying approaches to addressing this problem (see Robinson, 2004, and Appendix A). For example, in the Food and Drug Administration's (FDA's) analysis of its juice processing rule, the agency assumed that current conditions remained constant, so that both costs and benefits were the same in each future year (FDA, 1998, 2001). In addition to presenting this annual value, FDA calculated the present value of costs and benefits over an infinite time horizon. In contrast, in its analysis of emission controls for nonroad diesel engines, EPA limited the time period addressed to 20 years and presented costs and benefits on an annual basis as well as in present value terms (EPA, 2004b). These estimates took into account the phase-in of regulatory requirements as well as predicted changes over time in pollutant emissions and in the demographic characteristics of the affected population. As required by OMB (2003a), regulatory analyses generally also present the timing of the undiscounted impacts.

This presentation of both discounted and undiscounted results is particularly important when costs and benefits are widely separated in time. If there is a lag between the costs and the effects, the estimates of cost-effectiveness will vary depending on the length of time that elapses as well as the discount rate used, regardless of whether the benefits are measured in dollars, QALYs, life years, or cases avoided.[7] For example, if both costs and benefits are discounted, two regulatory options that differ only in the year in which benefits occur will have different present values if a positive discount rate is used. The regulatory option with the nearer term benefits will appear to be more cost effective. This outcome is derived from the underlying rationale for discounting, which reflects a general preference to receive benefits soon and delay costs.[8] Table 4-2 presents this issue in simplified form. As indicated in the table, the option without a lag between costs and benefits will be more cost-effective in present value terms when compared to another option with equivalent, but more delayed, benefits.[9] This difference in present values increases as the discount rate increases.[10]

Future Generations

When risks are imposed or benefits accrue in the distant future, the ethical concerns and issues related to discounting are more difficult and less satisfactorily addressed. Moral obligations to future generations should be considered separately from the question of discounting practices.[11] Present-

---

[7]In the majority of rules considered in the Committee's review of current practices (Robinson, 2004), costs and reduced incidence of illness, injury, or death occur in the same or relatively proximate time periods. FDA's analysis indicates that the reduction in the incidence of illness is likely to occur in the same year as the reduction in juice contamination. EPA makes the same assumption for changes in the incidence of the nonfatal effects of nonroad engine diesel emissions, while indicating that preventable mortality is distributed over a 5-year period after exposure.

[8]For example, most individuals generally would prefer to receive money today rather than at a later date because they can invest the money and earn interest. The present (discounted) value today of $100 received in a future year (t) is the amount that one would need to invest today to yield $100 in year (t).

[9]For simplicity, Table 4-2 assumes that the QALY losses all occur in a single year. However, for most chronic illnesses and for preventable mortality, a change in incidence in the current year will have future year effects, and these future year effects will also be discounted.

[10]See Portney and Weyant (1999), especially the essay by Weitzman (1999) for discussions of the interaction of the discount rate and the time period over which the discounting occurs.

[11]See, for example, "On Discounting Regulatory Benefits: Risk, Money, and Intergenerational Equity" (Sunstein and Rowell, 2005) for a discussion of this issue.

TABLE 4-2 Discounting and Timing of Impacts

Time Period	Regulatory Option 1	Regulatory Option 2
UNDISCOUNTED RESULTS		
Year 0	Costs = $100 million; benefits = 400 QALYs	Costs = $100 million
Year 10	—	—
Year 20	—	—
Year 30	—	Benefits = 400 QALYs
Cost per QALY	$100 million / 400 QALYs = $250,000 per QALY	$100 million/400 QALYs = $250,000 per QALY
RESULTS DISCOUNTED AT 3 PERCENT		
Present value in year 0	Costs = $100 million; benefits = 400 QALYs	Costs = $100 million; benefits = 165 QALYs
Cost per QALY	$100 million/400 QALYs = $250,000 per QALY	$100 million/165 QALYs = $610,000 per QALY
RESULTS DISCOUNTED AT 7 PERCENT		
Present value in year 0	Costs = $100 million; benefits = 400 QALYs	Costs = $100 million; benefits = 53 QALYs
Cost per QALY	$100 million/400 QALYs = $250,000 per QALY	$100 million/53 QALYs = $1.9 million per QALY

NOTES: For simplicity, this example assumes all the quality-adjusted life year (QALY) impacts occur in a single year and ignores the lifetime effects of chronic illness as well as the life years lost to premature mortality. It also does not provide information on the uncertainty in the estimates. All estimates are rounded to two significant digits.

ing undiscounted impacts, and their timing, along with a discussion of impacts on future generations, as OMB (2003a) advises, allows decision makers to identify situations where concerns about long-term impacts suggest that decisions should not be based simply on the discounted present value of the results.[12] Such presentation is necessary because otherwise, discounting may lead the present generation to impose extremely high costs on future generations, resulting in undesirable welfare losses as well as inequities between generations (Revesz, 1999). In addition, discounting

---

[12]Chapter 2 discusses other aspects of the OMB guidance on discounting, such as the selection of the appropriate discount rate and the need for sensitivity analysis. Circular A-4 also describes the rationale for discounting nonmonetary as well as monetary measures of benefits in regulatory analysis (see Appendix C). In the context of health and medicine, Gold et al. (1996b) provide a detailed discussion of discounting, and recommend discounting both costs and benefits at 3 percent in the reference case and conducting sensitivity analyses using rates ranging from 0 to 7 percent.

could give an undesirable priority to programs that would produce benefits more rapidly, but with substantially less overall improvement in health, when compared to programs that produce benefits later, but with substantially more overall improvement.

At the same time, a failure to discount could impose significant burdens on the present generation that regulatory interventions would alleviate. If regulators discount costs at a positive rate but value lives saved now and lives saved later equally, then the analysis paradoxically indicates that life-saving spending should be postponed indefinitely, because the net benefit becomes increasingly favorable into the future (Keeler and Cretin, 1983). Furthermore, because future generations can reasonably be expected to inherit a richer and more technologically advanced world, there may be less reason to protect future generations from present choices (Weitzman, 1999). Others have suggested that the discounting of benefits to future generations might be thought of as part of a mutually beneficial intergenerational trade or contract (Lind, 1982).

How future benefits and harms (costs) are viewed is likely to depend on the perspective adopted. For example, parents will likely take a more precautionary attitude toward protecting the world their children and grandchildren will inherit than might people unaffiliated with younger generations.

Representing the interests of future generations in current policy discussions is difficult but ethically obligatory. Future generations will be affected by current decisions, particularly if the consequences are not easily reversed. As those involved in such discussions consider the future effects of their choices, they should factor in the implications of their decisions for those who will live in the future. Alternative normative frameworks—the "just savings" principle of Rawls' social contract theory (1971, 1993), tort law, and utilitarianism—each can support a principle of compensation to guide discussion about the mix of benefits and costs that the present generation bequeaths to future ones (Sunstein and Rowell, 2005).

Comparing Cost-Effectiveness Ratios

The assumption underlying the use of CEA in regulation is that resources should be used to maximize the aggregate health status, or to minimize disease burdens, of a population. Some have suggested ranking regulatory programs from the lowest cost-per-QALY ratio to the highest, in order to identify better or more efficient investments in health production. Hahn (2005) has argued in favor of the use of such summary rankings, which he calls "regulatory scorecards" and which OMB has described as "league tables" (EOP, 2002). Although such scorecards enable comparisons across widely different interventions and provide useful information, they can mislead (Parker, 2003).

Given the many relevant features of decisions about the regulation of health and safety risks that are not part of the quantified economic analyses, and given considerable differences in the methodologies used to generate the summary results, the rankings of cost-effectiveness ratios are ambiguous. Furthermore, as discussed in Chapter 2, the legislative mandates and requirements for regulation vary across programs and agencies, making such comparisons less meaningful. Whether or not such cross-programmatic and interagency comparisons of CEAs might be helpful to decision makers, without being misleading, remains an open question. The Committee recommends against using summary rankings as the principal basis for policy decisions because the substance and methods of economic analysis do not support unqualified comparisons across widely different contexts.

IMPROVING REGULATORY DECISION MAKING

An important adjunct to the sorts of improvements in regulatory analyses discussed above is to strengthen the regulatory decision-making process itself. Such strengthening would involve greater transparency and ensuring a deliberative policy process that incorporates nonquantified information, including consideration of the distributive and ethical features of a proposed regulatory action. We discuss two fundamentally different strategies for introducing societal values and equity considerations into public policy decisions. One strategy is to incorporate information about distributive priorities directly into the CEA. This could either involve weighting health state index values to reflect priorities or stipulating values in the calculation of health-related effects. The other strategy is to pair the quantified economic analysis with qualitative information presented in a transparent and open process of regulatory development. The two approaches could also be combined.

Several approaches to societal weighting of health state index values have been proposed. First, standard index values could be modified with numerical factors or weights that convey priorities for age groups, severity of condition, or particularly vulnerable groups. These weights could be estimated by asking a representative sample of the general population to make PTOs between health improvements that are equal in terms of conventional index value gains, but different in terms of the characteristics of the people whose health is improved (Nord et al., 1999; Ubel et al., 2000). A variant on this approach would transform the health state index values into values that reflect societal values for giving priority to the worst off, which could be done by compressing the values of less severely impaired health states toward the upper end of the 0-to-1 scale (Nord, 2001). By locating moderate health states closer to the upper end of the HRQL scale, the value of improvements for the moderately ill is reduced relative to improvements for the severely ill.

Another approach to building equity considerations directly into the cost-effectiveness ratio is to value all reductions in preventable mortality at 1.0, rather than at the postregulatory health state index value that is actually expected to pertain. This is the approach EPA adopted in its pilot CEA in the Clean Air Interstate rule (EPA, 2005a), as described earlier in this chapter and more fully in Box 2-5.

Despite their apparent usefulness and appeal in combining distributive concerns with health production, formula-based approaches to incorporating societal values into CEA calculations are problematic. First, there is no consensus as to how equity weights should be calculated, or even whether their use is appropriate. It is also difficult to adjust health state index values for more than one dimension; should that adjustment be for age, severity of condition, or initial health status? Second, valuing all gains in longevity as life years in optimal health, as with EPA's Morbidity-Inclusive Life Year approach, changes the conventional relationship between morbidity and mortality effects and could lead to social choices that violate individual preferences in choices between quality and quantity of life (Johannesson, 2001). Finally, building equity considerations into the quantitative analysis in any of these forms makes the cost-effectiveness ratio less transparent, and therefore potentially more confusing and ambiguous for some.

In light of these concerns with adjusting health state index values to reflect distributional considerations, the Committee endorses a different strategy. In our view, standardizing the presentation of quantified analyses and their data inputs, assumptions, and methods offers the best chance for informed and transparent regulatory decision making. Presenting economic analyses in a common format and informing the deliberative process with alternative analyses helps to demonstrate how quantified results depend on value assumptions. Although we do not recommend that the CEA calculations be adjusted to incorporate distributional concerns quantitatively, we recognize that agencies might want to develop supplementary analyses using other measures and weighting schemes as sensitivity analyses. Such alternative quantifications could help to clarify the different implications of different regulatory strategies.

By including distributional and normative considerations in a public, transparent, and deliberative decision process, distinct concerns can remain separate. For example, how much should the fact that an auto safety requirement affects *children* count in judging the acceptability of its costs? A public and deliberative policy-making process permits the airing of reasonable disagreements about various priorities, rather than embedding one version of them in the CEA calculations. A fair and transparent process can resolve open questions of value in ways that achieve and maintain legitimacy.

Daniels and Sabin (1997, 2002) have characterized a fair process for decision making about health and health care as having certain central requirements or features. In the following summary, the Committee adapts these conditions for a fair process to the regulatory context.

- **Publicity:** The regulatory development process should be transparent and involve publicly available rationales for decisions affecting health and longevity. People have a basic interest in knowing the grounds for decisions that fundamentally affect their well-being.
- **Relevance:** Those who are affected by regulatory decisions, including those who bear the costs of regulations as well as those who realize the benefits, must agree that the rationales rest on relevant reasons, principles, and evidence.
- **Revisability and Appeals:** The regulatory process should make provisions for revisiting and revising decisions in light of new evidence and arguments.
- **Enforcement:** There should be a mechanism for ensuring that the previous three conditions are met.

These conditions hold decision makers accountable for the reasonableness of their choices in regulating health and safety risks. Decisions that meet these conditions provide a form of "case law" that helps make future reasoning more coherent. Many of the issues underlying regulatory interventions, both matters of fact and of values, are points of disagreement. A fair and transparent process of this sort adds legitimacy to the results. It also contributes to societal learning about the appropriate grounds for making the kinds of trade-offs involved and thus enhances broader democratic processes over time. The demand for fair process is a fundamental part of our political system. It is embedded in the statutory and administrative requirements for regulating risks, as discussed in Chapters 1 and 2. Further progress towards the goals of fair and transparent risk regulation is possible.

CONCLUSIONS

The Committee's key conclusions based on the discussion in this chapter follow.

CEA and BCA alike provide a useful but incomplete basis for informed societal decisions about reducing risks to human health and safety through regulation. The most feasible and desirable way to account for ethical and normative considerations in regulatory policy is to include them explicitly in the deliberative policy-making process.

The choice of QALYs as the basis for measuring the production of health through regulatory interventions entails certain value commitments and ignores others, and these limitations should be made explicit in regulatory analysis. While some societal values regarding the distribution of health benefits could be incorporated through quantitative modifications of health state values, such adjustments are of questionable validity and make the quantification of health improvements more difficult to interpret. However, presenting the quantitative results of such alternative measures as sensitivity analyses may help to highlight those distributive implications in a way that promotes consideration of them in the deliberative process.

Presenting the components of summary economic analyses individually is an important contribution to the transparency and accountability of regulatory decisions because such disaggregated information may be easier to understand and it conveys the relative contributions of various health impacts to the summary results.

Public participation in the development of regulatory priorities and specific regulations is vital to well-informed policy making. Existing administrative procedures that govern the issuance of regulations provide a framework for publicity, transparency, public involvement, and accountability. They do not guarantee adequate citizen participation in setting regulatory agendas and rulemaking, however. Greater public understanding of the environmental, health, and safety risks and the benefits and costs of strategies to mitigate such risks can be promoted by well-conducted and clearly presented regulatory impact analyses.

The next and final chapter presents the Committee's recommendations for regulatory analysis and policy development. Our recommendations reflect the conclusions above, as well as discussions and evidence that appeared earlier in this report.

5

Recommendations for Regulatory Cost-Effectiveness Analysis

This report responds to a charge from a consortium of federal agencies to make recommendations for conducting cost-effectiveness analysis (CEA) to assess regulatory interventions affecting human health and safety. In particular, the Committee was asked to consider the theoretical soundness, feasibility, and ethical implications of health-adjusted life-year (HALY) measures in making our recommendations. The previous chapters review a number of issues related to the use of these measures in regulatory analysis, including current federal guidelines and agency practices (Chapter 2), various HALY measures and strategies for applying them (Chapter 3), and ethical and contextual considerations related to the use of these measures in decision making (Chapter 4). This final chapter presents the Committee's conclusions based on the review and analysis described in the previous chapters, and its recommendations for conducting CEA in the regulatory setting.

The Committee drew on a variety of sources for insights, information, and evidence in determining how CEA could best inform regulatory decision making. These sources include:

- Interviews with policy and analytic staff at federal agencies about how they currently assess the economic costs and benefits of environmental, health, and safety regulations;
- Federal Executive Office of the President guidance on regulatory development, analysis, and reporting;
- Regulatory impact analyses for proposed and final regulations from

federal agencies, including the Environmental Protection Agency, the Food and Drug Administration, the Food Safety Inspection Service, the National Highway Traffic Safety Administration, the Federal Motor Carrier Safety Administration, the Occupational Safety and Health Administration, and the Consumer Product Safety Commission;

• Public workshop presentations by developers of health-related quality of life (HRQL) survey instruments and indexes, researchers in the fields of HRQL measurement and CEA, federal survey research officials, and ethicists;

• Three CEA case studies developed by the Committee in collaboration with federal agency staff, based on published regulatory impact analyses for final rules governing air quality, food safety, and children's car seat restraints; and

• Reviews of the peer-reviewed literature on the performance of HRQL measures and methods, methodological research on CEA using health-related effectiveness measures, and empirical and theoretical ethical analyses of the use of HRQL indexes and HALYs in CEA.

The Committee's investigations, analyses, and deliberations led us to the following overarching conclusions:

• *CEA, like benefit–cost analysis (BCA), offers a useful tool for the development and assessment of regulatory interventions to promote human health and safety. Different measures of effectiveness, including single-dimension measures such as life years and integrated metrics that combine estimates of HRQL and longevity such as HALYs, each provide useful and distinctive perspectives on regulatory impacts.*

• *As in the case of BCA, the results of CEA for regulatory interventions are not by themselves sufficient for informed regulatory decisions. The results of economic analyses are routinely supplemented with other types of analysis, and with information from the public, to provide a more comprehensive assessment of the advantages and disadvantages of different regulatory strategies. These other sources of information are a necessary part of the decision-making process because it is not possible to quantify all of the impacts of concern.*

• *It is feasible to apply CEA to regulatory interventions today, but additional data and improvements in the methods for measuring HRQL would make it more useful and reliable.*

• *Federal regulatory agencies analyze disparate data and contemplate widely varying interventions and types of impacts from their actions. They use diverse approaches to value health-related benefits, partly because of these differences in data sources and types of impact, but also for reasons related to institutional history and precedent. Greater consistency in the reporting of assumptions, data elements, analytic methods, and in the re-sulting estimates of costs, effectiveness, and benefits would increase the transparency and comparability of the results.*

*   *Presentations of cost-effectiveness ratios for diverse interventions can be misleading if they do not include information that highlights differ-ences in methods, unmeasured effects, and distributional impacts across interventions.*

Our recommendations for the use of CEA in regulatory analysis fall into four areas:

*   Selecting integrated measures of effectiveness;
*   Constructing and reporting cost-effectiveness ratios;
*   Providing additional information needed for decision making; and
*   Pursuing data collection and research necessary to improve HRQL measurement and regulatory CEA.

The recommendations are discussed in the following section and the chap-ter concludes with a brief summary.

RECOMMENDATIONS

Selecting Integrated Measures of Effectiveness

Because different effectiveness measures (e.g., deaths averted, life years saved, QALYs gained) have particular advantages and limitations, all regu-latory CEAs should report more than one measure of effectiveness. Report-ing a variety of measures provides decision makers with a richer under-standing of the impacts of different regulatory choices and responds to different questions.

The Committee's criteria for selecting integrated measures for use in regulatory CEA are summarized in Box 5-1.

Recommendation 1: Regulatory CEAs that integrate morbidity and mor-tality impacts in a single effectiveness measure should use the QALY to represent net health effects.

*   QALY estimates should be based, to the greatest possible extent, on research that considers the risk characteristics addressed and the popu-lation affected by the regulatory intervention.
*   The index values estimated for health conditions or health states of interest should be based on information from the population affected by the costs, benefits, or other impacts of the regulatory intervention,

BOX 5-1
Criteria for Selecting Integrated Effectiveness Measures
for Health-Related CEA

Choices Among Health-Adjusted Life Year (HALY) Measures

Because the requirements for regulatory CEA are already in effect and analysts need tools that are ready for application, the Committee's criteria for selecting among these HALY measures in the near term are largely practical ones:

• The HALY metric should be widely used, and methods for estimating the index values as well as estimates for specific health states should be available in the literature.
• The metric should be easy to understand and interpret.
• The metric should be comparatively inexpensive to use, in terms of both providing immediately applicable methods and values and facilitating the development of values for additional health states.

In addition to these practical considerations, measures must also provide valid and reliable estimates of the relative value of different health states.

Choices Among Generic Health-Related Quality of Life (HRQL) Indexes

Because generic indexes are well established and easy to use, the Committee expects that they will often be applied in regulatory analysis in the near term. The Committee's criteria for choosing among these indices focus on their suitability for regulatory analysis as well as the reliability and validity of the resulting estimates.

• The HRQL instrument must be applicable to the range of health-related effects being evaluated.
• The instrument should be sensitive enough to distinguish among health endpoints.
• The instrument should reflect the values or preferences for health of the population of interest.
• The instrument must be acceptable to and understandable by survey respondents, policy makers, and the general public.
• The instrument should be as inexpensive to use as is compatible with the other objectives.

which for most economically significant regulations will be best represented by the general U.S. population.

• In the absence of direct preference elicitation for health conditions of interest from the affected population, QALY estimates should be based on well-developed, generally accepted, and widely used generic HRQL indexes whose valuation is based on general population samples.

- The characterization of the health states or conditions of interest using generic HRQL indexes should be based on information obtained from people who are familiar with the conditions, such as patients.

The QALY is the best measure at present on which to standardize HALY estimation because of its widespread use, flexibility, and relative simplicity. As discussed in Chapter 3, alternatives to the QALY measure, including the healthy year equivalent, the saved young life equivalent, and the disability-adjusted life year, are either less feasible, have not been used extensively or evaluated, or incorporate features that render the measure not comparable with QALY results. For regulatory analysis, the QALY is best thought of in practical terms, as a measure of health improvement or production that allows analysts and decision makers to compare the impacts of different interventions. In short, we recommend the QALY as a useful construct on which to standardize the accounting of changes in health and longevity.

QALY estimates of regulatory effects may be based either on newly collected information or on previously conducted research. In both cases, the QALY estimates should address the same health states (i.e., the specific types of disease or injury) as identified in the risk assessment for the regulatory analysis. For example, the health states should be similar in terms of the severity and duration of the symptoms and of the effects of treatment. For chronic or long-term impacts, it may be desirable to separately assess different phases to reflect the variation in the HRQL impacts at different points in time. The QALY estimate also should reflect, to the extent possible, the effect of the health state on the particular population affected by the regulatory intervention in terms of characteristics such as age, preexisting conditions, income, and geographic location. If the HRQL estimate reflects a health state or scenario that differs from the regulatory health endpoint (i.e., addresses a somewhat different condition or affected population), these differences should, to the extent possible, be discussed and addressed in the uncertainty analysis. (See Recommendation 6.)

Chapter 3 discusses alternative strategies for developing QALY estimates for use in regulatory analysis. Briefly, these include:

- Eliciting preferences directly for the health states of interest, through a new valuation survey of the population that bears the costs and receives the benefits of the proposed regulation.
- Using generic health indexes to characterize and value the health states of interest. Health states may be characterized through surveys of patients or physicians knowledgeable about the condition of interest. This descriptive step is separate from the valuation of these health states, which

ideally should be derived from a survey of a representative sample of the population affected by the costs and benefits of the rule.

•   Using previously published health state and/or condition values. Such previously published values may have been either directly elicited or estimated with generic indexes.

Due to time and budget constraints, the Committee recognizes that, in the near term, regulatory analysts are likely to rely on published research and to adopt relatively simple approaches to assess health-related impacts in regulatory CEAs. Over the long term, the Committee hopes that investment in additional research will improve the information available for these assessments. (See Recommendations 11 and 12.)

Different approaches in different regulatory analyses may be required to pursue the dual objectives of (1) ensuring that the health states and populations addressed in the QALY analysis match those identified in the risk assessment and affected by the intervention, and (2) using ethically sound and robust societal valuations of health states. The best approach will depend on the time and resources available and the extent and quality of existing valuation research for the conditions of interest. Because these factors vary, it is not possible to specify one standard approach for QALY-based CEA that would apply in all cases. Regulatory analysts must exercise judgment in weighing the importance of different factors in choosing an approach to QALY estimation. The following discussion summarizes the Committee's conclusions from Chapter 3 and offers guidance regarding the use of existing HRQL research and generic indexes for QALY-based regulatory analysis.

Valuation. Health states can be valued directly in surveys of patients or the general population using elicitation techniques such as the standard gamble, time trade-off, category rating (e.g., visual analogue scale), and person trade-off. When a generic index is used, health states are described by locating their attributes within the functional categories or domains of the index. These domain attributes are then valued using a statistical model or algebraic formula based on a separate valuation survey that employed one or more elicitation methods. The underlying valuation surveys for the various generic indexes are based on general population surveys that differ in size and in the extent to which they represent the U.S. population as a whole (see Table 3-4).

For regulatory analysis, the population valuing different health states should include both those who will benefit from the intervention and those who will bear its costs. In the case of economically significant regulations that have relatively large costs and/or benefits, the affected population whose valuations are of interest is usually best represented by the U.S. population.

Elicitation methods that include an explicit choice, such as the standard gamble and time trade-off, would be preferred to other methods of preference assessment if they were more comprehensible and more easily administered. However, standard gamble and time trade-off methods are difficult for many respondents to understand, and often lead to inconsistent or poorly reproducible responses. Although category rating and visual analogue scale methods do not imply a direct trade-off between years of life and HRQL (a trade-off that is implicit in QALY-based CEA), they are generally easy to administer. Particularly if they are calibrated against trade-off methods to ensure that the same numerical rating means the same thing for both types of methods, rating scale elicitation methods can also play an important role.

Methods that elicit individual preferences for health have dominated QALY-based CEA. However, alternatives (such as the person trade-off method) that aim to elicit societal values for investments in health improvements more directly merit further development, as discussed in Recommendation 12. The aggregation of individual preferences for one's own health is but one approach to determining societal preferences for improved health, and evidence suggests that values for health states elicited in the standard way may not be well correlated with societal health resource allocation choices (Ubel et al., 1996).

Generic indexes. The Committee reviewed, and applied in its case studies, several generic HRQL indexes. These included the Quality of Well-Being Scale (QWB), the Health Utilities Index (HUI) Marks 2 and 3, the EuroQol-5D (EQ-5D), and the SF-6D. As discussed in Chapter 3, we concluded that no generic instrument is superior in all respects to the alternatives. All four of these instruments have well-developed and widely tested survey formats. Health state values based on the QWB, HUI, and EQ-5D are well represented in the published literature and, because the SF-6D can be calculated from SF-36 and SF-12 health profile data, it has the potential for extensive application.

Recent research suggests that these four generic instruments rank-order health states consistently, although the absolute values of individual health states differ depending on the instrument used (Franks, 2004; Franks et al., 2006). Furthermore, a growing research literature offers statistical conversions or translations of values from one instrument to another; see Table 3-7 for a summary of these studies.

These instruments do vary, however, in the representativeness of their underlying valuation surveys and in specific aspects of their methodology.

The QWB's valuation survey dates back to the mid-1970s, was based on a San Diego community sample, and uses a rating-scale methodology. The HUI attributes were valued by a sample from a metropolitan population in Ontario, Canada. The SF-6D values were derived from a U.K. population survey. The EQ-5D is the only generic instrument with a nationally representative U.S. valuation survey underlying its index values. In addition, some of the instruments (e.g., the HUI) require licensing fees, and others involve fees to access health profile data (e.g., as would be useful with the SF-6D). Given the current state of the art of HRQL measurement, the Committee recommends that agencies consider using the EQ-5D in their primary estimates for regulatory analyses at this time.

Characterizing health states with generic indexes. Using generic indexes to measure HRQL involves characterizing or locating the health states of interest according to the specific functional categories or domains of the index. In contrast with direct preference elicitation surveys, with generic indexes this *characterization* of health states is separate from the *valuation* of the generically described health states, where the latter is based on general population samples.

As described in Chapter 3, health states can be characterized using generic indexes either by patients or clinical experts who are familiar with the condition of interest. Published studies are one source of patient-based characterization or description of health states using these indexes. If original data collection for a regulatory analysis is contemplated, direct elicitation of health state index values for the conditions of interest, rather than patient characterization using a generic health index, should be considered. If neither of these approaches is feasible, then clinical experts could be asked to characterize the health conditions of interest using a generic index, similar to the approach used in the Committee's case studies. Good practices for expert assessment are discussed in Chapter 3.

HRQL measurement quality. Finally, the Committee recommends that sources of HRQL values for QALY-based CEA should be evaluated with specific and consistent criteria regarding:

- The quality of underlying valuation surveys; and
- The precision and reliability with which health states of interest are captured or located by direct elicitation or generic indexes, respectively.

Although it is not possible to develop absolute standards for assessing an existing study's quality and applicability for regulatory CEA, greater specification and standardization of quality review criteria in HRQL measurement will help analysts to (1) weigh the limitations of a study against the value of using it, and (2) determine when available valuation studies should not be used as a source of health state values in the context of a particular analysis.

There is a growing body of evidence on the quality of different valuation techniques and surveys, and formal criteria are being developed for judging quality in survey-based valuation research that addresses both willingness-to-pay and QALY estimation.[1] Such criteria for evaluating study quality should be further developed and applied to HRQL valuation research. For example, more attention should be given to internal consistency tests. Chapter 3 provides additional information on the research underlying generic indexes and these criteria.

Constructing and Reporting Cost-Effectiveness Ratios

The overarching objective of the Committee's recommendations is to improve the quality and comprehensiveness of the information available for regulatory decision making. We believe this objective can be advanced by standardizing, to the extent practical, the structure of CEAs within and across agencies, thus increasing the transparency of the presentation of analytic assumptions, methods, and results in regulatory analyses.

Recommendation 2: Regulatory analyses should report four measures of cost-effectiveness:

- *Compliance cost per death averted* using the net number of deaths averted as the outcome measure.
- *Compliance cost per life year gained* using the net change in years of preventable mortality as the outcome measure.
- A *health-benefits-only ratio* using the net change in QALYs as the outcome measure. Costs would include those associated with compliance, offset by estimates of the net changes in health care treatment costs associated with the outcomes included in the QALY measure.
- A *comprehensive ratio* using QALYs as the outcome measure and incorporating the value of other benefits as offsets to compliance costs. The cost measure would incorporate both net changes in health care treatment costs and the value of any monetized nonhealth benefits as offsets.

The components of these four ratios are illustrated in Table 5-1.

---

[1]See Freeman (2003, Chapter 6) and OMB (2003a) regarding criteria for willingness-to-pay studies and Chapman et al. (2000), Neumann et al. (2000), and AHRQ (2005) for criteria for QALY-based CEA.

TABLE 5-1 Components of Cost-Effectiveness Ratios

	Compliance Costs Per Death Averted	Compliance Costs Per Life Year Gained	Health-Benefits-Only Ratio	Comprehensive Ratio
Included in net costs				
Regulatory compliance costs	•	•	•	•
Health care treatment cost savings			•	•
Value of nonhealth benefits				•
Included in net effects				
Fatal effects: Deaths averted	•			
Fatal effects: Years of life gained		•	•	•
Fatal effects: Quality-adjusted life years gained			•	•
Nonfatal effects: Quality-adjusted life years gained			•	•

Ratios need not be reported if they do not provide additional information for decision making. For example, compliance cost per life year gained need not be presented when a regulation would have negligible impacts on longevity, and the comprehensive ratio need not be presented for regulations that do not provide monetized nonhealth benefits.

These ratios should be calculated over a time period selected to reflect the effects of the full implementation of the regulation. In addition, annualized impacts should also be reported and used to estimate expected cost-effectiveness on a yearly basis. The time periods within which the costs and savings and the health-related effects accrue should be reported using a time line to indicate the undiscounted impacts expected in each year. In addition, the present value of the impacts should be calculated using the same discount rate for both costs and effects (life years or QALYs). As discussed in Recommendations 8 and 9, agencies should also highlight information on distributional impacts and ethical considerations, on uncertainty in the estimates, and on any regulatory impacts not included in the cost-effectiveness measure.

A simplified example of the four recommended cost-effectiveness ratios, as well as the results of an accompanying BCA, is provided in Box 5-2.

The Committee recommends reporting all four cost-effectiveness ratios because no single formulation will be ideal in all circumstances. Different audiences will find different formulations more informative, more readily interpretable, or more comparable to other analyses. Furthermore, differ-

---

BOX 5-2
Example of Cost-Effectiveness Ratios

Values used in example:

Regulatory compliance costs: $100 million

Benefits values (willingness to pay)
for BCA: $60 million for averted mortality
     $30 million for averted morbidity
     $40 million for averted ecological impacts

Benefits values for CEA: 400 QALYs gained
     or
     100 life years saved
     or
     10 premature deaths averted

Health treatment cost savings
associated with reduced morbidity
and mortality: $20 million

Net benefits:

Net benefits = ($60 million + $30 million + $40 million) – $100 million = $30 million

Cost-effectiveness ratios:

- *Compliance costs per premature death averted* = $100 million / 10 lives = $10 million/death averted
- *Compliance costs per life year gained* = $100 million/100 life years = $1 million/life year
- *Costs per QALY, health benefits only* = ($100 million – $20 million) / 400 QALYs = $200,000/QALY
- *Costs per QALY, comprehensive* = ($100 million – $20 million – $40 million) / 400 QALYs = $100,000 / QALY

NOTES: For simplicity, this example provides the results for a single year and ignores the need to address the timing of the impacts. It also does not provide information on the uncertainty in the estimates. For simplicity we assume that the willingness-to-pay estimates used in the BCA calculation of net benefits encompass health treatment cost savings. See Chapter 2 and OMB, 2003a (Appendix C), for more discussion of this issue.

---

ences among potential interventions in the relative size or ranking of the four measures can highlight important aspects of the impact of alternative interventions. While agencies should report these four ratios at a minimum as relevant, they may also, at their discretion, provide additional comparisons that incorporate alternative perspectives if such comparisons are useful for decision making.

Each of the four formulations has particular advantages.

Compliance cost per death averted. This ratio focuses on the number of deaths averted, without regard for the expected years of life extended by a regulatory action. It is the simplest of the four ratios and excludes consideration of the HRQL for the life years gained, of nonfatal health impacts, of medical care savings, and of benefits that are not health related. This ratio avoids the criticism leveled at cost-effectiveness formulations that use some form of life years as the effectiveness measure, namely, that they discriminate against older people and those with lesser life expectancies. All preventable deaths count equally in this calculation.

Compliance cost per life year gained. This ratio is also limited to the mortality effects of a regulatory action and sets aside impacts on health status, but considers the years of life extension rather than simply the number of lives extended. It excludes consideration of the health-related quality of life for the life years gained, of nonfatal health impacts, of medical care savings, and of benefits that are not health related. This ratio may be more acceptable or understandable to those who find it difficult to interpret QALY measurement. It may be most important to those who are concerned primarily with the mortality impacts of the regulations or who are ethically opposed to reflecting HRQL differences in conveying information about preventable mortality.

Health-benefits-only ratio. This formulation is most comparable to and in harmony with the approach used as the reference case for CEAs that address public health and medical interventions. It answers the question of what it costs to produce a particular unit of health—that is, a QALY—that incorporates information on the HRQL impacts for both nonfatal illness and injury and life years lost. In this formulation, information about non-health benefits is not included in the ratio, but would be provided by listing and highlighting these effects in accompanying narrative.

Comprehensive ratio. For some regulations, the BCA will include the monetary valuation of benefits unrelated to health, such as ecological effects. In these cases, a comprehensive ratio should be reported. In most of these regulations, the costs of achieving the health and non-health benefits are not separable, and attributing all costs to the achievement of the health benefits can be misleading. Disregarding those impacts excluded from the previously described quantitative measures would result in decisions that underinvest in regulations that provide nonhealth as well as health benefits. The comprehensive ratio offers a more global perspective by incorporating a fuller set of implications of the regulatory action, and uses more of the available information about regulatory impacts.

When evaluating different regulatory options, analysts may find that the relative magnitudes of health and nonhealth benefits vary among options. If so, then the comprehensive ratio could lead to a different ordering (in terms of economic efficiency) of policy alternatives from the one that would emerge from the health-only ratio. The comprehensive approach is most consistent with the content of the accompanying BCA.

Definitions: The following definitions should be used in developing each component of the ratios:

- *Deaths averted:* the net change in the expected number of cases (sometimes referred to as "statistical cases") of preventable mortality attributable to the regulation, summed across the affected population.
- *Life years gained:* the net change in the predicted years of life extension attributable to the regulation, summed across the affected population.
- *Quality-adjusted life years gained:* the net change in health-related quality of life associated with morbidity, injury, and preventable mortality attributable to the regulation, summed across the affected population.
- *Regulatory compliance costs:* the net value of the materials, labor, and other inputs used to comply with the requirements of the regulation, and the impact of these net costs on related markets.
- *Regulatory benefits:* the net impacts related to the goals of, or rationale for, the regulation, including *health benefits* (averted morbidity, injury, and mortality) and *nonhealth benefits* (e.g., enhanced recreational value or increased protection of natural resources).
- *Health-care-treatment-cost impacts:* the net change in resource and time costs as a result of reduced need for medical treatment for the condition(s) affected by the regulatory intervention.

Sometimes it is difficult to make clear distinctions among these categories; however, they generally should include the following.

Deaths averted reflects the comparison of the predicted number of deaths in the population without the regulation to the number of deaths with the regulation. Conceptually, these deaths reflect the net number of people expected to live longer once the regulation is implemented. They are often calculated as statistical cases (changes in the risk of preventable mortality summed across a population). This measure should be calculated as the net change; that is, they should include both increases and decreases in the risks of preventable mortality attributable to the regulation, and information on related uncertainties should be presented along with the quantified estimates.

Life years gained reflects the comparison of life expectancy of the affected population in the absence of the regulation to life expectancy with the regulation in place. These estimates are not adjusted for the quality of life, and should reflect the actual predicted *change in the life expectancy of the affected population* to the maximum extent possible given available data. Any limitations of the data used to predict life expectancy should be included in the assessment of the uncertainty in the estimates and modeling.

QALYs gained reflects the net changes in HRQL and HRQL-adjusted life expectancy in the affected population without and with the regulation, including the HRQL impacts of morbidity, injury, and preventable mortality.

Regulatory compliance costs reflect the resources diverted from other purposes to meet the specific legal requirements established by the regulation. Costs may include, for example, those associated with testing for contamination, installing airbags in cars, or administering a new program. Where such costs lead to noticeable market impacts (e.g., decreased demand due to increased prices in the regulated industry and/or spillover effects in related sectors), these "second-order" consequences should also be included. In addition, compliance costs should include any significant savings that result. For example, if standards for vehicle engines result in fuel savings, these should be included as offsets to compliance costs.

Regulatory benefits generally relate to the goals of, or rationale for, the regulation. For health and safety regulations, these benefits will include the effects of the regulation on morbidity, injury, and preventable mortality, but may also include nonhealth benefits. Again, these effects may include "second-order" consequences if significant; for example, a chemical used to remove contaminants from drinking water may itself pose risks or can lead to additional risk reductions by removing co-occurring contaminants. Benefits may include some offsetting increases in risks.

Health-care-treatment-cost impacts are the net changes in health-care-related costs as a result of the regulation. These impacts are defined by the U.S. Panel on Cost-Effectiveness in Health and Medicine (PCEHM) as including "changes in the use of health care resources, changes in the use of non-health care resources, changes in the use of informal caregiver time, and changes in the use of patient time (for treatment)" (Gold et al., 1996b, p. 177).[2] In the case of regulations that prevent the occurrence of health conditions, these impacts are generally additional savings attributable to the regulations. In BCA, these impacts (if estimated) are usually counted as benefits to the extent that they do not double count other monetary estimates of impacts. In CEA, they should be counted as offsets to regulatory costs under both the health-only and comprehensive approaches.

---

[2]The PCEHM definition of treatment-related costs is discussed more fully in Chapter 1.

The Committee recognizes that in some cases the distinctions among the categories defined above may be difficult to determine, and analysts will need to rely on their own judgment. Judgment will also be needed to separate effects that are negligible and need not be quantified from effects that are significant and warrant inclusion in the analysis. Regardless, the rationale for including and excluding various impacts for each of these ratios, or for excluding impacts entirely from the quantitative assessment, should be included in the text of the regulatory analysis.

In reporting these measures, the agencies should make every effort to ensure that the results and limitations are reported clearly. Although OMB and agency guidance already emphasize the need for transparency, the Committee found that these qualities were lacking in many of the regulatory analyses it reviewed. To meet this goal, agencies should present summary materials describing the analyses in nontechnical language, including key definitions and assumptions, that can be easily understood by the general reading public. In addition, they should discuss data sources, calculations, results, and the implications of nonquantified effects as well as uncertainty in the quantified results.

Recommendation 3: The life-year and QALY estimates used in regulatory analyses should reflect actual population health as closely as possible, comparing the predicted HRQL and life expectancy of the affected population in the absence of the intervention (i.e., the regulatory baseline) to the predicted postintervention HRQL and health-adjusted life expectancy.

The economically significant regulations most directly affected by the Committee's recommendations will often have national impacts. However, the characteristics of the population affected by associated health risks may differ from the characteristics of the general U.S. population. For example, foodborne illness may be more severe in individuals with weakened immune systems; certain car safety problems may disproportionately affect children; and air emissions may lead to preventable mortality primarily among the elderly. In some cases, the analysis may not fully reflect the characteristics of these affected populations due to limitations in the available data. In these cases, the data limitations should be included in the uncertainty analysis discussed under Recommendation 6.

However, as discussed in Chapter 4, some practitioners have argued that the HRQL results should be adjusted to reflect equity issues; for example, higher QALY values could be assigned to subpopulations of concern such as the elderly, children, or those with preexisting conditions. The Committee believes that such approaches should be avoided for two reasons: (1) they lack transparency, and (2) they substitute the analyst's judgment about relative values for the deliberative process (see Recommendations 8 and 9).

The intent, as well as the underlying theory and methods, for preparing most components of regulatory CEAs (and BCAs) is to compare the relative economic efficiencies of alternative interventions. Equity weighting confuses the message; it becomes difficult to separate the extent to which a particular intervention appears preferable due to its economic efficiency from its equity impacts. In addition, there is no agreed-on set of weights for any subpopulation of concern. The Committee believes that the analysis should include the best available information about the impacts on groups of concern so that it can be incorporated into the deliberative decision-making process. Decision makers are better served by CEAs that clearly represent the actual impacts of regulations, supplemented by information that emphasizes the equity impacts.

The Committee's judgment is that the more comprehensive information needed to address equity considerations in policy decisions is not well suited for incorporation into cost-effectiveness ratios. The recommended formulations of cost-effectiveness ratios also reflect the value judgment implicit in the QALY measure to value life years rather than lives, and to adjust for quality. One consequence is that less weight is placed on permanent changes in HRQL for those with fewer remaining years of life, and on life extensions for those who have worse-than-average quality of life. Recognizing these concerns, we conclude that equity issues are better addressed as part of the discussion of distributive impacts of the intervention rather than by quantitative weighting of the QALY measure.

Age- and sex-specific U.S. population HRQL averages exist for four of the generic indexes used in the Committee's case studies. (See Hanmer et al., 2006, for population norms for several indexes.) For many regulations, these general population averages are likely to provide the best available estimates of the postregulatory (i.e., generally, improved) health of the affected population. Using age-specific population averages marks an advance over many studies published in the CEA literature that use an index value of 1.0 (perfect or optimal health) to assess health status in the absence of the condition of concern.

This practice could be further improved, however, by the development of better information on the extent to which persons who are likely to be affected by a regulatory intervention also have other health conditions or co-morbidities, on the extent to which these co-morbidities are affected (in terms of increases or decreases) by the regulations, and on the effect on HRQL of eliminating one health impairment when another remains.

Recommendation 4: Incremental cost-effectiveness ratios are generally the most useful summary measure for comparing different regulatory interven-

tions. Such ratios are not meaningful, however, for interventions that reduce both costs and risks. Options that are dominated (i.e., have higher
costs and lower effectiveness) also should not be included in the incremental comparisons.

Before incremental cost-effectiveness ratios are calculated, the analyst
should determine whether any of the options are both more costly *and* less
effective than other options. These options are *dominated* by the other
options. The dominance should be reported, but cost-effectiveness ratios
need not be calculated. Incremental cost-effectiveness ratios are usually
calculated relative to all other alternatives that are not dominated. The
determination of dominance may vary across the different ratios discussed
under Recommendation 2. For example, one ratio may dominate another
but still not be optimal if it is in turn dominated by, or at least broadly
considered inferior to, some third strategy. In addition, uncertainty must be
taken into account in determining dominance. If some elements of the CEA
are particularly variable, the analyst will need to consider the probability
that an alternative is dominated under different assumptions. The discussion of Recommendation 6 addresses this further.[3]

Whenever the value of a cost-effectiveness ratio is negative (i.e., it is
both cost saving and health enhancing, or both costly and results in net life
year or QALY losses), ratios should not be calculated or reported because
they are not meaningful and cannot be interpreted. The underlying estimates of net costs and net effects *are* informative, however, and should be
reported.

The results for each nondominated option should be independently
compared to each of the other nondominated options. The ranking of
interventions and whether they are dominated can vary among these ratios.
So, for example, in Table 5-2, intervention B dominates C on compliance
costs/life year saved, and is dominated by C on comprehensive costs/QALY
gained.

**Recommendation 5: In addition to reporting effects in the aggregate, regu-
latory analyses should report QALY impacts separately for each health
endpoint. Impacts should also be reported in terms of single-dimension
measures such as avoided cases of disease and cause-specific mortality
averted.**

To make the analysis more transparent and to provide more complete
information for decision making, the QALY gains attributable to each

---

[3]See Hunink et al. (2001, Chapter 9) and Drummond et al. (1997, Chapter 5) for extended
treatments of how to calculate and use incremental cost-effectiveness ratios.

TABLE 5-2 Comparison of Cost-Effectiveness Ratios

	Intervention A	Intervention B	Intervention C
Input data			
Compliance costs	$100 million	$140 million	$200 million
Health care cost savings	$10 million	$5 million	$10 million
Value of other (nonhealth) benefits	$40 million	$100 million	$200 million
Averted mortality	8 cases	10 cases	9 cases
Life years gained	250 life years	300 life years	280 life years
Quality-adjusted life years (QALYs) gained	2,000 QALYs	800 QALYs	1,000 QALYs
Cost numerators			
Compliance costs	$100 million	$140 million	$200 million
Compliance costs net of health care savings	$90 million	$135 million	$190 million
Compliance costs net of health care savings and other benefits	$50 million	$35 million	Savings of $10 million
Incremental cost-effectiveness			
Compliance costs per death averted	$13 million per case	$20 million per additional case	Dominated by B
Compliance costs per life year gained	$400,000 per life year	$800,000 per additional life year	Dominated by B
Compliance costs net of health care savings per QALY gained	$45,000 per QALY	Dominated by A	Dominated by A
Compliance costs net of health care savings and other benefits per QALY gained	$25,000 per QALY	Dominated by C	Cost saving

NOTES: For simplicity, this example provides the results for a single year and does not report information on the uncertainty in the estimates. All results are rounded to two significant figures. Estimates of life years and QALYs represent the discounted lifetime impacts of the new cases averted in a single year. For example, a case of premature mortality in the current year leads to life year losses equivalent to the individual's expected remaining life span.

regulatory option should be reported on a disaggregated basis. Detailed breakouts provide additional information for decision makers on the relative importance of different types of effects. Several types of disaggregation are desirable.

First, the QALY estimates should be reported separately for each health endpoint or condition, for example, preventable deaths, particular types of chronic health effects (e.g., heart disease, lung cancer), specific types of acute, time-limited health effects (e.g., gastrointestinal illness from a foodborne pathogen), and types of acute exacerbations of chronic conditions (e.g., an acute asthmatic episode). Net changes in expected life years should be calculated first and then adjusted for HRQL, so that only preventable mortality is reflected in the first estimate. Second, the analyses should report single-dimension estimates of impacts for each endpoint, for example, the estimated number of cases of illness, injury, or mortality averted and the number of life years saved. Table 5-3 illustrates these reporting recommendations.

Third, to the extent that the regulation is likely to disproportionately affect certain population subgroups of concern, impacts should be reported separately for each group (e.g., for children, elderly people, low-income populations, members of minority groups, and those with preexisting conditions, as relevant). The treatment of distributive impacts is discussed further under Recommendation 8.

Recommendation 6: The reporting of all CEA results should be accompanied by information on related uncertainties and on nonquantified effects.

Uncertainty in estimates of the costs and health-related effects of regulatory actions are attached to each component and accompany every step of

TABLE 5-3 Disaggregated Impacts

	Intervention A	Intervention B	Intervention C
Quality-adjusted life year (QALY) impacts			
Averted mortality	200 QALYs	240 QALYs	220 QALYs
Averted incidence of heart disease (morbidity only)	1,700 QALYs	520 QALYs	600 QALYs
Averted asthma exacerbations	100 QALYs	40 QALYs	180 QALYs
Total	2,000 QALYs	800 QALYs	1,000 QALYs
Single-dimension impacts			
Averted mortality	8 cases; 250 life years	10 cases; 300 life years	9 cases; 280 life years
Averted incidence of heart disease	85 cases	26 cases	30 cases
Averted asthma exacerbations	30,000 events	12,000 events	54,000 events

NOTES: For simplicity, this example provides the results for a single year and does not provide information on the uncertainty in the estimates. All results are rounded to two significant figures. Life-year and QALY estimates represent the discounted lifetime impacts of the new incidence. For example, the 26 to 85 new cases of heart disease are likely to lead to QALY impacts over each individual's remaining lifespan; hence the QALY impacts exceed the number of cases averted.

a CEA. Because BCA and CEA rely on much of the same data and employ many of the same tools, they face similar challenges in dealing with uncertainty in their results. For the common components of these analyses (e.g., the estimates of compliance costs and of cases of illness or injury averted), the treatment of uncertainty should be symmetrical across BCA and CEA. CEA, however, presents some particular challenges for analysis of uncertainty.[4]

Uncertainty means that regulatory alternatives that compare unfavorably in terms of both their costs and effectiveness (i.e., that are dominated) may still be worth considering if they involve substantially different technologies or intervention from the better performing alternatives. For example, when regulatory options differ only in stringency (e.g., a standard of 1 versus 5 parts per million), then dominated options should be excluded from the comparison. When options differ in other respects, such as warning labels versus mandatory processing standards for food contaminants, options that are only slightly dominated may be worth considering because the sources of uncertainty may be quite different for alternative interventions.

One common source of uncertainty is the inability to quantify or value in monetary or QALY terms some potentially important health and nonhealth impacts. Agencies should report these impacts, including, for example, preclinical physiological changes that are difficult to evaluate and effects on pregnant women that could affect fetal development. An example of a format for reporting these types of effects is provided in Table 5-4, from the Environmental Protection Agency's (EPA's) regulatory assessment of the nonroad diesel rule (EPA, 2004b).

In addition, the quantified estimates will often contain significant uncertainties. An earlier National Research Council committee reviewed EPA's work in estimating the health benefits of air pollution regulations. That committee recommended that the sources of uncertainty in impact analyses should be considered jointly in the primary analysis, rather than singly, so that the probability distributions describing ultimate effects (e.g., cases of illness avoided) and their values (e.g., QALY losses avoided) would be calculated correctly (NRC, 2002). The OMB 2003 guidelines for regulatory

---

[4]See Fenwick et al. (2004), Heitjan (2000), and Willan and O'Brien (1996) for discussions of these issues and of alternative approaches to statistical analysis of cost-effectiveness data. See also *Estimating the Public Health Benefits of Proposed Air Pollution Regulations* (NRC, 2002), which considers sources of uncertainty and offers guidance on the reporting of uncertainty in regulatory analysis. The use of ratios in CEA raises issues that do not occur in addressing uncertainty in BCA. For example, when zero is a possible value for the effectiveness measure, infinity becomes a possible value for the ratio, and the statistical expectation of the ratio is thus also infinite.

Valuing Health for Regulatory Cost Effectiveness Analysis

(Customers in North America Only)

Use this card to order additional copies of **Valuing Health for Regulatory Cost Effectiveness Analysis**. All orders must be prepaid. Please add $4.50 for shipping and handling for the first copy ordered and $0.95 for each additional copy. If you live in CA, DC, FL, MD, MO, TX, or Canada, add applicable sales tax or GST. Prices apply only in the United States, Canada, and Mexico and are subject to change without notice.

___ I am enclosing a U.S. check or money order.

___ Please charge my VISA/MasterCard/American Express account.

Number: _____

Expiration date: _____

Signature: _____

PLEASE SEND ME:

Qty.	Title	Price
___	Valuing Health	$59.95
		Subtotal ___
		Shipping ___
		Tax ___
		Total ___

Please print.

Name _____

Address _____

City _____ State _____ Zip Code _____ 10077

FOUR EASY WAYS TO ORDER

- **Electronically:** Order from our secure website at: www.nap.edu
- **By phone:** Call toll-free 1-888-624-8422 or (202) 334-3313 or call your favorite bookstore.
- **By fax:** Copy the order card and fax to (202) 334-2451.
- **By mail:** Return this card with your payment to NATIONAL ACADEMIES PRESS, 500 Fifth Street NW, Washington, DC 20001.

All international customers please contact National Academies Press for export prices and ordering information.

THE NATIONAL ACADEMIES PRESS

Publisher for The National Academies

National Academy of Sciences ◆ National Academy of Engineering ◆ Institute of Medicine ◆ National Research Council

THE NATIONAL ACADEMIES
Advisers to the Nation on Science, Engineering, and Medicine

Visit our web site at **www.nap.edu**

Use the form on the reverse of this card to order additional copies, or order online and receive a 10% discount.

TABLE 5-4 Nonmonetized Benefits of the Environmental Protection Agency's Nonroad Diesel Rule

Pollutant/ Type of Impact	Nonquantified Effects
Ozone health	Premature mortality. Respiratory hospital admissions. Minor restricted activity days. Increased airway responsiveness to stimuli. Inflammation in the lung. Chronic respiratory damage. Premature aging of the lungs. Acute inflammation and respiratory cell damage. Increased susceptibility to respiratory infection. Nonasthma respiratory emergency room visits. Increased school absence rates.
Ozone welfare	Decreased yields for commercial forests. Decreased yields for fruits and vegetables. Decreased yields for noncommercial crops. Damage to urban ornamental plants. Impacts on recreational demand from damaged forest aesthetics. Damage to ecosystem functions.
PM health	Low birth weight. Changes in pulmonary function. Chronic respiratory diseases other than chronic bronchitis. Morphological changes. Altered host defense mechanisms. Cancer. Nonasthma respiratory emergency room visits.
PM welfare	Visibility in many Class I areas. Residential and recreational visibility in non-Class I areas. Soiling and materials damage. Damage to ecosystem functions.
Nitrogen and sulfate deposition welfare	Impacts of acidic sulfate and nitrate deposition on commercial forests. Impacts of acidic deposition to commercial freshwater fishing. Impacts of acidic deposition to recreation in terrestrial ecosystems. Reduced existence values for currently healthy ecosystems. Impacts of nitrogen deposition on commercial fishing, agriculture, and forests.
CO health	Premature mortality. Behavioral effects.

continues

TABLE 5-4 Continued

Pollutant/ Type of Impact	Nonquantified Effects
HC health	Cancer (benzene, 1,3-butadiene, formaldehyde, acetaldehyde). Anemia (benzene). Disruption of production of blood components (benzene). Reduction in the number of blood platelets (benzene). Excessive bone marrow formation (benzene). Depression of lymphocyte counts (benzene). Reproductive and developmental effects (1,3-butadiene). Irritation of eyes and mucus membranes (formaldehyde). Respiratory irritation (formaldehyde). Asthma attacks in asthmatics (formaldehyde). Asthma-like symptoms in nonasthmatics (formaldehyde). Irritation of the eyes, skin, and respiratory tract (acetaldehyde). Upper respiratory tract irritation and congestion (acrolein).
HC welfare	Direct toxic effects to animals. Bioaccumulation in the food chain. Damage to ecosystem function. Odor.

NOTES: PM = particulate matter; CO = carbon monoxide; HC = hydrocarbons.
SOURCE: EPA (2004b, p. 39139, Table VI.E-6).

analysis make a number of recommendations for treating uncertainty in all economically significant rules, noting the need for qualitative discussion as well as quantitative assessment using sensitivity analysis or probabilistic modeling. This guidance now requires agencies to conduct formal probabilistic uncertainty analysis for all rules with impacts that exceed $1 billion annually (OMB, 2003a). Recommendation 10 of this report addresses the need for better information on the health effects of regulatory interventions, which is one major source of uncertainty.

At present there is also uncertainty about the correct health state index values to use in calculating QALYs due to several factors: (1) the lack of agreement on the concept of HRQL, (2) how it should be measured, and (3) measurement error. Different generic instruments and elicitation methods produce different results without a clear consensus on the theoretical or empirical superiority of one particular approach or model. Measurement error in estimating health state index values should be reported as credible intervals around point estimates and examined in the uncertainty analysis.

Recommendation 7: Regulatory analyses should not assign monetary values to estimates of health-adjusted life years as a method for valuing health states.

In the existing literature, monetary values have been applied to HALYs for two reasons. First, as discussed in Chapter 2, agencies often use monetized HALYs in their BCAs, apparently because suitable, high-quality willingness-to-pay estimates are lacking for many nonfatal health effects of concern. Health state index values are more plentiful, and address the shortcomings associated with reliance on other proxy measures (such as cost-of-illness estimates) for valuation.

Although the Committee recognizes that in the short term, regulatory agencies might continue this practice of using monetized HALY values in BCAs due to the lack of willingness-to-pay estimates for morbidity effects, we disapprove of and discourage this practice. As discussed in Chapter 1, willingness-to-pay and HRQL valuation and measurement have developed out of distinct disciplinary and methodological traditions. Given their different theoretical underpinnings and the different types of trade-offs they consider, it is misleading to combine them.

The second reason for assigning monetary values to HALYs is to provide a threshold for determining whether an intervention should be pursued. As discussed in Chapters 1 and 3, neither theoretical justification for nor evidence of a consensus about any particular threshold value exists. In the absence of any compelling rationale, the Committee concludes that the use of thresholds is inappropriate.

Information Needed for Regulatory Decision Making

Regardless of whether economic analysis takes the form of BCA or CEA, economic analysis is only one of many inputs into the policy-making process. Statutory requirements, judicial decisions, executive orders, and agency guidance all stress the importance of considering the distribution of a regulatory intervention's impacts, the ethical implications of different options, and the implications of nonquantifiable effects, some of which may be related to health and others not. The Committee endorses this multifaceted approach to decision making, and believes that the results of CEA should continue to be but one element in a deliberative policy development process that takes full account of both quantified and qualitative information.

Recommendation 8: The regulatory decision-making process should explicitly address and incorporate the distributional, ethical, and other implications of a proposed intervention along with the quantified results of BCA

and CEA. Comparisons of different interventions should highlight these distinctive features of the interventions and also any methodological differences, both in the case of cost-effectiveness ratios and of estimates of net benefits.

CEA plays an important role in regulatory development, providing a useful approach for collecting and organizing information, as well as for reporting the quantifiable results in summary form. Decision makers should, however, recognize the limitations of this and other approaches to economic analysis. Both BCA and CEA must be supplemented by other types of information.

Because both BCA and CEA focus on economic efficiency, they should be accompanied by a discussion that highlights distributional and ethical considerations that are not fully incorporated into the quantitative results. These concerns may relate to the disproportionate adverse effects of baseline (preregulatory) or postregulatory health conditions on subgroups of particular concern (e.g., very young and very old people, minority and/or low-income groups, or individuals with preexisting conditions). They also may relate to the characteristics of the risk itself, such as the extent to which those experiencing the risk do so voluntarily or involuntarily.

The Committee proposes that regulatory analysts and decision makers use a structured and systematic approach in the consideration of distributional and other ethical considerations raised by a particular regulatory action. By design, BCA and CEA aggregate benefits across the population. Their summary forms thus obscure important distributional effects that should be considered explicitly in the policy development process. In addition, they generally focus on the physiological consequences of the risk, and do not consider other characteristics of risk that may lead to different values. For example, the societal value placed on addressing two causes of preventable mortality—air pollution and car accidents, for example—may vary even if the probability of fatality is the same. A 1-in-100,000 chance of death may be valued differently depending on whether the risk is perceived as controllable or voluntary.

To help ensure that important concerns are not omitted, we have identified (in Box 5-3) features of a specific risk or regulatory intervention that should be considered, if applicable, in the regulatory impact analysis and in any summary comparison of CEAs. This itemization is not intended merely as a checklist, but rather as a framework for organizing important considerations not likely to be emphasized sufficiently in the CEA itself. Such distributional and other ethical considerations could be highlighted, for example, by presenting disaggregated quantified information about regulatory effects or by conducting sensitivity analyses with alternative valuation assumptions that reflect some of these considerations. As discussed in Chap-

BOX 5-3
Distributional and Other Aspects of Risk and Regulation

Distribution of Impacts

Do the baseline (preregulatory) or postregulatory costs or risks disproportionately affect certain segments of the population?

- The unborn or future generations
- Infants and young children
- Elderly people
- Persons with disabilities or preexisting health conditions
- Those particularly vulnerable to the risks of concern
- Members of minority groups
- Members of low-income groups
- Those residing in particular geographic locations

Characteristics of Risks

Do the risks have attributes that affect their value, but that are not reflected in the quantified valuation measures?

- Are the risks not subject to significant personal control?
- Are the risks particularly dreaded?
- Are the risks undetectable by the senses?
- Are the effects of the risks delayed, rather than immediate?
- Are the risks not well understood?

ter 4, agencies may want to conduct alternative quantitative analyses that use measures other than standard QALYs in uncertainty analyses. Such quantification of certain distributional effects could highlight the implications of particular value commitments.

Although comparisons of CEA ratios across different types of regulatory interventions can provide useful information on the relative impacts of different programs or policies, those using or reviewing these comparisons should recognize their limitations. Both policy makers and scholars are often interested in the relative effectiveness of different governmental or nongovernmental interventions aimed at achieving particular outcomes, such as the relative effectiveness of different programs for reducing preventable mortality. Those developing or using such comparisons, however, should recognize that economic evaluations in their summary forms (i.e., cost-effectiveness ratios and net benefits) are incomplete and may not be fully comparable due to differences in methodology as well as differences in the types of effects considered.

Different approaches to estimating risks or valuing effects may lead to differing estimates; the ranking of interventions may be affected by the lack of a standardized methodology rather than by real differences in effectiveness. Interventions that appear to differ significantly based on central tendency estimates may in fact be indistinguishable when the uncertainty in the estimates is considered. Thus it is important that such presentations of comparative information across interventions, such as relative cost-effectiveness or net benefit estimates, highlight these types of factors.

The Committee endorses the addition of QALY-based CEA to the other requirements for regulatory impact analysis. At the same time, we are concerned that presenting summary measures such as cost-effectiveness ratios in simple tables without reference to limitations of such comparisons or to their ethical and distributional implications could hinder—rather than help—the development of sound regulatory policy.

Recommendation 9: Because of the many value dimensions encompassed by societal decisions regarding the mitigation of risks to health and safety and the far-ranging impacts of such decisions, policy makers and program administrators should work to ensure the substantive involvement of a broad range of individuals and groups at all stages of policy development for regulating risks.

Regulatory agencies are, by definition, part of a political system designed to involve the public in decision making and balance competing views. Public outreach is mandated by several statutes and administrative orders and is a standard component of the regulatory development process. The Committee is concerned about the need to ensure that this outreach encourages widespread involvement and allows adequate consideration of the concerns voiced by diverse parties. Numbers can be very powerful in policy contexts; thus it is important that decision makers are presented not only with the results of economic analyses, but also have an opportunity to engage in deliberations with all constituencies and affected parties.

Although we did not evaluate the role of public participation in the regulatory development process in depth, we suggest that these activities merit further review and study. In particular, an effective deliberative process is needed to ensure that the appropriate weight is placed on those ethical, distributional, and nonquantifiable factors that are not included in the quantitative analysis.

Data Collection and Research Needed to Improve HRQL Measurement and CEA for Regulatory Decision Making

Although useful for regulatory analysis, the data and methods currently available for measuring and valuing health impacts in CEA have limitations that should be addressed by a long-term research agenda. As regulations become more stringent, or simply more costly, the importance of sound methods and accurate information for assessing societal priorities and values grows. Additional data collection and research to support regulatory analysis are costly undertakings that must be considered in the context of federal agencies' overall missions and priorities. Better planning and coordination among the relevant agencies could improve the cost-effectiveness of their investments in improved information.

For example, population HRQL norms for one or more generic indexes broken out by demographic characteristics (age, gender, race and ethnicity) have not been available in the past, and are not a standard component of periodic national health surveys. In addition, QALY-based CEAs may use any one of several generic HRQL indexes, and estimates based on different survey instruments are not readily combined or compared, because the relationships among the estimates produced by different instruments are not well understood. Perhaps most importantly, the data collection efforts for the risk assessments and epidemiological studies that underlie the economic analyses of regulations have not been designed with QALY-based analyses in mind, and the data are often inadequate for estimating HRQL impacts. The areas where additional routine data collection and research are most needed and likely to be fruitful include the following.

Recommendation 10: A high research priority should be improving the data used to assess the health risks (effects on incidence of particular types of illness, injuries, and deaths, and the duration and latency of effects) addressed by regulatory actions.

One significant source of uncertainty in estimating the economic impact of regulations is the information and modeling underlying the estimation of the type and magnitude of health-related effects on a population, that is, the risk assessment itself. Risk assessment is of fundamental importance because it supports BCA and CEA alike, as well as other aspects of the regulatory development process. Comparative risk assessment also helps set regulatory priorities. Greater precision and detail in the estimation of health effects would particularly improve QALY-based CEA because it provides more extensive information on the impact of the risk and its abatement on health status over time that are needed for this kind of analysis. As did the recent National Research Council Committee to Estimate the Public Health Benefits of Proposed Air Pollution Regulations, we recommend that federal agencies set as a high research priority improving the epidemiological and health status data used to model health and safety risks and the effects of interventions for reducing these impacts (NRC, 2002). For a discussion of methodological issues related to the calculation of attributable risk and population attributable fractions, see the Institute of Medicine workshop summary, *Estimating the Contributions of Lifestyle-Related Factors to Preventable Death* (IOM, 2005).

Recommendation 11: The Department of Health and Human Services (DHHS) and other federal agencies should collect HRQL information through routinely administered population health surveys and other major studies and data collection efforts related to risk assessment and monitoring.

DHHS should ensure that at least one population health survey—such as the National Health Interview Survey or the Medical Expenditure Panel Survey—incorporates on a periodic basis (e.g., every 3–4 years) at least one *complete* HRQL survey instrument that supports a preference-based measure in order to provide age- and sex-specific population HRQL norms or baselines. Survey questions regarding specific health conditions should be developed in consultation with regulatory agencies so that conditions that are common health endpoints for regulatory analyses or that are anticipated to be the targets of future regulatory action can be included. DHHS and its statistical agencies and programs should consult with regulatory agencies to identify these information needs and to reserve a portion of questionnaires and surveys for these purposes.

The sampling frames of these national health surveys are not ideally constructed for the collection of nationally representative HRQL information. People who reside in institutions, including those with severe mental and physical disabling conditions, and homeless people are systematically excluded from these household-based surveys. These exclusions may skew the statistical characterization of HRQL for the population overall and inhibit the ability of the agencies to assess HRQL impacts on these subgroups.

Regulatory agencies should consider including HRQL measures, as well as individual-level diagnostic and health profile information, in major data collection efforts and epidemiological studies undertaken as part of their risk monitoring systems and risk assessment research.

All federally supported research that includes HRQL measures and applications of any such measures should produce public access data sets.

DHHS should support the refinement and expansion of a catalogue of health state values derived from information in population health surveys, building on recent work to create a catalogue of preference-based chronic disease index values (see Sullivan et al., 2005). Such research should give special attention to the documentation of co-morbid conditions and the development of HRQL values for health states involving multiple impairments.

Recommendation 12: DHHS should coordinate, with the involvement of federal regulatory offices and agencies, the development of an integrated research agenda to improve the quality, applicability, and breadth of HRQL measures for use in regulatory CEA. The Committee identifies the following areas as priorities for research:

Current elicitation methods such as the standard gamble and time trade-off, while theoretically well founded, may be difficult for respondents to understand and prone to generate inconsistent responses. Research to facilitate improved methods is needed. In addition, methods for eliciting societal values for investments in health (in contrast to individual preferences for health states), such as person trade-off techniques, should also be investigated.

Despite widespread acceptance and endorsement by economists and decision theorists in the health field, preference elicitation methods based in utility theory have been criticized by behavioral scientists and survey researchers who have focused on the cognitive challenges, artificiality of choices posed, and susceptibility of responses to the framing of the choices (Fischhoff, 1991; Kahneman and Tversky, 2000). Research to refine survey practices for eliciting preferences for health states through standard gamble and time trade-off methods could improve the reliability, precision, and validity of survey results.

A more fundamental critique of using aggregate individual preferences to represent societal values in health policy has been offered by ethicists and political philosophers, among others (Nord, 1999; Ubel et al., 2000; Hausman, 2004). One approach to value elicitation that has attempted to capture judgments about societal investments in health has been the person trade-off method, either conducted individually or in consensus group settings. This method is still in a developmental phase. Although the person trade-off method will doubtless be tested and refined further to improve reliability and interpretability of results, other approaches to social valuation beyond the simple aggregation of individual preferences should also be explored.

Methods for measuring children's HRQL, including characterization of the impact of illness and injury and the valuation of these impacts, need continued development and refinement.

The Committee is particularly concerned about the adequacy of current metrics and methods for valuing health-related effects in children in two respects. First, the impacts of illness and injury on children are not well understood, due to limitations in the underlying health science research and in the methods used to describe these effects with HRQL instruments.

Existing instruments are limited in their capacity to capture important aspects of HRQL for children, such as impacts on cognitive abilities and social interactions. Second, the surveys used to assess societal values for changes in HRQL generally address impacts on adults. In reality, those affected by costs and benefits of economically significant regulations may assign a higher value to improving the HRQL and longevity of children than of adults. In addition, there are questions about when it may be desirable to include children's valuation of their own health states as one component of the total societal value of these effects.

Because children may lack the maturity and experience to evaluate their own health, and especially to provide informed responses to choice-based valuation questions, it may be appropriate to substitute the judgments of parents or other proxy respondents. Other questions include how to adapt preference elicitation techniques for use with children and young adolescents and how to include the effects of children's health on the well-being of parents and caretakers, effects that are not captured by individual-level HRQL measures. There appears to be no consensus on best practices for the measurement of children's HRQL and the conduct of CEA for pediatric interventions, and a concerted research and consensus development initiative on this topic is warranted. (See Griebsch et al., 2005, for a literature survey of pediatric CEAs and variability in valuation methods.)

Methods to correlate QALY estimates based on different generic HRQL indexes should be developed so that estimates from different underlying valuation studies are consistent and can be used in the same analysis.

As noted in Chapter 3, a federally supported survey effort with a nationally representative sample of noninstitutionalized adults is under way to collect HRQL information using several generic indexes, so that the relationships among the estimates produced by different indexes can be documented and conversion formulae developed. The results of this major data collection effort should make it possible to combine HRQL information based on different generic indexes, and could obviate the kinds of problems the Committee encountered in the air quality case study using published health state index values based on different generic instruments. (See Box 3-7 and Appendix A for discussions of this case study.)

SUMMARY

Regulatory decisions are, and should continue to be, based on a public and transparent deliberative process that includes consideration of a wide range of factors, including but not limited to the results of economic analyses using BCA and CEA. BCA and CEA are complementary tools in the development of major health and safety rules because they offer distinct perspectives and different types of information about regulatory impacts and effects. Both kinds of analyses provide a structured framework for collecting, analyzing, and presenting information on regulatory impacts. They do not, however, provide a complete accounting of all the effects and consequences that are important for policy-making purposes.

Given the substantial impact of major health and safety regulations on the national economy and societal welfare, it is imperative that related decisions be based on high-quality policy analysis, the results and limitations of which are clearly communicated in a form that is understandable by a wide variety of audiences. Because these rules vary significantly in the type of intervention, the characteristics of the affected population, and the characteristics of the risks addressed, benefits measures are needed that can be applied to a broad range of health scenarios. These measures should be supplemented by discussion of any attributes of the scenarios that cannot be fully captured in the quantitative measures. Furthermore, the substantial uncertainty that accompanies the risk analysis underlying the calculation of health-related effects, along with uncertainty about the preference weighting of QALYs due to alternative HRQL concepts and constructs and variability in measurement, should be conveyed in uncertainty analyses.

Finally, the process of developing and issuing regulations should:

- Be publicly accessible;
- Be based on information (including that used in BCA and CEA) that can be interpreted for and communicated to a wide audience;
- Facilitate the involvement of affected individuals, populations, and organizations in deliberations about health and safety risks and proposed interventions; and
- Be accountable for the policy choices made with reasons that are available to all participants and observers.

Appendixes

A

Summary of Case Studies

PURPOSE AND SCOPE

As part of the charge from its sponsors, the Institute of Medicine (IOM) Committee to Evaluate Measures of Health Benefits for Environmental, Health, and Safety Regulation was asked to conduct case studies that applied data from completed economic analyses to assess the impacts using different measures of effectiveness. The Committee chose to conduct three case studies that reflect the data and analytic approaches applied by different regulatory agencies as well as the diverse health impacts addressed. This appendix summarizes the case studies, which are described in more detail in three separate reports (Robinson et al., 2005a,b,c). The implications of these case studies for our deliberations are discussed in the main text of this report; some of the key conclusions are also summarized at the end of this appendix.

The case studies were a learning exercise for the Committee. They allowed us to examine in detail the data and methods currently applied by federal agencies when estimating the value of health and safety benefits. These case studies also permitted us to apply alternative quality-adjusted life-year (QALY) methods in the context of regulatory analysis and to examine the outcomes. Because the case studies were completed with limited resources and largely in advance of the Committee's deliberations, the case studies do not reflect in every respect the best practices ultimately recommended by the Committee, nor were they designed to replicate the complexity of a full regulatory analysis.[1] They do, however, provide a starting point for researchers interested in conducting more sophisticated versions of these types of analyses.

The Committee identified candidates for these case studies as part of a review of all major federal health and safety regulations finalized in recent years (Robinson, 2004). This review focused on those economically significant regulations that were supported by quantitative assessment of both costs and health or safety-related impacts, that is, the types of rules for which new Office of Management and Budget (OMB) guidance (2003a) now requires cost-effectiveness analysis (CEA) in addition to benefit–cost analysis (BCA). Based on this review and discussions with agency staff, we determined that the three rules listed below appeared to best illustrate the range of types of regulations, current practices, and health and safety impacts most likely to be significantly affected by the Committee's recommendations.

1. *The Food and Drug Administration's (FDA's) January 2001 juice processing rule:* This food safety regulation provides an example of FDA's use of monetized QALYs to value the impacts of acute and chronic illness in BCA. The health outcomes considered include acute gastrointestinal effects associated with exposure to four foodborne pathogens as well as chronic conditions stemming from these infections. Few cases of mortality were associated with these pathogens.

2. *The National Highway Traffic Safety Administration's (NHTSA's) March 1999 child restraint rule:* Because more recent rules were undergoing revision, we chose a somewhat older rule for the NHTSA case study. However, the data sources and analytic approach are similar to those currently used by NHTSA. NHTSA's approach to CEA involves converting nonfatal injuries to "equivalent lives saved" (ELS) based on the ratio of their costs to the value of a fatality; these costs include both expenditures and monetized QALY impacts. (See Chapter 2 and Box 2-4 for further detail on the ELS approach.) The health effects addressed by this rule include a variety of fatal and nonfatal crash-related injuries to children.

3. *The U.S. Environmental Protection Agency's (EPA's) June 2004 nonroad diesel rule:* Air pollution regulations account for a substantial

---

[1]One of the most important differences between these case studies and the Committee's recommendations is the limited information they provide on the range of possible values and associated uncertainties. We rely largely on mean or median estimates to assess QALY impacts, and also do not report uncertainties in each agency's characterization of the health effects averted by the regulations nor in their estimation of regulatory costs. The case studies also do not include detailed information on the distribution and equity of the impacts. In Chapter 4 of this report, however, we use the case studies to illustrate distributive and other concerns.

proportion of all major health and safety regulations finalized in recent years; this was the most recent of these rules. In its BCA, EPA used estimates of willingness to pay (WTP) to value benefits, supplemented by cost-of-illness estimates when suitable WTP values were not available. This case study provided an example of a rule that had several health-related impacts that could not be quantified, as well as both quantified and nonquantified nonhealth effects (e.g., on visibility, crop yields, and other ecosystem functions). The key health effects of concern include preventable mortality and a number of acute and chronic cardiovascular and respiratory conditions.

The following sections provide an overview of the general analytic approach for these case studies. We then discuss the details of the approaches applied in each case and report our results and conclusions. The final section summarizes the major lessons learned from these analyses.

GENERAL APPROACH

To estimate the QALY impacts of the regulations addressed by the case studies, we followed a three-part process.[2]

- First, we described each type of injury or illness averted by the rule, based (to the extent possible) on the materials the agency used to support its regulatory analysis.
- Second, we used several different approaches to estimate the impact of each condition on health-related quality of life (HRQL) over the affected individuals' lifespans. The methods used varied; each case study involved the application of three or four different approaches.
- Third, we determined the QALY losses averted by the regulation. This step involved estimating the change in HRQL attributable to the injury or illness under two scenarios: a base case analysis that assumed that affected individuals would be in average health (adjusted for age) over their remaining life expectancy in the absence of the condition of concern, and a sensitivity analysis that assumed that they would be in perfect or optimal health. For nonfatal effects, we then multiplied the resulting decrement by the expected duration of each illness. For preventable mortality, we estimated the change in life expectancy based on the average age of the affected individuals.

This process is illustrated in Figure A-1.

---

[2]The acknowledgments at the end of this appendix provide a complete list of those involved in each case study analysis.

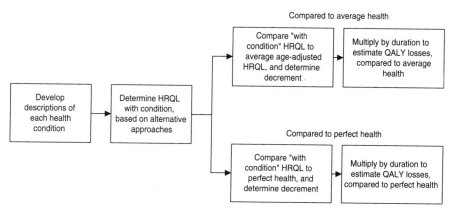

FIGURE A-1 Case Study Process

In these case studies, we focused on annual impacts for simplicity and comparability, assessing the change in disease or injury incidence attributable to a single year of the regulatory intervention. If the health effect is chronic or long-lived, however, the new cases of injury or illness prevented each year will have longer term impacts. We take these future year impacts into account and assess the lifetime effects of such cases, calculating the results both discounted and undiscounted. (We follow the discounting guidance in OMB, 2003a, as discussed in the main text of this report.) Agencies' regulatory analyses generally take a longer view and assess the impacts of the rulemakings over a multiyear period. We believe that this multiyear focus is appropriate; although the presentation of annualized impacts can provide useful information, it should be provided only as a supplement to an analysis that considers the implementation of the rule over a longer time horizon.

Below, we provide an overview of the methods we applied across all three case studies, focusing on the process used to describe the health endpoints and to compare HRQL with and without the condition of concern. In the health care field, "without condition" health (i.e., the health status of an individual in the absence of a particular illness or injury of concern) is often referred to as "baseline" health. We avoid this term because baseline means something different in regulatory analysis; it refers to the situation in the absence of the rule, which is equivalent to "with condition" health status.

Describing Health Endpoints

The first step in the case study analysis involved describing the health endpoints so that they could be valued under alternative HRQL approaches. To increase our understanding of the information typically available to regulatory agencies and for consistency with the agency analyses, we based these descriptions on the same information used by the agency in its risk assessment to the maximum extent possible. Because the original FDA analysis used an HRQL index in its BCA, it supplied most of the information needed for the case study. In contrast, the approach used in the NHTSA rule relied on broad standardized injury classifications that were not adequate for estimating HRQL impacts. Thus we used a different data set to develop descriptions of the injuries averted. For the EPA rule, we relied on a combination of the information provided in the agency's regulatory analysis and in a separate EPA analysis of the QALY impacts of air pollution-related health effects.

In each case study, we used at least one approach that involved expert assignment of the HRQL attributes for the illnesses or injuries of concern. Developing descriptions for these expert assignments involved several challenges. First, we needed to determine the appropriate level of detail. Our goal was to provide enough information so that medical experts could understand and distinguish between different health endpoints, without overwhelming them with unnecessary information. Our schedule precluded formal pretesting; instead, we consulted informally with individuals with relevant expertise to develop these descriptions.

Second, we wanted to avoid using language in the descriptions that could prejudice the assignment of the attribute levels included in each index (e.g., "little" or "no" difficulty in self-care; "moderate" pain). It was difficult to avoid this language completely, however; in some cases such terminology was part of the description used by the agencies to distinguish between different endpoints. For example, FDA distinguished between different types of long-term reactive arthritis based in part on the degree of pain experienced.

Finally, the agency regulatory assessments of the health endpoints were for predicted risks (or statistical cases) rather than for individual, identifiable patients, and cover time periods over which HRQL impacts may vary. In theory we could have developed longitudinal models that identified distinct phases of each condition, the duration of each phase, and its probability of occurrence. Such models are difficult to develop, however, and require substantially more time and resources than were available. Instead, we encouraged the experts to consider the average or typical patient with each illness or injury and to assess the expected average HRQL impact over the course of the condition. In some cases, we divided the health conditions into different phases. For the child restraints analysis, for example, we asked the experts to estimate the duration of the acute, rehabilitation, and long-term phases and to assign attribute levels separately to each phase. In the air quality case study, we split the cardiovascular disease endpoints into subcategories (based on age at incidence, severity, and disease progression), to better distinguish different health states.

Estimating "With Condition" HRQL

To estimate the HRQL impacts of each health condition averted by these regulations, we relied on several commonly used generic indexes: the EuroQol (EQ)-5D, the Health Utilities Index (HUI) Mark 2 and Mark 3, the SF-6D, and the Quality of Well-Being Scale (QWB).[3] In addition, for the NHTSA case study, we applied an instrument which is now being created specifically to assess the longer term impacts of traumatic injury, the Functional Capacity Index (FCI). Chapter 3 and Appendix B of this report provide detailed information on each of these indexes.

Applying these indexes entails two steps. First, the characteristics of each health condition are matched to (or assigned) attribute levels under each domain of each index. For example, for the EQ-5D, this process involves determining whether the disease or injury leads to "severe," "moderate," or "no" impairments within five domains—mobility, self-care, usual activities, pain/discomfort, and anxiety/depression. Second, the resulting attribute responses are weighted to reflect the value placed on different levels of impairment. Each generic index relies on a particular scoring algorithm to develop relative values for particular health states; this algorithm is based on statistical analyses of the results of a valuation survey developed especially for the classification system of that index. These valuation surveys are described in Chapter 3; see especially Table 3-4.

In each case study, at least one of the HRQL approaches involved expert assignment of the attributes defined under a particular generic index. Although it is generally preferable to ask patients to complete this step, expert judgment is often used to provide a faster and less costly assessment. For expediency, we followed a simple expert judgment process that was not fully consistent with the best practices described in Chapter 3. For example, we recruited volunteer experts through our informal professional networks based largely on their availability. Consequently, the resulting groups may not represent the full range of subspecialties or types of patients relevant to

---

[3]As discussed in Chapter 3 and shown in Appendix B, the HUI-2 and -3 include some differences in domains, in part because the HUI-2 was originally developed to assess health states among children.

the assessment.[4] A more sophisticated approach could use specific selection criteria to ensure a broad range of relevant expertise and experience as well as geographic stratification, and could involve asking specialty societies for nominations. We also did not work with the experts to ensure that they had a thorough or common understanding of the materials describing the health endpoints, the domain attributes, and the task itself. Nor did we attempt to resolve any inconsistencies either within the responses of an individual expert or across the responses from different experts. We used simple decision rules to fill in any missing data.

In a few cases, we relied on patient data from the available research literature rather than expert judgment. For the NHTSA study, we used QWB values from a study of trauma patients (Holbrook et al., 1999). For the EPA case study, we used preliminary condition-specific EQ-5D values estimated from the Medical Panel Expenditure Survey (MEPS) (Sullivan et al., 2005). In the EPA case study, we also transferred values from two patient studies selected from the Harvard School of Public Health's CEA Registry (http://www.hsph.harvard.edu/cearegistry/), based on a review by Brauer and Neumann (2005). The case study approaches are summarized in Table A-1.

Comparing to "Without Condition" HRQL

To represent likely HRQL in the absence of the conditions of concern (i.e., once the regulation has been implemented), we used estimates of average population health broken out by age from major national population health surveys that included the relevant generic index questionnaire. This approach is equivalent to assuming that, in the absence of the hazard addressed by the regulation, affected individuals on average would have the same health status as the average member of the U.S. population in the same age group. In sensitivity analysis, we also compared the "with condition" HRQL estimates to a value of 1.0. This latter comparison is equivalent to assuming that, in the absence of the illness or injury, the affected individuals would be in perfect or optimal health.[5]

These age-adjusted estimates of average population health use the same underlying community-based valuation survey for each index (as discussed in Chapter 3) and were based on unpublished analyses prepared for the

---

[4]The original construction and valuation of the FCI provides an example of a more formal expert judgment process in which multiple relevant clinical specialties and perspectives were represented.

[5]We provide this comparison because it is often found in the literature; however, the Committee does not recommend this approach. See Fryback and Lawrence (1997), for a discussion of the problems with calculating changes from optimal health (1.0).

TABLE A-1 Approaches for Determining "With Condition" HRQL

Rule	Approach	Indexes	Data Source
FDA Juice Processing	Expert assignment	EQ-5D, HUI-3, QWB, SF-6D	Analysis of data provided by medical experts contacted by case study team
NHTSA Child Restraints	Expert assignment	EQ-5D, HUI-2	Analysis of data provided by medical experts contacted by case study team
	Trauma patient survey	QWB	Analysis of patient data provided by Troy Holbrook, University of California, San Diego
	Expert judgment	FCI	Expert data and weighting formula provided by Ellen MacKenzie, Johns Hopkins University
EPA Nonroad Diesel Emissions	Expert assignment	EQ-5D	Analysis of data provided by medical experts contacted by case study team
	Population survey (MEPS)	EQ-5D	Preliminary analysis of self-reported HRQL provided by Patrick Sullivan, University of Colorado
	Transfer from Harvard Registry studies	EQ-5D, HUI-3	Analysis of patient data from Oostenbrink et al. (2001) and Torrance et al. (1999)

Committee's use in the case studies.[6] The estimates were provided by age and gender, and generally broken into 10-year age groups.

These population averages were missing estimates for very young and very old individuals. We assumed that, for ages 0 through 9 years, average health would equal perfect health (a value of 1.0); for ages 10 through 19, average health would be the midpoint between perfect health and the values estimated for ages 20 through 29; and for those older than the reported age

---

[6]*EQ-5D* estimated based on 2001 MEPS data by Dr. William Lawrence, Agency for Healthcare Research and Quality. *HUI-3* estimated based on 2002 Joint U.S.–Canada Survey of Health data by Barbara Altman, National Center for Health Statistics. (We used the HUI-3 estimates for the HUI-2 analysis, since the general populations averages are expected to be similar.) *SF-6D* estimated based on 2001 MEPS data by Janel Hanmer, University of Wisconsin-Madison. *QWB* estimated based on 2001 U.S. National Health Interview Survey data by John Anderson, University of California, San Diego. Updated estimates for the EQ-5D, SF-6D, and QWB are available in Hanmer et al. (2006). Population averages were not available for the FCI.

TABLE A-2 Without-Condition HRQL

	Age 20	Age 40	Age 60	Age 80
Mean Population Index Value (base case)				
EQ-5D	0.92	0.88	0.83	0.75
HUI-2 and 3	0.91	0.88	0.82	0.69
SF-6D	0.84	0.82	0.79	0.72
QWB	0.82	0.80	0.74	0.65
Perfect Health (sensitivity analysis)				
All indices	1.0	1.0	1.0	1.0

NOTES: See Hanmer et al. (2006) for updated estimates and information on uncertainty. Table presents results rounded to two significant figures for selected age groups. Unrounded estimates for each year of age are used in all calculations. SOURCES: EQ-5D: Unpublished analysis by William Lawrence, November 9, 2004. HUI-3: Unpublished analysis by Barbara Altman, January 7, 2005. SF-6D: Unpublished analysis by Janel Hanmer, January 24, 2005. QWB: Unpublished analysis by John Anderson, April 21, 2005.

ranges, average health would remain constant at the value reported for the eldest age group. This approach means that the HRQL impacts for young children will be the same regardless of whether the comparison is to perfect or average health, since a value of 1.0 is used for "without condition" HRQL in both cases.[7]

Table A-2 presents the estimates of average population health used in this analysis for selected ages, for males and females combined. These estimates are provided for illustrative purposes; the case study calculations used the full range of estimates available for each age group.

As is evident from the table, the estimates of average population health vary. This variation reflects several factors, including the differences in (1) the population surveyed to determine their health-related attributes; (2) the underlying valuation survey; and (3) the construction of indexes themselves. In combination, these factors generally lead to the highest average HRQL estimates under the EQ-5D and the lowest under the QWB. As expected, average HRQL declines with age under each index.

The comparison of HRQL with and without the conditions of concern is complicated by the assumptions that underlie the approach used to assign and value attributes under each index. In these comparisons, we adjusted the values depending on the source of the "with condition" esti-

---

[7]The assumption that average HRQL for infants and children is close to optimal and can be approximated by an index value of 1.0 may not be well founded, however. Some surveys of children's self-reported HRQL have reported lower values (Hennessy and Kind, 2002).

mates. We summarize these adjustments below; examples of the effects of these different adjustments are provided later in the summary of the EPA case study. Once we used these adjusted values to calculate the decrement in HRQL associated with each condition, we multiplied the decrement by the duration of the condition (taking longevity into account) to estimate QALY losses.

Comparison to "With Condition" Values Based on Expert Assignment

Many researchers hypothesize that experts responding to the sorts of questionnaires used in the case studies implicitly compare the condition to perfect health, rather than to average health for an individual of a given age. Our interviews of the experts involved in the case studies generally reinforced this impression; they reported that they considered the impacts of the illness or injury on someone who is otherwise in good health; i.e., does not have other conditions that affect their HRQL. To reflect this assumption, we adjusted the condition-specific HRQL results proportionately when comparing them to average health, which declines with age. For the comparison to perfect health in our sensitivity analysis, we use the unadjusted values based on the experts' attribute assignments.

For example, if the expert assessment results in a "with condition" value of 0.8, this value represents 80 percent of perfect health (i.e., of 1.0). If "without condition" health is 0.9 (based on the population average for an individual of the same age), then 80 percent of this value is 0.72. We would then use 0.72 as our estimate of "with condition" health when comparing to average health. This is equivalent to assuming that each expert was comparing the condition to perfect health and, if they had instead compared to age-adjusted average health, the HRQL with the condition would reflect the same proportionate reduction. While more sophisticated approaches could be developed for addressing this issue, we found that this approach was the most expedient option for the case studies.

Comparison to "With Condition" Values Based on Patient Self-Assessments

The NHTSA and EPA case studies also use patient data from previously completed studies. Three of these studies, the Holbrook et al. (1999) QWB estimates for injuries, the Torrance et al. (1999) HUI-3 estimates for chronic bronchitis, and the Oostenbrink et al. (2001) EQ-5D estimates for vascular disease, reflect all aspects of a patient's health, not only the effects of the illness or injury of concern. This raises two issues. First, because HRQL generally decreases with age, these estimates may reflect comorbidities that would not be present in younger populations but would increase in older populations. Second, the decrement in HRQL calculated from these estimates may overstate the effect of the condition, because the estimates may reflect health impairments that are not attributable to the condition of concern.

In these cases, we followed a two-step process. First, we compared the researcher's results to the estimate of average health for an individual of the same age as the average person in the researcher's sample, and determined the "with condition" HRQL as a percentage of the average ("without condition") HRQL for that age. Second, we applied this percentage reduction to the HRQL estimates for all ages as relevant. This approach is equivalent to assuming that the proportionate reduction in HRQL is the same for every age, and differs from the approach used in the expert assignments.

We do not adjust the researchers' values when comparing to perfect health; the decrement is the same in each year when compared to a constant value of 1.0. Thus, in this latter comparison, we are overstating the impacts of the health condition both because the values reflect HRQL decrements other than those related to the condition itself and because the affected individuals are not likely to be in perfect health throughout their lifetimes.

For example, the average age of the Holbrook et al. (1999) QWB sample of trauma patients was 36 years. If the Holbrook results for an injury were 0.7 and the estimate of average health for a 36-year-old was 0.8, then we assumed that HRQL with the injury was 87.5 percent of average health (0.7/0.8 = 0.875) regardless of the age of incidence. In the comparison to perfect health, we used the reported value of 0.7 without adjustment.

The preliminary EQ-5D estimates from MEPS used in the EPA case study are also based on data from persons reporting the condition; however, here we follow a different approach.[8] In this case, the researchers separated out the effects of co-morbidities from the effects of the condition of concern in their statistical analysis. We used the condition-specific decrements directly when comparing to average health without the condition. In the perfect health comparison, we added the difference between average health and perfect health at each age to the decrement provided by the researchers. (This process means that the "with condition" values are the same in both scenarios because we make the adjustment to the decrements.) This approach leads to decrements that increase with age because the difference between perfect health and average population health increases over time, as illustrated earlier in Table A-2.

---

[8]A different approach would be needed in applying the final results from this research, due to changes in how the decrements were calculated (see Sullivan et al., 2005).

FDA JUICE PROCESSING REGULATION

In this case study, we estimated the cost-effectiveness of FDA's 2001 juice processing rule. We selected this regulation as one of the Committee's case studies because it allowed us to explore the effects of applying different HRQL measures to both short-lived and lifelong illnesses. It also provides an example of a regulation where the issuing agency used a monetized QALY measure in its BCA. In this case study, we applied four indexes: the EQ-5D, the HUI-3, the SF-6D, and the QWB, asking clinical experts to determine the attributes that best match the expected impacts of each illness.

FDA Analysis

The starting point for our analysis was the research conducted by FDA to support its rulemaking efforts (FDA, 1998, 2001). In its BCA, FDA quantified the health impacts that were most significant in terms of severity and probability of occurrence, focusing on four microbial pathogens: *Bacillus cereus*, *Cryptosporidium parvum*, *Escherichia coli* O157:H7, and *Salmonella (non typhi)*. The effects of these pathogens include infections that result in gastrointestinal illness and may lead to reactive arthritis. Most effects are short-lived, lasting for a few days or weeks on average, although in a small number of cases the infection may lead to lifelong illness or death. FDA categorized these effects in terms of duration (i.e., average days of illness) and severity (i.e., mild, moderate, severe), determining severity based on whether the typical patient would be likely to seek medical attention and/or be hospitalized.

In its BCA, FDA valued these health impacts using a combination of approaches. Fatal cases were valued using a best estimate of $5 million per statistical life saved. (Statistical cases represent the aggregation of small risks across a large number of people; e.g., a fatality risk of 1 in 10,000 aggregated across 10,000 people would equal a statistical life.) Nonfatal cases were valued as follows (see also Box 2-3). First, FDA used a generic index, the QWB, to determine HRQL impacts. Analysts assigned the QWB attributes (which reflect functional status and include symptom/problem codes) that best corresponded to the HRQL impacts for each of the health endpoints considered. They then calculated the value of these impacts based on the standard QWB valuation formula. The index values were multiplied by the expected average duration of each health impact to estimate the quality-adjusted life-day (QALD) losses associated with each endpoint. These QALD losses were assigned a dollar value by converting the agency's value of statistical life estimate to a daily value of $630. Finally, FDA added the costs of medical treatment to these monetized QALD estimates. The resulting per-case values (monetized QALDs plus medical costs) were multiplied by the number of cases averted to determine the dollar value of the benefits of the rule. These results are summarized in Table A-3 below.[9]

As indicated by the table, FDA estimated that present value of the annual benefits would total $151 million, applying a discount rate of 7 percent to the future year effects of those illnesses with long-term impacts.[10] In comparison, FDA estimated that the annualized costs of the rule (including initial implementation and ongoing operations) would total $28 million. The rule thus results in monetized net benefits (benefits minus costs) totaling approximately $123 million per year. FDA noted that some, less significant, health effects were not quantified, such as those related to exposure to other pathogens and contaminants such as pesticides.

Case Study Analytic Approach

As discussed above, the Committee's approach to estimating QALY impacts for these case studies involved three steps: (1) developing descriptions of each health outcome assessed; (2) applying different approaches to estimate the HRQL impacts of each outcome; and (3) calculating the difference between "with condition" and "without condition" HRQL and multiplying the resulting decrement by the duration of the impact.

For this case study, the background materials for FDA's rulemaking (FDA, 1998, 2001) provided most of the information we needed to develop brief (one or two sentence) descriptions of each of the health endpoints listed in Table A-3. Our descriptions included information on the types of symptoms (e.g., diarrhea, abdominal pain, and nausea), indicated the pathogen causing the illness (*B. cereus, C. parvum, E. coli* O157:H7, or *Salmonella—non typhi*), noted the approximate duration of the symptoms (e.g., "expected to last less than one week," "typically lasting throughout the individual's remaining life span"), and indicated whether patients were likely to require medical attention or hospitalization.

We separated certain of the severe and chronic effects into subcategories to better reflect the varying health states that result, using data provided in FDA's analysis. This led to descriptions of 17 separate nonfatal endpoints, including 13 related to infections and 4 related to reactive arthritis, as listed in Table A-4 in the next section. Five of these endpoints involve chronic lifelong conditions; the remainder are of short-term dura-

---

[9]These estimates are for the selected policy only; FDA did not quantify the costs or benefits of alternative regulatory options in this analysis.

[10]This rate reflects the government-wide guidance in place at the time that the rule was promulgated; agencies are now required to discount the results using *both* 3 and 7 percent rates (OMB, 2003a). The year that was the basis for FDA's dollar estimates was not reported.

TABLE A-3 FDA Estimates of Annual Quantified Benefits

Endpoint	Avoided Incidence (cases/year)	Monetary Value
B. cereus		
Mild	340	$102,000
Moderate	<0.1	—
Severe	0.3	—
Death	0	—
Subtotal	340	$102,000
C. parvum		
Mild	2,890	$5,780,000
Moderate	290	1,450,000
Severe	20	360,000
Death	1	5,000,000
Subtotal	3,200	$12,590,000
E. coli O157:H7		
Mild	95	$190,000
Moderate	60	240,000
Severe-acute	5	165,000
Severe-chronic	10	12,210,000
Death	<0.1	—
Subtotal	160	$12,805,000
Salmonella (non typhi)		
Mild	1,590	$1,590,000
Moderate	730	1,460,000
Severe	20	320,000
Reactive arthritis–short-term	50	350,000
Reactive arthritis–long-term	120	117,120,000
Death	1	5,000,000
Subtotal	2,340	$125,840,000
Total	6,040	$151,337,000

NOTES: Dollar year not reported; long-term impacts discounted at 7 percent.
Detail does not add to total due to rounding; detailed break-outs do not add to total because they double-count cases that begin as acute and become chronic or long-term.

SOURCE: FDA (2001, pp. 6183–6184).

tion, lasting only a few days or weeks. The descriptions provided to the experts did not provide information on the average age of the affected individuals.

We then sent these descriptions to the medical experts, along with a list of the domain and attribute definitions for each generic index and instructions for characterizing each endpoint in terms of the attribute levels. We asked the experts to consider a "typical" patient with each type of illness in completing this exercise. The experts included eight infectious disease specialists and five rheumatologists, who were asked to characterize or assign the endpoints related to their area of expertise using each of the generic indexes.

Once we received the assignments, we entered the results into an Excel spreadsheet model to calculate the summary index values, to compare the "with condition" results to average age-adjusted HRQL and to perfect health, and to multiply the resulting decrements by the duration of the health effect, following the approaches summarized above. We used FDA's assumptions for average age at incidence and for the duration of the effects. Most of the effects are expected to occur on average in adulthood, except for severe *E. coli* infections, for which the average age at incidence was four years. For fatal cases and lifelong effects, we assumed that the average life expectancy of the affected individuals would extend with certainty to age 77, again consistent with FDA's approach.[11]

The FDA analysis (along with more recent studies) suggests that pathogen-related infections may be more common or more severe in individuals with suppressed immune systems. We were not, however, able to quantify the extent to which such individuals would be disproportionately affected, nor were we able to estimate the HRQL of these individuals with or without the illnesses of concern. Our assumption that, in the absence of the pathogen exposure, individuals with suppressed immune systems would have the same health status as the average member of the general population is likely to overstate their "without condition" HRQL. The impact of pathogen-related illness on HRQL may also differ for these individuals.

Estimates of QALY Gains

The expert assessment process resulted in identification of domain attributes under each of the four indexes for each of the 17 health endpoints assessed. In general, we found that endpoints of increasing severity were often assigned similar attributes, meaning that the descriptions and/or attribute levels offered by the several indexes did not distinguish sufficiently among severity levels. When attribute assignments varied, they usually followed the expected pattern in that the assignments for severe cases indicated greater problems than the assignments for mild cases. The range between the minimum and maximum values for each attribute suggested that the experts sometimes varied significantly in their judgments about the

---

[11]This differs from the other case studies which apply a preferred approach: using conditional survival rates to estimate life expectancy.

degree of problems imposed; however, we did not formally assess the extent or sources of this variation.

In Table A-4, we present the weighted values from the expert assignments, reporting median rather than average values as the estimate of central tendency because of the small number of experts involved. The results indicate the estimated HRQL with each condition (not the decrement from normal health), on a scale where one corresponds to perfect health and zero corresponds to death. This table excludes fatalities, which have a "with condition" value of zero.

The domain attributes assigned by the experts result in median index

TABLE A-4 Juice Processing Case Study: HRQL with Pathogen-Related Illness

Endpoint	HRQL with Pathogen-Related Illness (median)			
	EQ-5D	HUI-3	SF-6D	QWB
1. *B. cereus*, mild	0.82	0.76	0.74	0.59
2. *C. parvum*, mild	0.77	0.62	0.68	0.53
3. *C. parvum*, moderate	0.74	0.50	0.56	0.53
4. *C. parvum*, severe	0.44	0.35	0.47	0.49
5. *E. coli*, mild	0.74	0.64	0.65	0.56
6. *E. coli*, moderate	0.64	0.50	0.56	0.56
7. *E. coli*, severe-acute, with colitis	0.16	0.10	0.43	0.48
8. *E. coli*, severe-acute, with hemolytic uremic syndrome	(0.11)	0.04	0.37	0.44
9. *E. coli*, severe-chronic, with colitis	(0.11)	(0.08)	0.36	0.44
10. *E. coli*, severe-chronic, with hemolytic uremic syndrome	(0.11)	(0.10)	0.35	0.44
11. *Salmonella*, mild	0.80	0.71	0.69	0.53
12. *Salmonella*, moderate	0.60	0.58	0.57	0.53
13. *Salmonella*, severe	0.44	0.31	0.46	0.48
14. *Salmonella*, short-term reactive arthritis	0.71	0.73	0.80	0.64
15. *Salmonella*, long-term reactive arthritis, flares and remissions with some wellness	0.60	0.56	0.69	0.56
16. *Salmonella*, long-term reactive arthritis, waxes and wanes with no wellness	0.60	0.42	0.53	0.52
17. *Salmonella*, long-term reactive arthritis, chronic and unremitting	0.60	0.23	0.39	0.52

NOTES: With-illness values assumed to reflect comparison to perfect health. Values in parenthesis are negative; the experts assigned attributes indicating significant impairments.

SOURCE: Case study team analysis of expert assignments provided in February to March, 2005.

values that decrease with the increasing severity of the illness as expected, in some cases dropping below zero (indicating that the weighted attributes taken together result in a value considered worse than death). For mild cases, the EQ-5D generally results in the values closest to optimal or perfect health, while the QWB results in the lowest values, but this pattern is not constant across the different pathogen-related endpoints.

The next step involved estimating the QALY losses averted by FDA's juice processing rule. This included: (1) determining the decrement from "without condition" health for each condition; (2) multiplying the decrement by the duration of each condition to estimate the QALYs lost; and (3) multiplying the per-case values by the number of cases averted by the rule.[12] Table A-5 presents the resulting estimates of total QALYs lost for our base case scenario, where we assume that normal health (in the absence of the condition) would equal average age-adjusted health. As previously discussed, we assume that the expert assignment implicitly involved comparison to perfect health and that the decrement from average health would represent the same proportional reduction. This table presents the results discounted at both a 3 and 7 percent discount rate, reflecting current guidance for discounting in regulatory analysis (OMB, 2003a). Undiscounted, the total estimated losses range from 2,500 to 3,700 QALYs, depending on the index used.

This table indicates that the health effects that lead to the largest HRQL decrements (i.e., particularly severe *E. coli* cases, see Table A-4) are not necessarily the health effects that account for the largest proportion of the benefits of the rule.[13] When adjusted for duration and number of cases averted, prevention of long-term reactive arthritis accounts for the largest share of the overall benefits across all of the indexes, although the exact proportion varies. (FDA's original analysis was also dominated by the results for this endpoint, but these results are not included in the table because FDA did not compare their "with condition" results to an average health scenario.) In total, the HUI-3 leads to the largest estimate of QALY losses when compared to average health.

---

[12]We express these losses as QALYs (rather than as QALDs as in the FDA analyses) for consistency with how these losses are usually reported in the research literature.

[13]Because the experts assigned the lowest attribute level in more than one domain for severe *E. coli* infections under the EQ-5D and HUI-3, the resulting HRQL values are less than zero (see Table A-4). Hence the estimates of QALY losses are greater than the duration of the illness. For example, at the age of incidence (4 years), we assume that average HRQL without the illness is 1.0, and find that the HRQL with the illness is *negative* 0.11 under the EQ-5D, for a *decrement* of 1.11 from average health. If we multiply this decrement by 365 days to reflect the impacts of the first year of the illness (1.11*365), the QALDs lost total 405, exceeding the number of days in the year.

TABLE A-5 Juice Processing Case Study: QALY Losses, All Cases

Endpoint	Case Study Expert Assessment (median)							
	EQ-5D		HUI-3		SF-6D		QWB	
Discount Rate	3%	7%	3%	7%	3%	7%	3%	7%
1. *B. cereus*, mild	0.2	0.2	0.2	0.2	0.2	0.2	0.3	0.3
2. *C. parvum*, mild	15	15	25	25	19	19	27	27
3. *C. parvum*, moderate	3.2	3.2	6.2	6.2	5.0	5.0	5.0	5.0
4. *C. parvum*, severe	0.7	0.7	0.8	0.8	0.6	0.6	0.5	0.5
5. *E. coli*, mild	0.3	0.3	0.4	0.4	0.4	0.4	0.5	0.5
6. *E. coli*, moderate	0.5	0.5	0.7	0.7	0.5	0.5	0.5	0.5
7. *E. coli*, severe-acute, with colitis	0.3	0.3	0.3	0.3	0.2	0.2	0.1	0.1
8. *E. coli*, severe-acute, with hemolytic uremic syndrome	0.1	0.1	0.1	0.1	0.0	0.0	0.0	0.0
9. *E. coli*, severe-chronic, with colitis	242	120	234	116	134	67	108	53
10. *E. coli*, severe-chronic, with hemolytic uremic syndrome	61	30	60	30	34	17	27	13
11. *Salmonella*, mild	1.6	1.6	2.3	2.3	2.3	2.3	3.3	3.3
12. *Salmonella*, moderate	3.7	3.7	3.8	3.8	3.7	3.7	3.8	3.8
13. *Salmonella*, severe	0.5	0.5	0.6	0.6	0.4	0.4	0.4	0.4
14. *Salmonella*, short-term reactive arthritis	0.9	0.9	0.8	0.8	0.6	0.6	1.0	1.0
15. *Salmonella*, long-term reactive arthritis, flares and remissions with some wellness	601	327	663	360	432	233	574	313
16. *Salmonella*, long-term reactive arthritis, waxes and wanes with no wellness	246	134	353	192	272	147	256	140
17. *Salmonella*, long-term reactive arthritis, chronic and unremitting	246	134	472	257	348	187	256	140
18. Premature mortality	41	23	40	23	38	22	35	20
Total	1,463	794	1,864	1,019	1,293	706	1,298	721

NOTES: Assumes that, in the absence of illness, health status would equal the average for the U.S. population in the same age group. Represents HRQL decrement per case multiplied by duration and by number of new cases averted annually. Detail may not add to total due to rounding.

Although the table reflects the new cases of illness associated with a one-year decrease in exposure, in some cases the effects of the illness are lifelong, and we use discounting to adjust the value of future year impacts. Discounting the long-term impacts at a 3-percent annual rate, rather than at 7 percent, increases the present value of the results as expected. The relatively large difference in the results occurs because the 3-percent rate raises the contribution of the long-term impacts to the total present value; i.e., it discounts future impacts by a smaller amount. The undiscounted results are even larger, ranging from 2,500 to 3,700 QALYs, because the long-term impacts are not discounted to reflect their timing.

For preventable mortality, the estimates vary across indexes because we compare a "with condition" value of zero to the age-specific estimates of average population health, which differ across indexes (see Table A-2). Application of the QWB results in the lowest estimates of average health over time. Hence it also results in the lowest estimates of QALY losses for fatal cases. If we assess preventable mortality without adjusting the life years lost for HRQL, the two fatal cases averted annually lead to the loss of 84 life years undiscounted; 47 years if discounted at 3 percent, or 27 years if discounted at 7 percent.

In Table A-6, we compare the results of the above analysis to the results of our sensitivity analysis, which assumes that the affected individuals would be in perfect or optimal health (a value of 1.0) in the absence of the pathogen-related illness. This comparison overstates the actual impact of the rule because the affected individuals are unlikely to be in optimal health throughout their lifespan in the absence of these exposures. However, we include this perfect health comparison since it is often found in the literature and underlies the original FDA approach. The table includes the results

TABLE A-6 Juice Processing Case Study: Sensitivity Analysis for QALY Losses

Scenario	Discount Rate	Case Study Expert Assessment (median)				FDA QWB Results
		EQ-5D	HUI-3	SF-6D	QWB	
Total QALY losses compared to *average* age-adjusted health	3%	1,463	1,864	1,293	1,298	N/A
	7%	794	1,019	706	721	
Total QALY losses compared to *perfect* health	3%	1,659	2,121	1,563	1,700	
	7%	882	1,136	843	924	888*

N/A = not reported in FDA analysis (FDA, 2001).
*Adds life years lost for fatal cases to FDA's QALY estimate for nonfatal cases.

from FDA's 2001 analysis, which also applied the QWB in comparison to perfect health.

This table indicates that comparison to perfect health increases the estimates of QALYs across the different indexes, as expected. The difference between average health and perfect health rises with age (see Table A-2), and hence has the largest impact on the results for illnesses with lifelong effects. The differences between the median results from the case study's expert assignment using the QWB and the original FDA analysis (also based on the QWB) appear to stem largely from differences in the attributes assigned to the individual health endpoints. The FDA results are, however, within the same general range as the other estimates.

Cost-Effectiveness Ratios

Our final step involved reporting the cost-effectiveness ratios described in the Committee's recommendations (see Chapter 5). We include three of the four recommended ratios because the fourth (comprehensive) ratio is not relevant in this case; the rule does not lead to quantified benefits other than those health risk reductions included in the effectiveness measure.

In these calculations, we use FDA's estimates of annualized regulatory costs and health treatment cost savings. In both cases, FDA applies a discount rate of 7 percent. While we were able to recalculate the estimate of regulatory costs to reflect a 3 percent discount rate, we lacked the data necessary to recalculate the estimates of medical cost savings. Thus we use the same estimates of medical cost savings under both discounting scenarios, which understates these savings under the 3-percent scenario. In addition, the FDA estimates include medical expenditures only and do not include the other types of health treatment cost savings recommended for inclusion in these calculations. Hence the net costs used in these ratios are higher than they would be if we had been able to follow all of the Committee's recommendations.

In Table A-7, we first report the costs per life saved and per life year saved, discounted at 3 and 7 percent. The cost estimate in each of these calculations reflects compliance costs only, including both recurring costs and the annualized value of the initial costs.[14] Medical cost savings are not considered. We then report the health-benefits-only ratio using each of the alternative approaches to estimating QALY losses; in this case, we net out the medical costs savings from the regulatory costs. In all cases, this exhibit

---

[14]Annualization spreads initial costs over the estimated lifetime of the investment, similar to the process of determining loan payments (with an interest rate that equals the discount rate). In this case, we annualized the costs over 20 years.

TABLE A-7 Juice Processing Case Study: Cost-Effectiveness Ratios

	3% Discount Rate				7% Discount Rate			
Averted deaths	2 deaths				2 deaths			
Averted life-year losses	47 years				27 years			
Regulatory compliance costs	$26 million				$28 million			
Compliance cost per fatality averted	$13 million				$14 million			
Compliance cost per life year gained	$560,000				$1.0 million			
	EQ-5D	HUL-3	SF-6D	QWB	EQ-5D	HUL-3	SF-6D	QWB
Averted QALY losses	1,500 QALYs	1,900 QALYs	1,300 QALYs	1,300 QALYs	790 QALYs	1,000 QALYs	700 QALYs	720 QALYs
Regulatory compliance costs, net of health treatment savings	$22.0 million				$23.4 million			
Health-benefits-only ratio	$16,000 per QALY	$13,000 per QALY	$18,000 per QALY	$18,000 per QALY	$29,000 per QALY	$23,000 per QALY	$33,000 per QALY	$32,000 per QALY

NOTES: Reflects new incidence averted by a single year of full implementation of the rule, dollar year not reported. Assumes that, without the pathogen-related illness, health status will be the same as the average for the U.S. population in the same age group. Rounded to two significant figures; calculations are based on unrounded results.

reports QALY losses calculated as a decrement from average population health.

This table indicates that the costs per life saved and per life year saved are relatively high, because this rule averts only two cases of mortality per year. Once we add in the impacts of the nonfatal effects, as well as the associated medical cost savings, the ratios result in much smaller values. In general, the HUI-3 leads to the lowest cost per QALY, and the SF-6D leads to the highest, although the results for the EQ-5D, the SF-6D, and the QWB are very similar. Because a higher discount rate reduces the impact of future year QALY losses, the costs per QALY are higher under a 7 percent discount rate than under the 3-percent rate. All of these ratios would show lower costs per QALY if the results of our sensitivity analysis were used, because the comparison to perfect health increases the estimates of QALY gains.

FDA's QWB results lead to estimates of cost-effectiveness within the same general range. FDA's estimates compare to perfect health and are discounted at 7 percent. If we add the effects of preventable mortality (which FDA excluded from the QALY estimate) to the estimates for nonfatal effects, the result is a value of $26,000 per QALY. This estimate is similar to the cost-effectiveness ratios that result if we use the QALY estimates (from Table A-6) that compare to perfect health discounted at the same rate.

As noted earlier, this analysis does not follow some of the Committee's recommendations. We did not assess the distributional and ethical implications of these regulations in detail, and the FDA analysis provides only limited information on these impacts. An example of the type of information that could be highlighted in such an assessment is provided in Chapter 4 of this report.

In addition, our analysis does not fully address the uncertainty in these estimates, as required under current government-wide guidance (OMB, 2003a) and as recommended by the Committee. Uncertainty is inherent in all the components of the analysis, regardless of whether the assessment is in the form of a CEA or BCA. Further investigation would be needed to determine which aspects of the analysis are most uncertain and to estimate the extent to which such uncertainty varies depending on the HRQL valuation approach used.

We did, however, explore the experts' views on the assessment process in a series of brief phone interviews. The experts noted that the assessment was more difficult in cases for which a single endpoint represented an illness that has changing symptoms over time and that varies in its impacts across patients. In some cases, the experts found that the endpoints were not sufficiently distinguished to allow for level differences on the attribute scales, and the indexes included some attributes that appeared irrelevant or were improperly described for these particular health effects. Several experts thought that asking clinical experts to act as proxies for patients was problematic.

Other sources of uncertainty in our HRQL assessment relate to the indexes themselves. For example, the developers of each index calculated relative health state index values using different population surveys (see Table 3-4), and another set of population surveys were the basis for the Committee's estimates of average age-specific health under each index (see Table A-2). Hence some of the variation in our results may reflect differences in the data sources used rather than solely reflecting differences in the indexes themselves.

Across all of the HRQL approaches, the estimates of the decrements associated with the conditions also may be misstated if a significant portion of those affected are in less good health than the general population, due, for example, to immune system problems. For these individuals, the difference between "with pathogen-related illness" and "without pathogen-related illness" HRQL may be different than assumed in our analysis, and the duration of the condition may also vary.

NHTSA CHILD RESTRAINTS REGULATION

Our second case study addressed an NHTSA regulation requiring anchoring systems for child restraints. We selected this regulation to explore issues related to valuing effects on children as well as alternative approaches for assessing the HRQL impacts of injuries. This case study also provided an example of NHTSA's approach to regulatory analysis, which relies on estimates of ELS to value nonfatal health impacts.

We were unable to use injury data from NHTSA's analysis of the child restraints rule for this case study, however. NHTSA used very broad injury categories that did not provide the descriptive information needed for characterizing HRQL impacts. Because the estimates of the number and types of injuries used in our analysis are quite different from the estimates in the child restraints rule and reflect a high level of uncertainty, the case study results are not comparable to the results of NHTSA's original analysis and we do not present cost-effectiveness ratios.

In this case study, we first applied the EQ-5D and the HUI-2, asking medical experts to match the characteristics of each injury to the relevant attribute levels. We then used data from previously completed research to apply the QWB and the FCI to the same set of injuries.

NHTSA Analysis

We began this case study with a review of the analysis NHTSA completed for its child restraints rule (NHTSA, 1999a,b). This rule requires the use of standardized anchor systems in motor vehicles and on child restraints. In its economic analysis, NHTSA quantified the costs and benefits of both rigid and flexible anchor systems, assessing two regulatory options that represented alternate approaches to complying with the final rule and a third option that it ultimately rejected.

To estimate the benefits of the rule, NHTSA combined data on deaths and injuries to children in seat restraints with data on the impacts of child restraint misuse from several sources, focusing on children ages zero to six. NHTSA made several modifications to these data, first adjusting for the number of injuries that would have occurred in the absence of restraints, then estimating the percent of all injuries associated with restraint misuse and the fraction of this misuse that would be eliminated by the anchor rule. The data on injuries and fatalities were reported by KABCO category, which classifies injuries based on the degree of incapacitation (killed (K), incapacitating injury (A), nonincapacitating injury (B), possible injury (C), and no injury (O)). NHTSA converted the estimates from the KABCO categories to the Abbreviated Injury Scale (AIS), using a standard algorithm that reflects the distribution of all crash-related injuries (not solely injuries to restrained children).

The AIS is a simple numerical system for ranking and comparing the severity of injuries based on the probability that the injury could be fatal. A score of 0 indicates that there were no injuries, whereas a score of 6 indicates that the injury was likely to be immediately fatal; intermediate scores of 1 through 5 indicate injuries of increasing threat to life. When multiple injuries occur, they are scored according to the most life-threatening injury; i.e., the Maximum AIS or MAIS. Examples of the types of injuries that fall into each category are provided in Chapter 2, Table 2-6.

To value these injuries, NHTSA applied its ELS approach, which first involves determining the costs and monetized QALY impacts for nonfatal injuries in each AIS category.[15] See Box 2-4 for a description of the ELS approach. These monetary estimates are converted to ELS fractions by dividing the value for each injury category by the value of a fatality (estimated by NHTSA as roughly $3 million). These fractions are then multiplied by the number of injuries averted in each category and added to the number of fatalities, to determine the total ELS value for each regulatory option. The ELS values for each AIS category are calculated periodically based on data for all types of crashes nationally, then applied across the

---

[15]The QALY losses are based on an index adapted especially for crash-related injuries (Miller et al., 1991), rather than on one of the generic indexes used elsewhere in this case study.

subsequent regulatory analyses.[16] More information on this approach is provided in Chapter 2.

For the child restraints rule, the results imply that, on average, 58 injuries were equivalent to one fatality, given the severity of the injuries produced by NHTSA's standard conversion formula. The results for each of the options assessed are reported in Table A-8 below; the table suggests that the regulatory options considered led to almost identical ranges of benefits.

NHTSA determined that the national costs of the final rule were most likely to average $152 million annually (in 1996 dollars), with a range from $123 to $167 million. This best estimate reflects the less expensive of the two implementation options (a nonrigid restraint attachment and rigid vehicle anchor). The alternative option permitted (both rigid) was estimated to cost $217 to $256 million annually, while the rejected approach (both nonrigid) was between these two estimates, at $149 to $196 million per year.

NHTSA then calculated the cost-effectiveness of the final rule by dividing the compliance costs by the ELS estimates reported in Table A-8. The results indicated that the costs per ELS ranged from $1.5 to $2.7 million, without discounting. NHTSA also presented several sensitivity analyses, including several that discounted the estimates of equivalent fatalities at different rates. (This discounting reflects the fact that the costs of the rule would be incurred in the year in which the vehicle or car restraint is purchased, while the benefits accrue over the several-year period for which the vehicle or car restraint is used.) At the time that the analysis was completed, OMB recommended application of a 7-percent discount rate, which led to a cost per ELS ranging from $2.1 to $3.7 million.

In this analysis, NHTSA did not report a total dollar value for all of the injuries and fatalities averted by the rule, and hence did not calculate net benefits (benefits minus costs). In more recent analyses, NHTSA has used its estimates of the dollar value of injuries and fatalities in each AIS category (including expenditures and monetized QALY impacts) in both BCA and CEA to determine net benefits as well as cost-effectiveness.

Case Study Analytic Approach

For this case study, the analysis of QALY impacts was more complicated than in the FDA analysis. Our first step involved identifying a readily accessible source of more detailed injury descriptions that could be valued

---

[16]The data used in the child restraints rule were derived from NHTSA's report on 1994 crashes; NHTSA is now using updated values for the year 2000 (NHTSA, 1996, 2002a).

TABLE A-8 NHTSA Estimates of Annual Quantified Benefits

Type of Anchor	Endpoint	Avoided Incidence (cases/year)	Equivalent Fatalities (undiscounted)
Options permitted in final rule:			
Rigid restraint attachment/	Lives saved	36–47	36–47
Rigid vehicle anchor	Injuries prevented	1,231–2,893	21–50
	Total	N/A	57–97
Nonrigid restraint attachment/	Lives saved	36–50	36–50
Rigid vehicle anchor	Injuries prevented	1,235–2,929	21–50
	Total	N/A	57–101
Option not permitted in final rule:			
Nonrigid restraint attachment/	Lives saved	36–50	36–50
Nonrigid vehicle anchor	Injuries prevented	1,235–2,929	21–50
	Total	N/A	57–101

NOTE: Detail does not add to total due to rounding.

SOURCE: NHTSA (1999a), p. i, Table S-1, p. 49, Table 17.

using generic HRQL indexes. Based on advice from NHTSA staff, we relied on data from the agency's National Automotive Sampling System, Crashworthiness Data System (NASS-CDS) for the years 1999–2003. While this system includes data on thousands of crash victims, only 22 of the sampled cases involved injuries to children in child restraints. These sample cases represent roughly 1,752 cases nationwide (including 160 that are immediately fatal); however, NHTSA staff caution that the standard error associated with extrapolating from this small number of sample cases is quite large. As a result, we did not adjust our estimates for comparability with the estimates of cases averted for the different injury classes in the NHTSA child restraints analysis. (The regulation was not expected to prevent all injuries to restrained children, even after all vehicles and restraints in use are equipped with the anchors.)

The injuries reported for these 22 cases are provided in Table A-9 below. For each case, the table indicates the sample weight, or multiplier, that is applied to the sample values to extrapolate to the national population. In addition, the exhibit indicates the status of the child immediately after the accident and lists the individual injuries incurred. The final column reports the AIS classification for the case; the MAIS for cases with multiple injuries is marked with an asterisk (*).[17]

---

[17]Cases with injuries in AIS categories 0 or 1 only were excluded from this analysis because they are not expected to noticeably impact HRQL.

TABLE A-9 Child Restraints Case Study: Injuries to Restrained Children, Ages 0–6, 1999–2003

Case Number	Weighting Factor	Injury Description	MAIS
1	21.29	Nonfatal (hospitalized) a. Blunt, traumatic abdominal injury b. Vault skull fracture NFS*	2
2	54.34	Fatal a. Humerous fracture open/displaced/comminuted b. Vault skull fracture comminuted	3
3	18.81	Nonfatal (hospitalized) a. Cerebrum contusions—multiple NFS* b. Cerebrum subarachnoid hemorrhage c. Vault skull fracture closed	3
4	411.33	Nonfatal (hospitalized) a. Vault skull fracture NFS	2
5	85.65	Fatal a. Head crush b. Lung contusion bilateral with or without hemo-/pneumothorax c. Rib cage fracture >3 ribs on one side and <4 ribs on either side d. Tibia fracture NFS	6
6	3.41	Fatal a. Brain stem injury involving hemorrhage b. Vault skull fracture complex (open with loss of brain tissue) c. Cerebrum hematoma/hemorrhage NFS—extra axial d. Cerebrum hematoma/hemorrhage subdural NFS e. Subclavian vein laceration NFS f. Cerebrum subarachnoid hemorrhage g. Vault skull fracture comminuted	5
7	124.43	Nonfatal (hospitalized) a. Cerebrum hematoma/hemorrhage epidural or extradural small bilateral* b. Vault skull fracture complex (open with loss of brain tissue) c. Cerebrum hematoma/hemorrhage subdural small d. Unconscious post resuscitation on admission or initial observation at scene (GCS <9), appropriate movements with painful stimuli no matter e. Cerebrum contusion multiple, at least one on each side small f. Cerebrum subarachnoid hemorrhage	5
8	8.39	Nonfatal (transported and released) a. Lethargic, stuporous, obtunded post resuscitation on admission or initial observation at scene (GCS 9-14) NFS	2

continues

TABLE A-9 Continued

Case Number	Weighting Factor	Injury Description	MAIS
9	50.12	Nonfatal (hospitalized) a. Unconscious post resuscitation on admission or initial observation at scene (GCS <9), inappropriate movements no matter length of unconsciousness* b. Lung contusion bilateral with or without hemo-/pneumothorax c. Cervical spine cord contusion incomplete cord syndrome with dislocation d. Spleen laceration moderate (OIS Grade III)	5
10	8.24	Nonfatal (transported and released) a. Tibia fracture shaft	2
11	37.29	Nonfatal (hospitalized) a. Cerebrum contusion single small* b. Orbit fracture open/displaced/comminuted c. Vault skull fracture closed	3
12	75.56	Nonfatal (hospitalized) a. Awake post resuscitation on admission or initial observation at scene (GCS 15), prior unconsciousness, but length of time NFS	2
13	16.03	Fatal a. Cerebrum hematoma/hemorrhage epidural or extradural small b. Cerebrum hematoma/hemorrhage subdural small c. Cerebrum brain swelling/edema NFS d. Cerebrum subarachnoid hemorrhage e. Base (basilar) skull fracture NFS f. Vault skull fracture comminuted g. Vault skull fracture closed	4
14	145.31	Nonfatal (transported and released) a. Leg or ankle fracture NFS	2
15	1	Nonfatal (hospitalized) a. Clavicle fracture (OIS Grade I or II)	2
16	128.9	Nonfatal (hospitalized) a. Unconscious post resuscitation on admission or initial observation at scene (GCS <9) appropriate movements with painful stimuli no matter* b. Cerebrum subarachnoid hemorrhage	4
17	61.87	Nonfatal (transported and released) a. Clavicle fracture (OIS Grade I or II)	2
18	85.65	Nonfatal (hospitalized) a. Base (basilar) skull fracture NFS* b. Orbit fracture NFS	3
19	1	Fatal a. Thoracic spine cord laceration incomplete cord syndrome with fracture	5

continues

TABLE A-9 Continued

Case Number	Weighting Factor	Injury Description	MAIS
		b. Lung contusion bilateral with or without hemo-/pneumothorax	
		c. Cerebrum hematoma/hemorrhage subdural NFS	
		c. Jejunum-ileum laceration perforation (OIS Grade III)	
		f. Cerebrum subarachnoid hemorrhage	
		g. Cervical spine dislocation	
		h. Humerus fracture NFS	
20	7.75	Nonfatal (hospitalized)	3
		a. Femur fracture NFS*	
		b. Pelvis fracture NFS	
21	382.64	Nonfatal (hospitalized)	2
		a. Maxilla fracture NFS	
22	23.03	Nonfatal (hospitalized)	
		a. Awake post resuscitation on admission or initial observation at scene (GCS 15) amnesia	2

NOTES: Injury descriptions are transferred verbatim from the NHTSA file without editing.
NFS = Not further specified; GCS = Glasgow Coma Scale; OIS = Organ Injury Score.
*indicates MAIS injury for multiple injury cases that are not immediately fatal.
Case 11 included two MAIS 2 injuries; we identify the first (injury 11a) as the MAIS because it generally results in larger HRQL decrements.

SOURCE: NASS-CDS data provided by Jim Simons, NHTSA, December 7, 2004.

The NASS-CDS data did not include information on the duration of the injury or on life expectancy (NHTSA, 2002b). We estimated duration using the same data sources as used to assess HRQL, as described below. To estimate life expectancy without the injury or fatality, we used conditional survival rates, similar to the approach NHTSA uses in its ELS assessment.[18] For the case study, we relied on data on average U.S. mortality rates for each year of life from detailed life tables (CDC, 2002), and calculated the probability of surviving to each year of age conditional on having survived to the previous age. With the exception of the five immediately fatal cases and two of the 17 nonfatal sampled cases, the injuries were not expected to affect life expectancy. For the traumatic brain injury in case 7, we used data from Harrison-Felix et al. (2004) to assess the reduction in life expectancy; for the spinal cord injury in case 9, we relied on data from Frankel et al. (1998).

---

[18]Conditional survival rates take this form: conditional survival rate for current year = survival rate for prior year * (1 − current year death rate).

In completing the analysis, we applied some simplifying assumptions due to data and time constraints. First, we assumed that the average age of the affected children was 3 years, and that they reflected the same gender distribution as the general population of the same age. Although injuries to a newborn could have quite different effects than would the same injury for a 3- or 6-year-old, the sources used in our analysis did not provide information on age-related HRQL differences for young children. Second, we treated these injuries as if they all occurred in a single year, rather than spread out over a 5-year period. We used discounting only to reflect the time value of averting the future year HRQL impacts associated with an injury that occurs in the current year; we did not discount the different years of incidence in the NASS-CDS data set.

Our assessment of HRQL impacts involved the use of four generic indexes. For two of these indexes, the EQ-5D and the HUI-2, we asked five medical experts to match the characteristics of each injury to the relevant index attributes, following a process similar to that applied in the FDA case study. We also asked the experts to assess duration, breaking each case into three time periods: the acute, rehabilitation, and long-term phases. We requested that they assess each injury separately and assess the combined effects of all injuries for each of the multiple injury cases.

For the other two indexes, we used values from previously completed research. For the QWB, we relied on data provided by Troy Holbrook of the University of California, San Diego. Holbrook's team used patient self-assessments to determine the attributes associated with various injuries, for individuals age 18 or older (Holbrook et al., 1999).[19] The resulting HRQL estimates are available by body region and injury severity (based on the six major AIS categories) for four time periods: predischarge, and at 6, 12, and 18 months. We matched these data with the body regions and AIS scores for each injury in our data set, focusing on the injury identified as the MAIS in multiple injury cases. We applied the Holbrook predischarge values to the hospitalization period, then applied the 6-month values from discharge (or injury date, if not hospitalized) to 6 months, the 12-month values from 6 to 12 months, and the 18-month values from 12 months through the remaining lifespan.

The fourth index used was the FCI, which is currently being developed (with NHTSA support) to measure the impacts of nonfatal injuries on functional status. It differs from the other indexes in that it is not intended to reflect all aspects of HRQL. Furthermore, it is not yet widely validated or

---

[19]Holbrook also provided adolescent data, but we used the adult values because of the small size of the adolescent sample. Comparison of the adolescent and adult values showed a lower "with injury" HRQL for adults, as expected, given that adolescents are likely to be in better health, on average, absent injury.

used. Ellen MacKenzie of Johns Hopkins University provided predicted 12-month FCI scores based on the AIS descriptions for each injury contained in our database. For most of the nonfatal injuries, the scores indicated that the individual would have returned to normal functioning at the 12-month mark; functional limitations persisted in only 5 of the 17 sampled cases with nonfatal injuries. MacKenzie reported FCI values for each individual injury in each of these five cases. Values for multiple injury cases were based on the worst score in each domain across all of the injuries incurred.

Because the FCI only provides 12-month scores at this point in its development, we did not use it to assess lifetime impacts. Instead, we compared the 12-month FCI values to the values for the same time under the EQ-5D, HUI-2, and QWB. For each index, we use the "with injury" values that reflect comparison to perfect health (a value of 1.0), because average population values were not available for the FCI.

Estimates of QALY Gains

The first step in applying the above indexes involved determining HRQL with the injuries. As discussed above, for the EQ-5D and HUI-2 we asked medical experts to determine the duration and attribute descriptions that best matched the likely impacts of each of the injuries listed in Table A-9. To better understand the variability in these estimates, the Committee commissioned a statistical analysis of the expert ratings to determine the extent of agreement both within and across the different indexes (Mason, 2005). The results indicated that, while the experts differed in the attributes they selected, the extent of these differences was not significantly affected by which index was used. The major differences in the results were due to the varying estimates of duration rather than to the differences in the estimates of HRQL in each injury phase.

For the QWB, the attribute data were provided by adult patients and reflected all aspects of their health, not simply the effects of the injury. Inspection of the resulting HRQL estimates suggests that the QWB results appear more uniform across cases than the estimates using the other indexes. At least some of this difference results from disparities in the data sources; for example, the QWB data set includes injury cases that may vary less in severity than the NASS-CDS cases assessed by the experts (e.g., it includes only hospitalized patients), and it used a more aggregated categorization scheme (i.e., classification by body part and AIS rather than by individual injury).

The next step in the analysis involved estimating the QALY losses that could be avoided if all of these injuries were averted by a hypothetical regulation. This step included (1) determining the decrement from "without condition" health for each phase of each injury; (2) multiplying the decrement by duration and summing across the phases for each injury to estimate QALY losses; and (3) multiplying these per case values by the sample from Table A-9.

Table A-10 provides the resulting estimates of total QALY losses for the EQ-5D, HUI-2, and QWB, assuming that normal health (in the absence of the injury) would equal average population health for an individual of the same age, and applying both 7 and 3 percent discount rates. Undiscounted, the results range from 21,000 to 27,000 QALYs. If we consider only the

TABLE A-10 Child Restraints Case Study: QALY Losses, All Cases

Case Number	Mais	Case Study Expert Assessment (median)				Holbrook QWB Patient Data (median)	
		EQ-5D		HUI-2			
		3% Discount Rate	7% Discount Rate	3% Discount Rate	7% Discount Rate	3% Discount Rate	7% Discount Rate
1	2	1.6	1.6	2.2	2.2	98	53
2	3 (fatal)	1,517	783	1,511	780	1,421	748
3	3	105	55	47	25	91	50
4	2	7.5	7.5	11	11	1,886	1,027
5	6 (fatal)	2,392	1,235	2,381	1,230	2,240	1,180
6	5 (fatal)	95	49	95	49	89	47
7	5	2,437	1,237	2,178	1,100	556	269
8	2	18	9.6	15	7.7	38	21
9	5	925	458	881	432	277	119
10	2	0.3	0.3	0.3	0.3	41	22
11	3	172	89	46	25	181	99
12	2	0.002	0.002	0.1	0.1	347	189
13	4 (fatal)	448	231	446	230	419	221
14	2	6.3	6.3	5.0	5.0	724	393
15	2	0.03	0.03	0.02	0.02	4.1	2.3
16	4	824	431	650	341	543	299
17	2	2.0	2.0	1.1	1.1	256	140
18	3	2.6	2.6	1.4	1.4	416	226
19	5 (fatal)	28	14	28	14	26	14
20	3	1.2	1.2	1.1	1.1	44	24
21	2	15	15	5.5	5.5	1,431	791
22	2	0.00	0.00	0.00	0.00	106	58
	Total	8,998	4,629	8,305	4,263	11,236	5,992

NOTES: Assumes that, in the absence of injury, health status would equal the average for the U.S. population in the same age group. Represents HRQL decrement per case for each phase multiplied by duration and sample weight. Detail may not add to total due to rounding.

160 cases nationally that are immediately fatal, the life-year losses (unadjusted for HRQL) total 12,000 life years undiscounted; 4,800 years if discounted at 3 percent, or 2,400 years if discounted at 7 percent.

The table indicates that the QALY losses for each endpoint vary in the extent to which they are similar across the three indexes; the QWB results in the largest estimates of total losses, followed by the EQ-5D and then the HUI-2. Not surprisingly, the largest values are generally associated with those fatal cases and severe injuries with the largest sample weights, reflecting their comparatively high per-case values and the number of cases represented nationally.[20] However, under the QWB, some of the more minor (e.g., MAIS 2) injuries also have relatively large values, reflecting the lower variability of the QWB estimates, which are magnified in cases where the sample is large. Several cases have very small values, usually because they reflect injuries with only short-term impacts. The cases with values of 0 represent those where the experts believed that any impairments would not be noticeable, given the attribute definitions used under the relevant index.

Discounting the long-term impacts at a 3-percent rate, rather than at 7 percent, increases the present value of the totals, as expected. It does not affect the values for the short-term effects because we did not discount the first-year values. Larger differences occur for the long-term impacts because the 3 percent rate increases the contribution of future year effects to the total present value.

Our sensitivity analysis, presented in Table A-11, indicates that comparison to perfect health (a value of 1.0) rather than average health increases the estimates of QALY losses across the different approaches, as expected. This difference is moderated, however, by the fact that we assume that HRQL is 1.0 for the young children considered in this analysis under both the average health and perfect health scenarios. Average HRQL decreases with age (see Table A-2) and hence has the largest impact on the results for those injuries that have lifelong effects. The difference between the average and perfect health results is larger under the QWB because the sensitivity analysis does not include adjustment for the use of adult values, which include decrements unrelated to the injury. In contrast, the expert assignment approach used with the EQ-5D and HUI-2 reflects injuries to children. The results for individual endpoints show similar patterns to the results reported in Table A-10 and continue to be dominated largely by those fatal and severe cases with the highest sample weights.

---

[20]For one injury (case 9, a severe spinal cord injury), the attribute assignments lead to a negative HRQL value under the EQ-5D. As discussed in the FDA case study, multiplying this negative value by duration leads to a undiscounted QALY estimate that exceeds the actual duration of the effect.

TABLE A-11 Child Restraints Case Study: Sensitivity Analysis for QALY Losses

Scenario	Discount Rate	Case Study Expert Assessment (median)		Holbrook QWB Results (median)
		EQ-5D	HUI-2	
Total QALY losses compared to *average* age-adjusted health	3%	8,998	8,305	11,236
	7%	4,629	4,263	5,992
Total QALY losses compared to *perfect* health	3%	9,717	9,040	19,862
	7%	4,832	4,469	9,822

Because of the data limitations discussed earlier, for the FCI we compare the 12-month values to the 12-month values for the other three indexes, rather than using it to assess lifetime effects. We focus on the five cases with injuries that were identified (by MacKenzie) as affecting functioning at the 12-month mark.[21] (Under the FCI, the remaining 12 nonfatal injury cases are expected to result in full recovery by this time.) The results of the comparison are provided in Table A-12, based on the perfect health scenario for consistency with the FCI estimates.

The estimates vary in the extent to which they appear consistent across indexes, due to differences between the indexes themselves as well as in the data sources and methods used in the analyses. For example, the characterization of injuries according to the FCI resulted from a more extensive and collaborative expert process than used by case study team for the EQ-5D and HUI-2. The FCI and QWB estimates are based on injuries to adults, while the EQ-5D and HUI-2 attribute assignments reflect injuries to children. In addition, the QWB patient assessments do not separate the impact of these injuries from other factors affecting HRQL, and the data are reported for broad injury categories. For all indexes, the estimates used reflect values for adults rather than children.

As noted earlier, we did not compare these results to the results of NHTSA's regulatory analysis because our estimates of the numbers and types of injuries differ significantly from the data used to support the rule

---

[21]The median results from the expert assessment suggest that six cases would have long-term HRQL effects: the five in Table A-12 plus case number 8.

TABLE A-12 Child Restraints Case Study: HRQL with Injury, 12 Months after Injury

IOM Case Number	MAIS	HRQL with Injury at 12 Months			
		FCI	EQ-5D	HUI-2	QWB
3	3	0.86	0.80	0.91	0.68
7	5	0.66	0.32	0.39	0.71
9	5	0.60	0.39	0.42	0.71
10	2	0.92	1.00	1.00	0.67
16	4	0.68	0.77	0.82	0.70

NOTES: With-illness values assumed to reflect comparison to perfect health. FCI, EQ-5D, and HUI estimates include only the impact of the injuries; QWB estimates include all aspects of health. FCI and QWB based on injuries to adults, EQ-5D and HUI-2 reflect injuries to children. Includes only those nonfatal cases with FCI estimates less than 1.0 at 12 months.

SOURCES: Case study team analysis of data from the following sources: FCI: Ellen MacKenzie, February 2 and March 16, 2005. QWB: Troy Holbrook, January 21, 2005. EQ-5D and HUI-2: Expert assignment, December 2004 to January 2005.

and reflect a very high degree of uncertainty. We were unable to investigate the reasons for the differences between our estimates and those used in the NHTSA analysis, and hence did not attempt to adjust our data to better reflect the rule's likely impacts.

Similar to the FDA case study, the Committee did not conduct a detailed assessment of the distributional and ethical implications of these findings, nor did we formally address the uncertainty in the estimates. However, we believe that one of the major sources of uncertainty in this case study relates to the use of adult health state index values for children. While the use of adult values is often necessitated by limitations in the available data, it raises difficult practical and ethical questions as discussed in more detail in the main text of this report.

We also discussed the attribute assignment process with the experts involved in this case study, who indicated that it was difficult and time consuming due to need to assess a large number of injuries. Estimating duration was particularly challenging. The experts' experience with this task suggests that it may be preferable to use estimates from the research literature (similar to the approach used in the other case studies), or to ask the experts to assess HRQL at prespecified intervals (e.g., at 3, 6, 12, and 18 months postinjury). In addition, the experts received relatively little descriptive information and indicated that more information on the injuries would have been helpful. They also observed that medical specialization affects how one classifies health impacts; a larger and more broadly representative panel would have been desirable.

The experts' comments on the domains and attribute scales used in the different indexes were similar to those raised in the FDA case study, but the problems appeared to be exacerbated by the need to apply the indexes to children. The experts noted that the attribute scales do not provide enough variation within each domain to describe some injuries adequately. In addition, the scales are not always applicable to young children, who are not likely to engage in some of the activities described. Finally, the experts indicated that using these indexes to assess the long-term effects of injuries incurred in childhood is particularly difficult.

EPA NONROAD ENGINE AIR EMISSIONS REGULATION

The third case study was based on an EPA regulation establishing air emissions standards for nonroad engines as well as standards for diesel fuel. This regulation enabled the Committee to explore issues related to valuing the effects of chronic illness and preventable mortality. In addition, it provided insights into the data and methods EPA uses in its analysis of air pollution rules, which account for a sizable fraction of the regulations likely to be affected by the Committee's recommendations. This case study also provided an example of a rule with quantified nonhealth (visibility) benefits, as well as significant health and environmental benefits that could not be quantified.

In this case study, we considered a subset of the cardiovascular and respiratory effects included in EPA's analysis, focusing on those endpoints that account for the majority of the monetized benefits of the rule: preventable mortality, chronic bronchitis, and cardiac disease following nonfatal acute myocardial infarction (AMI). For simplicity, we omitted the less significant endpoints from our comparison of HRQL approaches. While these other endpoints involve short-lived events and exacerbations of preexisting illnesses that pose a number of conceptual and analytic challenges, evaluation of their HRQL impacts may be desirable within the framework of a regulatory CEA.

We used three approaches to estimate QALY losses in this case: (1) asking clinical experts to assign EQ-5D attributes; (2) applying EQ-5D index values based on statistical analysis of MEPS data; and (3) transferring estimates from selected studies in the CEA Registry. The approaches vary only in the valuation of nonfatal effects. Under all three approaches, we use identical values for averted mortality, comparing a "with condition" value of zero to the EQ-5D index value that would be otherwise expected at each age over the remaining lifespan.

EPA Analysis

The foundation of our case study was the analysis supporting EPA's final nonroad diesel rule (EPA, 2004a,b). EPA's BCA quantified the impact of reduced fine particulate matter (PM) emissions on a number of respiratory and cardiovascular health effects as well as preventable mortality. To predict cases averted and assess benefit values, EPA relied on its BenMAP model (http://www.epa.gov/ttn/ecas/benmodels.html), which it developed to support a wide range of air pollution rules. This model combines estimates from selected epidemiological studies with detailed data on population characteristics and emissions changes to provide both summary and disaggregate estimates of impacts. It also supports probabilistic analysis of uncertainty.

To value averted cases of mortality, EPA applied a range of estimates of the value of statistical life, with a mean of $5.5 million. EPA adjusted these estimates to reflect the effects of real income growth over time and the lag between exposure reduction and reduction in mortality rates. For chronic bronchitis and restricted activity days, EPA adapted dollar values from stated preference studies of individual WTP. For other nonfatal effects, EPA relied on data on the medical costs of illness and lost earnings due to the lack of suitable WTP estimates. EPA also used WTP estimates to value changes in visibility at selected recreational areas.

EPA's primary estimates of health and other impacts are provided in Table A-13. The table reports annual impacts as of the year 2030, when virtually all engines in use are expected to meet the standards. As indicated by the table, EPA estimates that annual monetized benefits will total $80 billion or $83 billion, depending on which discount rate is used.[22] The dollar value of these benefits is determined largely by the impact of averted mortality, which represents over 90 percent of the monetized effects.[23]

EPA's cost analysis addressed the short- and long-term impacts of the rule on the costs of producing and operating engines of various types as well as refining and distributing fuel. EPA then used a multimarket model to assess the economic impacts of these cost changes. The results indicated that the social welfare costs of the final rule would total approximately $2.0 billion annually as of 2030.

---

[22]Although the estimates presented in the table are for a single year of the regulatory intervention, discounting is used to adjust some of the monetary values to better reflect the timing of the impacts (e.g., the lag between exposure reduction and reduction in incidence).

[23]These estimates are for the final rule; EPA did not quantify the cases averted or other impacts for alternative regulatory options in this analysis.

TABLE A-13 EPA Estimates of Annual Quantified Benefits

Endpoint	Avoided Incidence (cases/year)	Monetary Value (in millions)
Premature mortality: Long-term exposure (adults, 30 and over)	12,000	$72,000–$77,000
Infant mortality (infants, under one year)	22	$150
Chronic bronchitis (adults, 26 and over)	5,600	$2,400
Nonfatal myocardial infarctions (adults, 18 and older)	15,000	$1,200
Hospital admissions—Respiratory (adults, 20 and older)	5,100	$92
Hospital admissions—Cardiovascular (adults, 20 and older)	3,800	$83
Emergency room visits for asthma (18 and younger)	6,000	$1.7
Acute bronchitis (children, 8–12)	13,000	$5.2
Asthma exacerbations (asthmatic children, 6–18)	200,000	$9.2
Lower respiratory symptoms (children, 7–14)	160,000	$2.7
Upper respiratory symptoms (asthmatic children, 9–11)	120,000	$3.2
Work loss days (adults, 18–65)	1,000,000	$130
Minor restricted activity days (adults, 18–65)	5,900,000	$320
Recreational visibility impairment (86 areas)	N/A	$1,700
Total	N/A	$80,000–$83,000

NOTES: Primary estimates for the year 2030; excludes nonmonetized health and welfare benefits and EPA's analyses of uncertainty. 2000 dollars, ranges reflect results discounted at 3 and 7 percent.

EPA reports all figures rounded to two significant digits; detail does not add to total due to rounding. Respiratory hospital admissions for PM include admissions for chronic obstructive pulmonary disease, pneumonia, and asthma. Cardiovascular hospital admissions for PM include total cardiovascular admissions and admissions subcategories for ischemic heart disease, dysrhythmias, and heart failure, excluding myocardial infarction to avoid double-counting.

SOURCE: EPA (2004b, pp. 39134–39135, Tables VI.E-1 and VI.E-2).

The monetized net benefits (benefits minus costs) of the final rule will thus total approximately $78 to $81 billion annually as of 2030, depending on the discount rate used. EPA accompanied these estimates with a discussion of the distribution of the impacts as well as quantified analyses of different sources of uncertainty. Because EPA was not able to quantify a number of other health and ecological benefits associated with reductions in a variety of pollutants, EPA concluded that the monetized benefits may significantly understate the total benefits of the regulations.

Case Study Analytic Approach

This case study follows the same general approach as the other case studies. We began by developing disease descriptions, relying primarily on EPA's regulatory impact analysis and the epidemiological studies EPA used in its risk assessment (Pope et al., 2002, for preventable mortality; Abbey et al., 1995, for chronic bronchitis; and Peters et al., 2001, for nonfatal AMI). As needed, we supplemented these data with information from a 2004 CEA of a one-microgram reduction in PM prepared by Bryan Hubbell of EPA (which EPA subsequently updated and applied in its Clean Air Interstate Rule (EPA, 2005), as discussed in Chapter 2). While the Hubbell analysis considered a different reduction in pollution levels and used population data for a different year (2000 rather than 2030) than used in the nonroad rule analysis, it reflects the same underlying risk studies and the same general modeling approach.

We used the descriptions from the EPA data sources directly in the case study approaches that relied on existing research; i.e., the MEPS-based EQ-5D and the transfer of values from the Harvard Registry. The expert assignment approach required more detailed condition descriptions. For chronic bronchitis, we described three severity categories and instructed the experts to assume that the patient is in middle age. In our calculations, we assumed the chronic bronchitis would last for the remainder of the affected individuals' lifespan but did not consider its effects on life expectancy nor model the likely worsening of symptoms over time.[24] Our assessment of life expectancy used conditional survival rates as in the NHTSA case study, similar to the approach used in Hubbell (2004) and other EPA analyses.

For AMI, the development of disease descriptions for the expert assignment process was more complicated. First, to assess the likelihood that AMI survivors would develop angina and/or congestive heart failure, we used the approach in Hubbell (2004), which assumed that 10.2 percent of survivors would experience congestive heart failure and angina, 9.8 percent would experience congestive heart failure without angina, 40.8 percent would experience angina only, and 39.2 percent would experience neither congestive heart failure or angina. We then split the cases in each of these categories into severity classes and further subdivided them by whether the age at incidence was above or below 65 years. These steps resulted in 22 subcategories for the post-AMI progression of heart disease.

For these post-AMI disease states, we assumed that cardiac disease would last for the remainder of the affected individuals' lifespan and again

---

[24]Hubbell (2004) assessed reduced life expectancy associated with chronic bronchitis based on data on the effects of all chronic lower respiratory disease. We did not make this adjustment in the case study.

did not model the likely worsening of symptoms over time. We did, however, consider the effects of cardiac disease on life expectancy. We adjusted the population average conditional survival rates using different factors for AMI cases with and without congestive heart failure. Consistent with Hubbell (2004) and EPA's 2004 regulatory analysis, we assumed that the years lost to preventable mortality from cardiac disease were included in the separate estimates of fatal cases and (to avoid double-counting) did not assess them as part of the cardiac disease scenario. Hence the reduction in HRQL associated with the nonfatal endpoints is assessed only for the affected individuals' remaining lifespans.

For mortality, no disease descriptions were needed because "with condition" HRQL is zero in all cases. However, assessing PM-related mortality requires addressing a number of other issues. A key question raised in EPA's analysis is whether the affected individuals would have had the same remaining lifespan as the general population in the absence of the pollution. This issue has been the subject of some debate; however, EPA generally assumes that the distribution of underlying conditions is the same as for the overall population of the same age. (Exposure to PM most affects the risk of death among elderly individuals—age 74 on average, and there is a high prevalence of preexisting heart disease and other illnesses among the general population at this age.) EPA also adjusts for the time lag between pollution reductions and reductions in mortality among the adult population; this adjustment is not made in assessing infant mortality. In general, we followed the same base case assumptions as used in EPA's primary benefits estimates but do not replicate the sensitivity analyses that EPA reports.

Once we had developed the descriptive information needed for the assessment of each endpoint, we implemented three approaches for estimating "with condition" HRQL. Our first approach, expert assignment, was similar to that used in the FDA and NHTSA case studies. For the EPA study, we asked two groups of experts (six respiratory disease specialists and five cardiologists) to apply the EQ-5D attributes to those endpoints related to their area of specialization.

In the second approach, we applied preliminary estimates of HRQL decrements from a recently developed catalogue of EQ-5D values. This catalogue has since been published by Patrick Sullivan and colleagues (2005) and used a population survey (MEPS) to develop EQ-5D for a number of chronic conditions. (The catalogue is described in Chapter 3.) The researchers first calculated EQ-5D index values for those respondents reporting each condition, then used regression analysis to determine the marginal impact of the condition of interest alone, separating out the effects of any comorbidities. We used preliminary estimates of these marginal decrements in our analysis for chronic bronchitis, AMI, angina pectoris, and heart failure, based on data provided by Sullivan for each condition (reported by three-digit International Classification of Disease Version 9 (ICD-9) code), and combined the decrements as needed to reflect each of the health endpoints assessed. These preliminary estimates differ from the updated estimates provided in the published study.

The third approach involved the transfer of estimates from studies selected from the CEA Registry, based on a review conducted by Brauer and Neumann (2005). Brauer and Neumann identified 127 respiratory and cardiovascular health states with index values in the database, focusing on studies published after 1994. They identified those estimates most suitable for application to this case study based on the similarity of the health state and appropriateness of the methodology, as discussed in Chapter 3.

Based on our review of these studies, we identified two that appeared to provide the most suitable estimates for this case study. For chronic bronchitis, we used a Canadian study that compared alternative medications and applied the HUI-3 to develop one-year average HRQL values covering both chronic and acute phases of the condition (Torrance et al., 1999). For post-AMI health states, we used a Dutch study (Oostenbrink et al., 2001) that employed the EQ-5D to estimate HRQL in patients after infrainguinal bypass surgery. This study included HRQL estimates for a subset of patients who suffered an AMI during the follow-up period.[25]

The two studies selected from the CEA Registry use different indexes, raising questions about the appropriate index to use for preventable mortality. It was difficult to find a justification for using either the EQ-5D (consistent with the AMI study) or the HUI-3 (consistent with the chronic bronchitis study), or for averaging the results under each index to establish "without condition" HRQL. For simplicity and comparability, we applied the same EQ-5D estimates to assess mortality for the CEA Registry analysis as in the other two HRQL approaches used in this case study.

Estimates of QALY Gains

The three approaches applied in this case study addressed different respiratory and cardiovascular endpoints broken out in different ways. Our expert assignment approach used 25 subcategories characterized by severity and symptoms; our application of the MEPS-based catalogue used four ICD codes (one for chronic bronchitis and three for cardiac disease) in

---

[25]Although we considered using different estimates for cases with and without congestive heart failure or angina (as in the expert assignment and application of values from the MEPS catalogue), we were unable to find an internally consistent set of index values that addressed all of the combinations of the conditions of interest.

various combinations; and our benefits transfer from the CEA Registry studies used one estimate for chronic bronchitis and one estimate for all post-AMI conditions.

In the expert assignment, we found that the results did not always vary across the severity categories. The EQ-5D allows a choice of three attribute levels within each domain. In some cases, individual experts assigned the same attribute levels to cases of differing severities. The assignments also indicated that the experts disagreed about whether certain conditions would impose no, moderate, or severe problems in a particular domain. Where the estimates varied across endpoints, they generally followed the expected pattern, showing increasing problems for cases with increasing severity. Mild cases resulted in median HRQL values close to 1.0, indicating a negligible effect on the quality of life. In contrast, the most severe form of congestive heart failure led to HRQL values close to zero, with median estimates of 0.05 or less. In general, the median values were identical for the two age groups specified in the AMI scenarios (those above and below 65 years).

The QALY estimates varied across the three approaches. In Table A-14, we provide the results for the average age at incidence under each approach, in comparison to both average and perfect health. (The adjustments made in these comparisons are described in the "General Approach" section, above.) While these adjustments seem sensible within the context of each approach, they lead to inconsistencies in the relationships across the results.

As illustrated by the table, for the expert assessment, the "with condition" values (and the decrement from normal health) are consistently lower under the average health scenario than under the perfect health scenario; we applied the same percentage reduction to a lower value (average "without condition" HRQL is less than perfect HRQL). For the MEPS-based EQ-5D catalogue, the "with condition" values are the same under both scenarios, but the decrement is larger under the perfect health scenario and increases with age (because we add the difference between average and optimal health, which grows with age). For the values taken from the CEA Registry studies, which scenario results in larger estimates depended on age, because we anchored the percentage reduction from average population health at the average age of the underlying study samples. The average age in the chronic bronchitis study is 55 years, slightly higher than the average age at incidence used in our analysis (Torrance et al., 1999). For the AMI study, the average age of the study sample is 69 years (Oostenbrink et al., 2001).

We multiplied the estimates of decrements from "without condition" health by duration (taking life expectancy into account) to determine the QALY losses associated with each nonfatal endpoint as well as with pre-

TABLE A-14 Nonroad Diesel Emissions Case Study: HRQL with Illness, at Average Age of Incidence

Endpoint	Average Age at Incidence	Base Case, Compared to Average Health				Sensitivity Analysis, Compared to Perfect Health			
		Without Condition[a]	With Condition			Without Condition[a]	With Condition		
			EQ-5D Expert Assessment[b]	EQ-5D MEPS Catalogue[c]	Transfer from Selected Studies[d]		EQ-5D Expert Assessment[b]	EQ-5D MEPS Catalogue[c]	Transfer from Selected Studies[d]
Nonfatal chronic bronchitis	49	0.88	0.34-0.88	0.81	0.82	1.00	0.39-1.00	0.81	0.78
Nonfatal acute myocardial infarction	53	0.85	0.03-0.85	0.70-0.81	0.60	1.00	0.03-1.00	0.70-0.81	0.58
	78	0.78	0.02-0.78	0.63-0.74	0.55	1.00	0.03-1.00	0.63-0.74	0.58
Preventable mortality—adults	74	0.78	0.00	0.00	0.00	1.00	0.00	0.00	0.00
Preventable mortality—infants	0	1.00	0.00	0.00	0.00	1.00	0.00	0.00	0.00

NOTES: Ranges reflect the results for the different health state subcategories assessed for each endpoint.

[a]Without condition values for average health are based on the EQ-5D, except for the values for chronic bronchitis under the Harvard Registry approach, which are based on the HUI-3. At age 49, the value for average population health is 0.88 under both indices.

[b]For the expert assignment, "with condition" health is assumed to be the same fraction of average health as of perfect health for all years of age affected.

[c]For the EQ-5D MEPS catalogue, numerical decrements from average health are assumed to be constant across all years of age, and the difference between "without condition" average and perfect health is added to this decrement for the perfect health comparison.

[d]For the transfer from the CEA Registry studies, "with condition" health is assumed to be a constant fraction of "without condition" health; this fraction is calculated based on the average age of the samples used in each study.

SOURCES: Case study team analysis of data from the following sources.
Expert assignment: Data provided February to April, 2005.
MEPS data: preliminary results provided by Patrick Sullivan, April 4, 2005.
CEA Registry: Torrance et al. (1999) and Oostenbrink et al. (2001).

ventable mortality. We report the results of these calculations in Table A-15. The results reflect the losses for all cases, assuming that the health status of affected individuals would be the same as the population average for individuals of the same age in the absence of the pollution-related health effects. These estimates represent the lifetime losses for all cases averted by the annual reduction in pollution levels as of the year 2030; using discounting to reflect the future year impacts of the new cases, i.e., their lifetime effects. Undiscounted, the results range from 160,000 to 170,000 QALYs. Without adjustment for HRQL, the life-year losses associated with the cases of preventable mortality (including fatalities for 12,000 adults and 22 infants) total 130,000 life years undiscounted; 93,000 life years if discounted at 3 percent; and 64,000 life years discounted at 7 percent.

As shown in Table A-15, the three approaches to estimating HRQL impacts yield differing results. Because the estimates for mortality are identical under all three approaches, these differences are driven by the approaches used to value the nonfatal endpoints. The expert assignment yields values for chronic bronchitis that are more than twice as large as the estimates from the EQ-5D MEPS catalogue or CEA Registry studies. For

TABLE A-15 Nonroad Diesel Emissions Case Study: QALY Losses, All Cases

HRQL Approach/Endpoint	3% Discount Rate	7% Discount Rate
Expert Assignment of EQ-5D Attributes		
Nonfatal chronic bronchitis	16,245	9,966
Nonfatal AMI	10,259	7,823
Preventable mortality	92,852	63,605
Total	119,356	81,395
EQ-5D MEPS Catalogue		
Nonfatal chronic bronchitis	7,136	4,341
Nonfatal AMI	8,848	6,402
Preventable mortality	92,852	63,605
Total	108,837	74,349
Transfer from Selected Studies		
Nonfatal chronic bronchitis	6,028	3,699
Nonfatal AMI	15,246	10,782
Preventable mortality	92,852	63,605
Total	114,126	78,086

NOTES: Assumes that, in the absence of illness, health status would equal the average for the U.S. population in the same age group. Represents HRQL decrement per case multiplied by duration and by number of new cases averted annually. Detail may not add to total due to rounding.

the AMI endpoints, the CEA Registry studies lead to estimates of QALY losses that are greater than the results under the expert assessment or the EQ-5D catalogue, possibly because that study addressed more severe cases than the average post-AMI population. The estimates of the number of cases avoided, age at incidence, and life expectancy are constant across all three approaches; hence these results reflect the differing estimates of the HRQL decrement associated with each condition.

Table A-16 provides the estimates of QALY losses that result when the "with condition" HRQL is compared to perfect health rather than to average age-adjusted HRQL. As noted earlier and illustrated in Table A-14, the approach that produces the largest estimates of "with condition" HRQL varies due to the differing adjustments used in these comparisons. As expected, the results are larger in the perfect health comparison because perfect health is represented by a constant value of 1.0 across all years of age, while average health declines with age.

Cost-Effectiveness Ratios

Our final step involved reporting the four cost-effectiveness ratios discussed in Chapter 5 of this report, based on the data available for this case study. In these calculations, we use EPA's estimates of annualized regulatory costs, which are reported as $2.0 billion per year regardless of whether a 3 or 7 percent discount rate is used. For health care treatment costs, we use the per-case medical cost estimates for treatment of chronic bronchitis and nonfatal AMIs provided in Hubbell (2004), which round to $1.1 billion regardless of which discount rate is applied. This estimate will understate total health care cost savings because it excludes other types of costs (such as health care-related time losses) associated with treatment of the conditions.

TABLE A-16 Nonroad Diesel Emissions Case Study: Sensitivity Analysis for QALY Losses

Scenario	Discount Rate	EQ-5D Expert Assignment	EQ-5D MEPS Catalogue	Transfer from Selected Studies
Total QALY losses compared to *average* age-adjusted health	3%	119,356	108,837	114,126
	7%	81,395	74,349	78,086
Total QALY losses compared to *perfect* health	3%	154,447	186,785	173,160
	7%	104,666	125,292	116,638

In the comprehensive ratio, we net out the value of the benefits not addressed in the effectiveness measure; i.e., the short-lived health impacts and the environmental effects. According to EPA's analysis, the total value of these additional benefits is about $2.3 billion annually as of the year 2030. In other words, the combined value of these other benefits exceeds the costs of the regulations. Thus netting these benefit values out of the regulatory costs led to negative costs, or savings.

In Table A-17, we report the results for each of the ratios recommended by the Committee. The costs per QALY are less than the costs per life year saved in part because the estimate of costs in the former ratio is lower due to the netting out of medical cost savings. The ratios are within the same order of magnitude across the different approaches used to assess HRQL, and in some cases appear indistinguishable. For the comprehensive ratio, we do not report the results of the calculations because the netting out of other benefits leads to cost savings. All of the cost per QALY estimates would be lower if we used the results of our sensitivity analysis, since the comparison to perfect health yields larger estimates of QALY losses.

Again, this case study does not fully reflect certain of the Committee's recommendations. While we did not fully assess the distributional or ethical implications of this regulation, Chapter 4 provides an example of a summary of these impacts, and EPA's analysis provides more detailed information on related topics. In addition, our analysis relies on mean or median values and provides only limited assessment of uncertainty. More extensive uncertainty analysis is required by both the Committee's recommendations and the existing government-wide guidance. EPA's BCA provides substantial discussion of this issue, including various assessments of the degree of uncertainty in both the cost and benefit estimates.

In this case study, the experts involved in determining the EQ-5D attributes raised several issues similar to those raised by the experts involved in the FDA and NHTSA studies. These concerns related to the relationship between the disease descriptions and the attribute descriptions, the differences between expert and patient judgments about disease impacts, and the difficulties inherent in considering an "average" or "typical" case rather than an individual patient. As noted earlier, there are a number of steps that analysts can take to develop a more thorough assessment process; e.g., pre-testing the approach, working with the experts to ensure that they have a common understanding of the health conditions, index attributes, and the task itself, and following the initial assignment with a process for resolving (or better understanding) any inconsistencies in the results. Relying on patient, rather than expert, assignments was not possible given the time and resources available for this case study, but could significantly alter the findings.

For the other two approaches used in this case study, related uncertain-

TABLE A-17 Nonroad Diesel Emissions Case Study: Cost-Effectiveness Ratios

	3% Discount Rate			7% Discount Rate		
	EQ-5D Expert Assignment	EQ-5D MEPS Catalogue	Transfer from Selected Studies	EQ-5D Expert Assignment	EQ-5D MEPS Catalogue	Transfer from Selected Studies
Averted deaths	12,000 deaths			12,000 deaths		
Averted life-year losses	93,000 years			64,000 years		
Regulatory compliance costs	$2.0 billion			$2.0 billion		
Compliance cost per fatality averted	$170,000			$170,000		
Compliance cost per life-year gained	$22,000			$31,000		
Averted QALY losses	120,000 QALYs	109,000 QALYs	114,000 QALYs	81,000 QALYs	74,000 QALYs	78,000 QALYs
Regulatory compliance costs, net of health treatment savings	$ 0.9 billion					
Regulatory compliance costs, net of health treatment savings and value of additional benefits	($1.4 billion)					
Health-benefits-only ratio	$7,500 per QALY	$8,300 per QALY	$7,900 per QALY	$11,000 per QALY	$12,000 per QALY	$12,000 per QALY
Comprehensive ratio	Cost-Saving					

NOTES: Reflects new incidence averted in the year 2030; 2000 dollars. Assumes that, without the pollution-related illness, health status would be the same as the average for the U.S. population in the same age group. Rounded to two significant figures, numbers in parentheses are negative, calculations are based on unrounded results.

ties are discussed in the background documents. The MEPS-based EQ-5D analysis (Sullivan et. al, 2005) includes a variety of data that could be used in more formal, quantitative analysis of uncertainty. In applying estimates from the CEA Registry studies, we rely on a single study for each endpoint. However, other studies report varying results for similarly defined health conditions (see Brauer and Neumann, 2005). A more comprehensive approach would consider the full range of values reported; similar, for example, to the approach used in Hubbell (2004).

CONCLUSION

These case studies demonstrated that it is possible to apply a number of approaches to assess the cost-effectiveness of economically significant health and safety regulations. While the Committee was not able to conduct new primary research on the HRQL impacts of the health effects considered, we were able to examine the consequences of applying expert judgment processes and information from different types of existing studies. Although more sophisticated application of these approaches is desirable in the context of actual regulatory analyses, all appear feasible and provide information of interest for decision making.

The case studies also aided us in identifying areas where more research would be useful. For example, the experts involved in the assignment process noted that the generic indexes did not always provide attribute descriptions that were applicable to the health conditions being characterized, and better tailored approaches might be desirable. This was particularly true when the indexes were applied to children. In addition, our review of existing studies in the CEA Registry indicated gaps and inconsistencies in the HRQL values currently available for application to regulatory analysis. Meta-analysis or other approaches that combine results of different studies, as well as additional analysis of uncertainties, also could be helpful. In addition, further development of criteria and best practices for transferring estimates from existing studies would be desirable. We also found that the MEPS catalogue used in the EPA case study was quite useful for this sort of analysis; it provides U.S. population health state index values for a variety of conditions encountered in many regulatory analyses.

The case studies suggested that the types of health risk information available to regulatory analysts pose challenges not necessarily present in clinical outcomes studies or medical technology assessments. In particular, regulatory agencies generally work with risk estimates that reflect small changes in the probability of injury, illness, or death spread throughout a large population. This focus on expected or statistical cases often may require assessing HRQL and longevity impacts for an average or typical case (or range of cases) of each condition averted by a rule. While some of the health risk information needed to implement a QALY-based CEA is not needed for a BCA, many agencies have developed this additional data in the context of implementing their own approaches to CEA. We faced the most significant data constraints in the NHTSA case study because of the broad injury categories used by that agency. More detailed data on the injuries averted by a particular rule would allow more accurate assessment of HRQL impacts.

The cost-of-illness estimates currently used by the agencies are not entirely compatible with the definition of health treatment costs developed for the reference case by the U.S. Panel on Cost Effectiveness in Health and Medicine (Gold et al., 1996b) and discussed in the Committee's recommendations. In many cases, these estimates only include direct medical costs. When lost productivity estimates were available, they addressed the long-term impacts of the health condition, not solely the impacts of medical treatment. As noted in the main text of this report, such estimates of lost productivity are likely to double count impacts included in the effectiveness measure, and hence are not suitable for this type of analysis. Development of standard estimating practices for the health care treatment costs to be used in CEA would be useful.

The case studies also provide examples of the implications of a number of the Committee's recommendations. For instance, the FDA and EPA rules differ significantly in terms of the importance of preventable mortality to the results. For the EPA rule, which averts a relatively large number of deaths, the cost per life year and cost per QALY gained are much more similar than in the case of the FDA rule, which prevents very few deaths. The EPA rule also illustrates the potential for significant changes in the cost-effectiveness measure when other benefits are considered in a comprehensive ratio. Furthermore, the analyses show the importance of comparing "with condition" values to measures of expected *actual* "without condition" health; comparisons to *perfect* health lead to estimates of QALY losses that are misleadingly large in some cases.

Finally, we were not able to assess whether alternative HRQL approaches would change regulatory decisions. The final rules used in these case studies lacked information on the impacts of the wide range of regulatory options required by the OMB guidance, so we could not compare the results of different HRQL approaches across regulatory options. However, the cost-per-QALY estimates appear relatively similar across the different HRQL approaches used in the case studies. For example, using a 3 percent discount rate, the range for the health-benefits-only ratio was $13,000 to $18,000 per QALY in the FDA case study, and $7,500 to $8,300 in the EPA case study.

ACKNOWLEDGMENTS

This appendix represents the collaborative efforts of the IOM Committee members, advisers, consultants, and staff with federal agency staff and consultants. The case studies could not have been completed without the exceptional efforts of a great many people. The goal of these studies was to enhance the Committee's understanding of current practices and of the issues that arise in applying different measures of benefits in a regulatory context, and they were an important source of information and insights that contributed significantly to our deliberations.

In a very real sense, everyone who contributed to these case studies was a volunteer. The scope of effort to produce these analyses exceeded the time and money originally budgeted for the task, and the case study teams worked beyond all original expectations. The Committee is indebted to all those who have contributed their time and expertise to gather information, explain agency policies and practices, and complete a daunting array of analytic tasks. The Committee thanks the following individuals for their advice, generosity, and hard work.

Juice Processing Regulation Case Study

Lead authors: Lisa A. Robinson, Independent Consultant; Wilhelmine Miller, Institute of Medicine; Robert Black, Independent Consultant.

IOM Committee advisers: Alan Garber (lead); Judith Wagner.

Other advisers: Clark Nardinelli, Food and Drug Administration; Sajal Chattopadhyay, Centers for Disease Control and Prevention.

Contributors: John Anderson, University of California, San Diego; Barbara Altman, National Center for Health Statistics; Fred Angulo, Centers for Disease Control and Prevention; Lawrence Deyton, M.D., Veteran's Administration; Sherine Gabriel, M.D., Mayo Clinic; Janel Hanmer, University of Wisconsin-Madison; William Lawrence, M.D., Agency for Healthcare Research and Quality; Gwen Wanger, M.D., Beth Israel Deaconess Medical Center.

Expert application of generic indexes: *Infectious disease*—Claire Panosian, M.D., David Geffen School of Medicine, University of California, Los Angeles (UCLA); David A. Pegues, M.D., David Geffen School of Medicine, UCLA; Matthew Leibowitz, M.D., David Geffen School of Medicine, UCLA; Glenn Mathisen, M.D., Olive View-UCLA Medical Center; Sherwood L. Gorbach, M.D., Tufts New England Medical Center; David R. Snydman, M.D., Tufts New England Medical Center; Mark Holodniy, M.D., Veteran's Administration Palo Alto Health Care System; Victoria

Davey, R.N., M.P.H., U.S. Department of Veterans Affairs. *Rheumatology*—Lenore Buckley, M.D., Virginia Commonwealth University School of Medicine; Gene G. Hunder, M.D., Mayo Clinic (retired); Eric L. Matteson, M.D., Mayo Clinic College of Medicine; Daniel H. Solomon, M.D., Harvard Medical School; Elizabeth A. Tindall, M.D., Oregon Health and Science University.

Child Restraints Regulation Case Study

Lead authors: Lisa A. Robinson, Independent Consultant; Phaedra Corso, Centers for Disease Control and Prevention; Xiangming Fang, Centers for Disease Control and Prevention; Robert Black, Independent Consultant; Wilhelmine Miller, Institute of Medicine.

IOM Committee advisers: Emmett Keeler (lead); Henry Anderson; Lisa Iezzoni; Alan Krupnick.

Other advisers: Larry Blincoe, National Highway Traffic Safety Administration; Jim Simons, National Highway Traffic Safety Administration; Carmen Brauer, M.D., Harvard School of Public Health.

Contributors: John Anderson, University of California, San Diego; Barbara Altman, National Center for Health Statistics; Nancy Bondy, National Highway Traffic Safety Administration; David Feeny, Kaiser Permanente; Janel Hanmer, University of Wisconsin-Madison; Troy Holbrook, University of California, San Diego; Robert Kaplan, University of California, Los Angeles; William Lawrence, M.D., Agency for Healthcare Research and Quality; Ellen MacKenzie, Ph.D., Johns Hopkins University; Bryce Mason, Rand Corporation; Ted Miller, Pacific Institutes for Research and Evaluation; Ryan Palugod, Institute of Medicine; William Rhoads, Centers for Disease Control and Prevention; Jon Walker, National Highway Traffic Safety Administration.

Expert application of generic indexes: Carmen Brauer, M.D., Harvard School of Public Health; Kristine Campbell, M.D., Children's Hospital of Pittsburgh; Tim Davis, M.D., Centers for Disease Control and Prevention; Arlene Greenspan, Ph.D., Centers for Disease Control and Prevention; David Mooney, M.D., Children's Hospital, Boston.

Nonroad Engine Air Emissions Regulation Case Study

Lead authors: Lisa A. Robinson, Independent Consultant; Wilhelmine Miller, Institute of Medicine; Robert Black, Independent Consultant.

IOM Committee advisers: Maureen Cropper (lead); Richard Burnett; James Hammitt; Alan Krupnick.

Other advisers: Carmen Brauer, M.D., Harvard School of Public Health; Bryan Hubbell, U.S. Environmental Protection Agency; Tursynbek Nurmagambetov, Centers for Disease Control and Prevention; Seymour Williams, Centers for Disease Control and Prevention.

Contributors: Adam Atherly, Centers for Disease Control and Prevention; Sarah Brennan, Industrial Economics Incorporated; Jim DeMocker, U.S. Environmental Protection Agency; Chris Dockins, U.S. Environmental Protection Agency; Janel Hanmer, University of Wisconsin-Madison; Fernando Holguin, Centers for Disease Control and Prevention; William Lawrence, M.D., Agency for Healthcare Research and Quality; Darwin LaBarthe, Centers for Disease Control and Prevention; Jim Neumann, Industrial Economics, Incorporated; Peter Neumann, Harvard School of Public Health; Nathalie Simon, U.S. Environmental Protection Agency; Patrick Sullivan, University of Colorado.

Expert application of generic indexes: *Respiratory disease*—David M. Mannino, M.D., University of Kentucky School of Medicine; Peter Barkin, M.D., Emerson Hospital; R. Graham Barr, M.D., Presbyterian Hospital, Columbia University; Scott D. Ramsey, M.D., Fred Hutchinson Cancer Research Center; Mark J. Utell, M.D., University of Rochester; Roger Yusen, M.D., Washington University School of Medicine. *Cardiovascular disease*—Harlan M. Krumholz, M.D., Yale Medical School; Russell V. Luepker, M.D., Mayo Clinic; John Rumsfeld, M.D., University of Colorado; Douglas D. Schocken, M.D., University of South Florida; John Spertus, M.D., University of Missouri-Kansas City.

B

Health Indexes

TABLE B-1 The Quality of Well-Being Scale (QWB)

Domains	Attribute Levels	Description
MOBILITY SCALE	5	No limitations for health reasons.
	4	Did not drive a car, health related; did not ride in a car as usual for age (younger than 15 years), health related.
	3	Did not use public transportation, health related.
	2	Had or would have used more help than usual for age to use public transportation, health related.
	1	In hospital, health related.
PHYSICAL ACTIVITY SCALE	4	No limitations for health reasons.
	3	In wheelchair, moved or controlled movement of wheelchair without help from someone else.
	2	Had trouble or did not try to lift, stoop, bend over, or use stairs or inclines, health related; limped, used a cane, crutches, or walker, health related; had any other physical limitation in walking; or did not try to walk as far or as fast as others the same age are able, health related.
	1	In wheelchair, did not move or control the movement of wheelchair without help from someone else, or in bed, chair, or couch for most or all of the day, health related.
SOCIAL ACTIVITY SCALE	5	No limitations for health reasons.
	4	Limited in other (e.g., recreational) role activity, health related.
	3	Limited in major (primary) role activity, health related.
	2	Performed no major role activity, health related, but did perform self-care activities.
	1	Performed no major role activity, health related, and did not perform or had more help than usual in performance of one or more self-care activities, health related.

continues

TABLE B-1 Continued

Domains	Attribute Levels	Description
SYMPTOM/ PROBLEM COMPLEX	23	Trouble sleeping; intoxication; problems with sexual interest or performance; *or* excessive worry.
	22	No symptoms or problem.
	21	Breathing smog or unpleasant air.
	20	Wore glasses or contact lenses.
	19	Taking medication or staying on a prescribed diet for health reasons.
	18	Pain in ear, tooth, jaw, throat, lips, tongue; several missing or crooked permanent teeth—includes wearing bridges or false teeth; stuffy, runny nose; or any trouble hearing—includes wearing a hearing aid.
	17	Overweight for age and height or skin defect of face, body, arms, or legs, such as scars, pimples, warts, bruises, or changes in color.
	16	Pain or discomfort in one or both eyes (such as burning or itching) or any trouble seeing after correction.
	15	Trouble talking, such as lisp, stuttering, hoarseness, or being unable to speak.
	14	Burning or itching rash on large areas of face, body, arms, or legs.
	13	Headache, or dizziness, or ringing in ears, or spells of feeling hot, or nervous or shaky.
	12	Spells of feeling upset, being depressed, or of crying.
	11	Cough, wheezing, or shortness of breath, with or without fever, chills, or aching all over.
	10	General tiredness, weakness, or weight loss.
	9	Sick or upset stomach, vomiting or loose bowel movement, with or without fever, chills, or aching all over.
	8	Pain, burning, bleeding, itching, or other difficulty with rectum, bowel movements, or urination (passing water).
	7	Pain, stiffness, weakness, numbness, or other discomfort in chest, stomach (including hernia or rupture), side, neck, back, hips, or any joints or hands, feet, arms, or legs.
	6	Any combination of one or more hands, feet, arms, or legs either missing, deformed (crooked), paralyzed (unable to move), or broken—includes wearing artificial limbs or braces.
	5	Trouble learning, remembering, or thinking clearly.
	4	Pain, bleeding, itching, or discharge (drainage) from sexual organs—does not include normal menstrual (monthly) bleeding.
	3	Burn over large areas of face, body, arms, or legs.
	2	Loss of consciousness such as seizure (fits), fainting, or coma (out cold or knocked out).
	1	Death.

Scoring algorithm: See Kaplan and Anderson (1988) or Patrick and Erickson (1993, pp. 389–391).

TABLE B-2 The Health Utilities Index Mark 2 (HUI-2)

Domains	Attribute Levels	Description
SENSATION	1	Able to see, hear, and speak normally for age.
	2	Requires equipment to see or hear or speak.
	3	Sees, hears, or speaks with limitations even with equipment.
	4	Blind, deaf, or mute.
MOBILITY	1	Able to walk, bend, lift, jump, and run normally for age.
	2	Walks, bends, lifts, jumps, or runs with some limitations but does not require help.
	3	Requires mechanical equipment (such as canes, crutches, braces, or wheelchair) to walk or get around independently.
	4	Requires the help of another person to walk or get around and requires mechanical equipment as well.
	5	Unable to control or use arms and legs.
EMOTION	1	Generally happy and free from worry.
	2	Occasionally fretful, angry, irritable, anxious, depressed, or suffering "night terrors."
	3	Often fretful, angry, irritable, anxious, depressed, or suffering "night terrors."
	4	Almost always fretful, angry, irritable, anxious, depressed.
	5	Extremely fretful, angry, irritable, anxious, or depressed usually requiring hospitalization or psychiatric institutional care.
COGNITION	1	Learns and remembers school work normally for age.
	2	Learns and remembers school work more slowly than classmates as judged by parents and/or teachers.
	3	Learns and remembers very slowly and usually requires special educational assistance.
	4	Unable to learn and remember.
SELF-CARE	1	Eats, bathes, dresses, and uses the toilet normally for age.
	2	Eats, bathes, dresses, or uses the toilet independently with difficulty.
	3	Requires mechanical equipment to eat, bathe, dress, or use the toilet independently.
	4	Requires the help of another person to eat, bathe, dress, or use the toilet.
PAIN	1	Free of pain and discomfort.
	2	Occasional pain. Discomfort relieved by nonprescription drugs or self-control activity without disruption of normal activities.
	3	Frequent pain. Discomfort relieved by oral medicines with occasional disruption of normal activities.

continues

TABLE B-2 Continued

Domains	Attribute Levels	Description
	4	Frequent pain; frequent disruption of normal activities. Discomfort requires prescription narcotics for relief.
	5	Severe pain. Pain not relieved by drugs and constantly disrupts normal activities.
FERTILITY	1	Able to have children with a fertile spouse.
	2	Difficulty in having children with a fertile spouse.
	3	Unable to have children with a fertile spouse.

Scoring algorithm: See Torrance et al. (1996). Also available at http://www.fhs.mcmaster.ca/hui2.htm.

TABLE B-3 The Health Utilities Index Mark 3 (HUI-3)

Domains	Attribute Levels	Description
VISION	1	Able to see well enough to read ordinary newsprint and recognize a friend on the other side of the street, without glasses or contact lenses.
	2	Able to see well enough to read ordinary newsprint and recognize a friend on the other side of the street, but with glasses.
	3	Able to read ordinary newsprint with or without glasses but unable to recognize a friend on the other side of the street, even with glasses.
	4	Able to recognize a friend on the other side of the street with or without glasses but unable to read ordinary newsprint, even with glasses.
	5	Unable to read ordinary newsprint and unable to recognize a friend on the other side of the street, even with glasses.
	6	Unable to see at all.
HEARING	1	Able to hear what is said in a group conversation with at least three other people, without a hearing aid.
	2	Able to hear what is said in a conversation with one other person in a quiet room without a hearing aid, but requires a hearing aid to hear what is said in a group conversation with at least three other people.
	3	Able to hear what is said in a conversation with one other person in a quiet room with a hearing aid, and able to hear what is said in a group conversation with at least three other people, with a hearing aid.
	4	Able to hear what is said in a conversation with one other person in a quiet room, without a hearing aid, but unable to hear what is said in a group conversation with at least three other people even with a hearing aid.
	5	Able to hear what is said in a conversation with one other person in a quiet room with a hearing aid, but unable to hear what is said in a group conversation with at least three other people even with a hearing aid.
	6	Unable to hear at all.
SPEECH	1	Able to be understood completely when speaking with strangers or friends.
	2	Able to be understood partially when speaking with strangers but able to be understood completely when speaking with people who know me well.
	3	Able to be understood partially when speaking with strangers or people who know me well.

continues

TABLE B-3 Continued

Domains	Attribute Levels	Description
	4	Unable to be understood when speaking with strangers but able to be understood partially by people who know me well.
	5	Unable to be understood when speaking to other people (or unable to speak at all).
AMBULATION	1	Able to walk around the neighborhood without difficulty, and without walking equipment.
	2	Able to walk around the neighborhood with difficulty; but does not require walking equipment or the help of another person.
	3	Able to walk around the neighborhood with walking equipment, but without the help of another person.
	4	Able to walk only short distances with walking equipment, and requires a wheelchair to get around the neighborhood.
	5	Unable to walk alone, even with walking equipment. Able to walk short distances with the help of another person, and requires a wheelchair to get around the neighborhood.
	6	Cannot walk at all.
DEXTERITY	1	Full use of two hands and ten fingers.
	2	Limitations in the use of hands or fingers, but does not require special tools or help of another person.
	3	Limitations in the use of hands or fingers, is independent with use of special tools (does not require the help of another person).
	4	Limitations in the use of hands or fingers, requires the help of another person for some tasks (not independent even with use of special tools).
	5	Limitations in use of hands or fingers, requires the help of another person for most tasks (not independent even with use of special tools).
	6	Limitations in use of hands or fingers, requires the help of another person for all tasks (not independent even with use of special tools).
EMOTION	1	Happy and interested in life.
	2	Somewhat happy.
	3	Somewhat unhappy.
	4	Very unhappy.
	5	So unhappy that life is not worthwhile.

continues

TABLE B-3 Continued

Domains	Attribute Levels	Description
COGNITION	1	Able to remember most things, think clearly and solve day-to-day problems.
	2	Able to remember most things, but have a little difficulty when trying to think and solve day-to-day problems.
	3	Somewhat forgetful, but able to think clearly and solve day-to-day problems.
	4	Somewhat forgetful, and have a little difficulty when trying to think or solve day-to-day problems.
	5	Very forgetful, and have great difficulty when trying to think or solve day-to-day problems.
	6	Unable to remember anything at all, and unable to think or solve day-to-day problems.
PAIN	1	Free of pain and discomfort.
	2	Mild to moderate pain that prevents no activities.
	3	Moderate pain that prevents a few activities.
	4	Moderate to severe pain that prevents some activities.
	5	Severe pain that prevents most activities.

Scoring algorithm: Available at http://www.fhs.mcmaster.ca/hug/hui3.htm.

TABLE B-4 The EuroQol-5D (EQ-5D)

Domains	Attribute Levels	Description
MOBILITY	1	I have no problems in walking about.
	2	I have some problems in walking about.
	3	I am confined to bed.
SELF-CARE	1	I have no problems with self-care.
	2	I have some problems washing or dressing myself.
	3	I am unable to wash or dress myself.
USUAL ACTIVITIES	1	I have no problems with performing my usual activities (e.g., work, study, housework, family or leisure activities).
	2	I have some problems with performing my usual activities.
	3	I am unable to perform my usual activities.
PAIN/ DISCOMFORT	1	I have no pain or discomfort.
	2	I have moderate pain or discomfort.
	3	I have extreme pain or discomfort.
ANXIETY/ DEPRESSION	1	I am not anxious or depressed.
	2	I am moderately anxious or depressed.
	3	I am extremely anxious or depressed.

Scoring algorithm: See Shaw et al., 2005, for U.S. population-based preference weights. Scoring algorithms for statistical applications (SPSS, Stata, SAS) are available at the Agency for Healthcare Research Quality website, http://www.ahrq.gov/rice/.

TABLE B-5 The SF-6D (SF-12 version)

Domains	Attribute Levels	Description
PHYSICAL FUNCTIONING	1	Your health does not limit you in *moderate activities.*
	2	Your health limits you a little in *moderate activities.*
	3	Your health limits you a lot in *moderate activities.*
ROLE LIMITATIONS	1	You have no problems with your work or other regular daily activities as a result of your physical health or any emotional problems.
	2	You are limited in the kind of work or other activities as a result of your physical health.
	3	You accomplish less than you would like as a result of emotional problems.
	4	You are limited in the kind of work or other activities as a result of your physical health and accomplish less than you would like as a result of emotional problems.
SOCIAL FUNCTIONING	1	Your health limits your social activities *none of the time.*
	2	Your health limits your social activities *a little of the time.*
	3	Your health limits your social activities *some of the time.*
	4	Your health limits your social activities *most of the time.*
	5	Your health limits your social activities *all of the time.*
PAIN	1	You have pain that does not interfere with your normal work (both outside the home and housework) *at all.*
	2	You have pain that interferes with your normal work (both outside the home and housework) *a little bit.*
	3	You have pain that interferes with your normal work (both outside the home and housework) *moderately.*
	4	You have pain that interferes with your normal work (both outside the home and housework) *quite a bit.*
	5	You have pain that interferes with your normal work (both outside the home and housework) *extremely.*
MENTAL HEALTH	1	You feel downhearted and low *none of the time.*
	2	You feel downhearted and low *a little of the time.*
	3	You feel downhearted and low *some of the time.*
	4	You feel downhearted and low *most of the time.*
	5	You feel downhearted and low *all of the time.*
VITALITY	1	You have a lot of energy *all of the time.*
	2	You have a lot of energy *most of the time.*
	3	You have a lot of energy *some of the time.*
	4	You have a lot of energy *a little of the time.*
	5	You have a lot of energy *none of the time.*

Scoring algorithm: See Brazier and Roberts, 2004. Scoring algorithm and software are available from the authors.

TABLE B-6 The Functional Capacity Index (FCI) Version 2.1 Final

Domains	Attribute Levels	Description
EXCRETORY FUNCTIONS	A	No limitations No accidents and no use of medication or devices
	B	Controllable excretory difficulty (bowel and bladder) No accidents with use of medication or devices* or accidents once per week or less with or without use of medication or device*
	C2	Severe incontinence (bowel and bladder); Accidents every day or continuous use of catheter or colostomy pouch *device does not include catheter or colostomy pouch*
EATING	A	No limitation No limitations in chewing, swallowing, or digesting food that require restrictions in diet or special preparation of foods
	B	Minor to moderate limitation Restrictions in diet or special preparation of foods required
	C	Tube feeding and/or gastrostomy required
SEXUAL FUNCTION	A	No limitations due to physical limitation
	B	Some difficulty due to physical limitation
	C	A lot of difficulty due to physical limitation including not being able to do it at all
AMBULATION (MAY INCLUDE LIMITATIONS DUE TO PAIN)	A	No limitations walking, running, walking briskly, or standing for long periods No limitations walking without help from another person or device* No limitations running or walking briskly or standing for long periods
	B	Some limitations running or walking briskly or standing for long periods No limitations walking without help from another person or device* But has some limitations running, walking briskly, or standing for long periods
	C1	Some limitations walking but independent (independent community ambulator) Has some limitations walking But can walk at least 150 yards (length of city block) without help from another person or device*
	C2	Can walk long distances but only with device or help (community ambulator with assistance) Has some limitations walking Can walk at least 150 yards (length of city block) but only with help from another person or device*

continues

TABLE B-6 Continued

Domains	Attribute Levels	Description
	D	Walking limited to short distances with or without device or help (home ambulator)
		Cannot walk 150 yards even with help or device*
		But can walk shorter distances (i.e. < 150 yards) with or without help from another person or device*
	E	Cannot walk at all
		Cannot walk even short distances; requires wheelchair all the time to get around
		Device includes walking aids (e.g. cane, crutch, walker) or prosthesis/orthosis
BENDING, STOOPING, AND LIFTING (MAY INCLUDE LIMITATIONS DUE TO PAIN)	A	No difficulty bending, stooping, lifting and no difficulty lifting arms over head
		No difficulty lifting and carrying weights up to 50 lbs (a small child)
		No difficulty lifting arms over head
	B	Minor difficulty bending, stooping, lifting, and/or difficulty lifting arms over head
		Has difficulty lifting and carrying 50 lbs (a small child), but can lift at least 10 lbs (a bag of groceries) with no or little difficulty *and/or*
		Has difficulty lifting arms over head but can do it at least 5 times in a row
	C	Major difficulty bending, stooping, lifting
		Has a lot of difficulty lifting and carrying at least 10 lbs (a bag of groceries), including not being able to do it at all
		May or may not have difficulty lifting arms over head but can do it at least 5 times in a row
	D	Complete or near complete loss of upper body function
		Has difficulty lifting and carrying at least 10 lbs (a bag of groceries), including not being able to do it at all
		Has difficulty lifting arms over head at least 5 times in a row, including not being able to do it at all
HAND AND WRIST FUNCTION (MAY INCLUDE LIMITATIONS DUE TO PAIN)	A	No limitations
		No difficulty grasping and handling small or large objects with either hand
		No difficulty twisting and turning doorknob or key with either hand
	B1	Minor difficulty in hand and/or wrist function—one hand
		Difficulty grasping and handling small objects with one hand but no difficulty with large objects *and/or*
		Difficulty twisting and turning doorknob or key with one hand

continues

TABLE B-6 Continued

Domains	Attribute Levels	Description
		May use special tool but does not require the help of another person
	B2	Minor difficulty in hand and/or wrist function—both hands
		Difficulty grasping and handling small objects with both hands but no difficulty with large objects *and/or*
		Difficulty twisting and turning doorknob or key with one or both hands
		May use special tool but does not require the help of another person
	C1	Major difficulty in hand function—one hand
		Difficulty grasping and handling large *and* small objects with one hand
		May or may not have difficulty twisting and turning doorknob or key with one or both hands
		May use special tool but does not require the help of another person
	C2	Major difficulty in hand function—both hands
		Difficulty grasping and handling large *and* small objects with both hands
		May or may not have difficulty twisting and turning doorknob or key with one or both hands
		May use special tool but does not require the help of another person
	D	Near complete loss of hand function (including paralysis)
		Difficulty grasping and handling large and small objects
		Requires the help of another person for some, but not all tasks necessary for daily living
	E	Complete loss of function (including paralysis) in both hands
		Difficulty grasping and handling large and small objects
		Requires the help of another person for all or nearly all tasks necessary for daily living
SPEECH	A	No limitations
	B	Minor limitations in everyday situations
		Can be understood by most everyone; may get stuck, stutter, stammer, slur
	C	Major limitations
		Can only be understood by people who know person well
	D	Cannot speak and/or be understood by others or requires voice box to speak
HEARING	A	No limitations hearing without hearing aid
	B1	Minor difficulty hearing

continues

TABLE B-6 Continued

Domains	Attribute Levels	Description
	B2	With or without hearing aid has some difficulty hearing, but only when listening conditions are less than ideal Moderate difficulty With or without hearing aid has difficulty hearing under everyday listening conditions
	C	Profound to total loss of hearing; noncorrectable Cannot hear even with the use of a hearing aid
VISION	A	No limitations; No difficulties reading small and large print, driving and going about daily activities with or without glasses/contacts
	B	Minor or moderate limitations Minor or moderate difficulty reading small and large print, driving and going about daily activities with or without glasses/contacts
	C	Severe limitations Severe difficulty reading small and large print, driving and going about daily activities with or without glasses/contacts; includes blind with light perception only
	D	Blind without light perception
COGNITIVE FUNCTION	A	No limitations
	B	Minor limitations Minor difficulties with reasoning/solving problems, memory, concentration/thinking and/or attention; can live independently (i.e. does not require assistance with either ADL or IADL activities due to cognitive deficits)
	C	Moderate to severe limitations Moderate to severe difficulties with reasoning/solving problems, memory, concentration/thinking and/or attention; can live independently (i.e. does not require assistance with ADL activities) but (due to cognitive deficits) may need assistance with some IADL activities of daily living
	D	Unconfined dependence Cannot live independently due to cognitive deficits but 24-hour supervision is not required
	E	Confined dependence Cannot live independently due to cognitive deficits; 24-hour supervision is required
	F	Minimally responsive or vegetative state Cannot respond to simple commands except possibly with eye movement

Scoring algorithm: See MacKenzie et al. (1996), for original FCI scores and classifications; contact author for current scoring algorithm.

C

OMB Circular A-4

September 17, 2003

TO THE HEADS OF EXECUTIVE AGENCIES
AND ESTABLISHMENTS

Subject: **Regulatory Analysis**

This Circular provides the Office of Management and Budget's (OMB's) guidance to Federal agencies on the development of regulatory analysis as required under Section 6(a)(3)(c) of Executive Order 12866, "Regulatory Planning and Review," the Regulatory Right-to-Know Act, and a variety of related authorities. The Circular also provides guidance to agencies on the regulatory accounting statements that are required under the Regulatory Right-to-Know Act.

This Circular refines OMB's "best practices" document of 1996 (http://www.whitehouse.gov/omb/inforeg/riaguide.html), which was issued as a guidance in 2000 (http://www.whitehouse.gov/omb/memoranda/m00-08.pdf), and reaffirmed in 2001 (http://www.whitehouse.gov/omb/memoranda/m01-23.html). It replaces both the 1996 "best practices" and the 2000 guidance.

In developing this Circular, OMB first developed a draft that was subject to public comment, interagency review, and peer review. Peer reviewers included Cass Sunstein, University of Chicago; Lester Lave, Carnegie Mellon University; Milton C. Weinstein and James K. Hammitt of the Harvard School of Public Health; Kerry Smith, North Carolina State University; Jonathan Weiner, Duke University Law School; Douglas K. Owens, Stanford University; and W. Kip Viscusi, Harvard Law School. Although these individuals submitted comments, OMB is solely responsible for the final content of this Circular.

A. Introduction

This Circular is designed to assist analysts in the regulatory agencies by defining good regulatory analysis—called either "regulatory analysis" or "analysis" for brevity—and standardizing the way benefits and costs of Federal regulatory actions are measured and reported. Executive Order 12866 requires agencies to conduct a regulatory analysis for economically significant regulatory actions as defined by Section 3(f)(1). This requirement applies to rulemakings that rescind or modify existing rules as well as to rulemakings that establish new requirements.

The Need for Analysis of Proposed Regulatory Actions[1]

Regulatory analysis is a tool regulatory agencies use to anticipate and evaluate the likely consequences of rules. It provides a formal way of organizing the evidence on the key effects—good and bad—of the various alternatives that should be considered in developing regulations. The motivation is to (1) learn if the benefits of an action are likely to justify the costs or (2) discover which of various possible alternatives would be the most cost-effective.

A good regulatory analysis is designed to inform the public and other parts of the Government (as well as the agency conducting the analysis) of the effects of alternative actions. Regulatory analysis sometimes will show that a proposed action is misguided, but it can also demonstrate that well-conceived actions are reasonable and justified.

Benefit-cost analysis is a primary tool used for regulatory analysis.[2] Where all benefits and costs can be quantified and expressed in monetary units, benefit-cost analysis provides decision makers with a clear indication of the most efficient alternative, that is, the alternative that generates the largest net benefits to society (ignoring distributional effects). This is useful information for decision makers and the public to receive, even when economic efficiency is not the only or the overriding public policy objective.

---

[1] We use the term "proposed" to refer to any regulatory actions under consideration regardless of the stage of the regulatory process.

[2] See Mishan EJ (1994), *Cost-Benefit Analysis*, fourth edition, Routledge, New York.

It will not always be possible to express in monetary units all of the important benefits and costs. When it is not, the most efficient alternative will not necessarily be the one with the largest quantified and monetized net-benefit estimate. In such cases, you should exercise professional judgment in determining how important the non-quantified benefits or costs may be in the context of the overall analysis. If the non-quantified benefits and costs are likely to be important, you should carry out a "threshold" analysis to evaluate their significance. Threshold or "break-even" analysis answers the question, "How small could the value of the non-quantified benefits be (or how large would the value of the non-quantified costs need to be) before the rule would yield zero net benefits?" In addition to threshold analysis you should indicate, where possible, which non-quantified effects are most important and why.

Key Elements of a Regulatory Analysis

A good regulatory analysis should include the following three basic elements: (1) a statement of the need for the proposed action, (2) an examination of alternative approaches, and (3) an evaluation of the benefits and costs—quantitative and qualitative—of the proposed action and the main alternatives identified by the analysis.

To evaluate properly the benefits and costs of regulations and their alternatives, you will need to do the following:

- Explain how the actions required by the rule are linked to the expected benefits. For example, indicate how additional safety equipment will reduce safety risks. A similar analysis should be done for each of the alternatives.
- Identify a baseline. Benefits and costs are defined in comparison with a clearly stated alternative. This normally will be a "no action" baseline: what the world will be like if the proposed rule is not adopted. Comparisons to a "next best" alternative are also especially useful.
- Identify the expected undesirable side-effects and ancillary benefits of the proposed regulatory action and the alternatives. These should be added to the direct benefits and costs as appropriate.

With this information, you should be able to assess quantitatively the benefits and costs of the proposed rule and its alternatives. A complete regulatory analysis includes a discussion of non-quantified as well as quantified benefits and costs. A non-quantified outcome is a benefit or cost that has not been quantified or monetized in the analysis. When there are important non-monetary values at stake, you should also identify them in your analysis so policymakers can compare them with the monetary benefits and costs. When your analysis is complete, you should present a summary of the benefit and cost estimates for each alternative, including the qualitative and non-monetized factors affected by the rule, so that readers can evaluate them.

As you design, execute, and write your regulatory analysis, you should seek out the opinions of those who will be affected by the regulation as well as the views of those individuals and organizations who may not be affected but have special knowledge or insight into the regulatory issues. Consultation can be useful in ensuring that your analysis addresses all of the relevant issues and that you have access to all pertinent data. Early consultation can be especially helpful. You should not limit consultation to the final stages of your analytical efforts.

You will find that you cannot conduct a good regulatory analysis according to a formula. Conducting high-quality analysis requires competent professional judgment. Different regulations may call for different emphases in the analysis, depending on the nature and complexity of the regulatory issues and the sensitivity of the benefit and cost estimates to the key assumptions.

A good analysis is transparent. It should be possible for a qualified third party reading the report to see clearly how you arrived at your estimates and conclusions. For transparency's sake, you should state in your report what assumptions were used, such as the time horizon for the analysis and the discount rates applied to future benefits and costs. It is usually necessary to provide a sensitivity analysis to reveal whether, and to what extent, the results of the analysis are sensitive to plausible changes in the main assumptions and numeric inputs.

A good analysis provides specific references to all sources of data, appendices with documentation of models (where necessary), and the results of formal sensitivity and other uncertainty analyses. Your analysis should also have an executive summary, including a standardized accounting statement.

B. The Need for Federal Regulatory Action

Before recommending Federal regulatory action, an agency must demonstrate that the proposed action is necessary. If the regulatory intervention results from a statutory or judicial directive, you should describe the specific authority for your action, the extent of discretion available to you, and the regulatory instruments you might use. Executive Order 12866 states that "Federal agencies should promulgate only such regulations as are required by law, are necessary to interpret the law, or are made necessary by compelling need, such as material failures of private markets to protect or improve the health and safety of the public, the environment, or the well being of the American people . . . ."

Executive Order 12866 also states that "Each agency shall identify the problem that it intends to address (including, where applicable, the failures of private markets or public institutions that warrant new agency action) as well as assess the significance of that problem." Thus, you should try to explain whether the action is intended to address a significant market failure or to meet some other compelling public need such as improving governmental processes or promoting intangible values such as distributional fairness or privacy. If the regulation is designed to correct a significant market failure, you should describe the failure both qualitatively and (where feasible) quantitatively. You should show that a government intervention is likely to do more good than harm. For other interventions, you should also provide a demonstration of compelling social purpose and the likelihood of effective action. Although intangible rationales do not need to be quantified, the analysis should present and evaluate the strengths and limitations of the relevant arguments for these intangible values.

Market Failure or Other Social Purpose

The major types of market failure include: externality, market power, and inadequate or asymmetric information. Correcting market failures is a reason for regulation, but it is not the only reason. Other possible justifications include improving the functioning of government, removing distributional unfairness, or promoting privacy and personal freedom.

1.   Externality, common property resource and public good

An externality occurs when one party's actions impose uncompensated benefits or costs on another party. Environmental problems are a classic case of externality. For example, the smoke from a factory may adversely affect the health of local residents while soiling the property in nearby neighborhoods. If bargaining were costless and all property rights were well defined, people would eliminate externalities through bargaining without the need for government regulation.[3] From this perspective, externalities arise from high transactions costs and/or poorly defined property rights that prevent people from reaching efficient outcomes through market transactions.

---

[3]See Coase RH (1960), *Journal of Law and Economics*, 3, 1–44.

Resources that may become congested or overused, such as fisheries or the broadcast spectrum, represent common property resources. "Public goods," such as defense or basic scientific research, are goods where provision of the good to some individuals cannot occur without providing the same level of benefits free of charge to other individuals.

2. Market Power

Firms exercise market power when they reduce output below what would be offered in a competitive industry in order to obtain higher prices. They may exercise market power collectively or unilaterally. Government action can be a source of market power, such as when regulatory actions exclude low-cost imports. Generally, regulations that increase market power for selected entities should be avoided. However, there are some circumstances in which government may choose to validate a monopoly. If a market can be served at lowest cost only when production is limited to a single producer—local gas and electricity distribution services, for example—a natural monopoly is said to exist. In such cases, the government may choose to approve the monopoly and to regulate its prices and/or production decisions. Nevertheless, you should keep in mind that technological advances often affect economies of scale. This can, in turn, transform what was once considered a natural monopoly into a market where competition can flourish.

3. Inadequate or Asymmetric Information

Market failures may also result from inadequate or asymmetric information. Because information, like other goods, is costly to produce and disseminate, your evaluation will need to do more than demonstrate the possible existence of incomplete or asymmetric information. Even though the market may supply less than the full amount of information, the amount it does supply may be reasonably adequate and therefore not require government regulation. Sellers have an incentive to provide information through advertising that can increase sales by highlighting distinctive characteristics of their products. Buyers may also obtain reasonably adequate information about product characteristics through other channels, such as a seller offering a warranty or a third party providing information.

Even when adequate information is available, people can make mistakes by processing it poorly. Poor information-processing often occurs in cases of low probability, high-consequence events, but it is not limited to such situations. For instance, people sometimes rely on mental rules-of-thumb that produce errors. If they have a clear mental image of an incident which makes it cognitively "available," they might overstate the probability that it will occur. Individuals sometimes process information in a biased manner, by being too optimistic or pessimistic, without taking sufficient account of the fact that the outcome is exceedingly unlikely to occur. When mistakes in information processing occur, markets may overreact. When it is time-consuming or costly for consumers to evaluate complex information about products or services (e.g., medical therapies), they may expect government to ensure that minimum quality standards are met. However, the mere possibility of poor information processing is not enough to justify regulation. If you think there is a problem of information processing that needs to be addressed, it should be carefully documented.

4.   Other Social Purposes

There are justifications for regulations in addition to correcting market failures. A regulation may be appropriate when you have a clearly identified measure that can make government operate more efficiently. In addition, Congress establishes some regulatory programs to redistribute resources to select groups. Such regulations should be examined to ensure that they are both effective and cost-effective. Congress also authorizes some regulations to prohibit discrimination that conflicts with generally accepted norms within our society. Rulemaking may also be appropriate to protect privacy, permit more personal freedom or promote other democratic aspirations.

Showing That Regulation at the Federal Level Is the Best Way to Solve the Problem

Even where a market failure clearly exists, you should consider other means of dealing with the failure before turning to Federal regulation. Alternatives to Federal regulation include antitrust enforcement, consumer-initiated litigation in the product liability system, or administrative compensation systems.

In assessing whether Federal regulation is the best solution, you should also consider the possibility of regulation at the State or local level. In some cases, the nature of the market failure may itself suggest the most appropriate governmental level of regulation. For example, problems that spill across State lines (such as acid rain whose precursors are transported widely in the atmosphere) are probably best addressed by Federal regulation. More localized problems, including those that are common to many areas, may be more efficiently addressed locally.

The advantages of leaving regulatory issues to State and local authorities can be substantial. If public values and preferences differ by region, those differences can be reflected in varying State and local regulatory policies. Moreover, States and localities can serve as a testing ground for experimentation with alternative regulatory policies. One State can learn from another's experience while local jurisdictions may compete with each other to establish the best regulatory policies. You should examine the proper extent of State and local discretion in your rulemaking context.

A diversity of rules may generate gains for the public as governmental units compete with each other to serve the public, but duplicative regulations can also be costly. Where Federal regulation is clearly appropriate to address interstate commerce issues, you should try to examine whether it would be more efficient to retain or reduce State and local regulation. The local benefits of State regulation may not justify the national costs of a fragmented regulatory system. For example, the increased compliance costs for firms to meet different State and local regulations may exceed any advantages associated with the diversity of State and local regulation. Your analysis should consider the possibility of reducing as well as expanding State and local rulemaking.

The role of Federal regulation in facilitating U.S. participation in global markets should also be considered. Harmonization of U.S. and international rules may require a strong Federal regulatory role. Concerns that new U.S. rules could act as non-tariff barriers to imported goods should be evaluated carefully.

The Presumption Against Economic Regulation

Government actions can be unintentionally harmful, and even useful regulations can impede market efficiency. For this reason, there is a presumption against certain types of regulatory action. In light of both economic theory and actual experience, a particularly demanding burden of proof is required to demonstrate the need for any of the following types of regulations:

- price controls in competitive markets;
- production or sales quotas in competitive markets;
- mandatory uniform quality standards for goods or services if the potential problem can be adequately dealt with through voluntary standards or by disclosing information of the hazard to buyers or users; or
- controls on entry into employment or production, except (a) where indispensable to protect health and safety (e.g., FAA tests for commercial pilots) or (b) to manage the use of common property resources (e.g., fisheries, airwaves, Federal lands, and offshore areas).

C. Alternative Regulatory Approaches

Once you have determined that Federal regulatory action is appropriate, you will need to consider alternative regulatory approaches. Ordinarily, you will be able to eliminate some alternatives through a preliminary analysis, leaving a manageable number of alternatives to be evaluated according to the formal principles of the Executive Order. The number and choice of alternatives selected for detailed analysis is a matter of judgment. There must be some balance between thoroughness and the practical limits on your analytical capacity. With this qualification in mind, you should nevertheless explore modifications of some or all of a regulation's attributes or provisions to identify appropriate alternatives. The following is a list of alternative regulatory actions that you should consider.

Different Choices Defined by Statute

When a statute establishes a specific regulatory requirement and the agency is considering a more stringent standard, you should examine the benefits and costs of reasonable alternatives that reflect the range of the agency's statutory discretion, including the specific statutory requirement.

Different Compliance Dates

The timing of a regulation may also have an important effect on its net benefits. Benefits may vary significantly with different compliance dates where a delay in implementation may result in a substantial loss in future benefits (e.g., a delay in implementation could result in a significant reduction in spawning stock and jeopardize a fishery). Similarly, the cost of a regulation may vary substantially with different compliance dates for an industry that requires a year or more to plan its production runs. In this instance, a regulation that provides sufficient lead time is likely to achieve its goals at a much lower overall cost than a regulation that is effective immediately.

Different Enforcement Methods

Compliance alternatives for Federal, State, or local enforcement include on-site inspections, periodic reporting, and noncompliance penalties structured to provide the most appropriate incentives. When alternative monitoring and reporting methods vary in their benefits and costs, you should identify the most appropriate enforcement framework. For example, in some circumstances random monitoring or parametric monitoring will be less expensive and nearly as effective as continuous monitoring.

Different Degrees of Stringency

In general, both the benefits and costs associated with a regulation will increase with the level of stringency (although marginal costs generally increase with stringency, whereas marginal benefits may decrease). You should study alternative levels of stringency to understand more fully the relationship between stringency and the size and distribution of benefits and costs among different groups.

Different Requirements for Different Sized Firms

You should consider setting different requirements for large and small firms, basing the requirements on estimated differences in the expected costs of compliance or in the expected benefits. The balance of benefits and costs can shift depending on the size of the firms being regulated. Small firms may find it more costly to comply with regulation, especially if there are large fixed costs required for regulatory compliance. On the other hand, it is not efficient to place a heavier burden on one segment of a regulated industry solely because it can better afford the higher cost. This has the potential to load costs on the most productive firms, costs that are disproportionate to the damages they create. You should also remember that a rule with a significant impact on a substantial number of small entities will trigger the requirements set forth in the Regulatory Flexibility Act. (5 U.S.C. 603(c), 604).

Different Requirements for Different Geographic Regions

Rarely do all regions of the country benefit uniformly from government regulation. It is also unlikely that costs will be uniformly distributed across the country. Where there are significant regional variations in benefits and/or costs, you should consider the possibility of setting different requirements for the different regions.

Performance Standards Rather than Design Standards

Performance standards express requirements in terms of outcomes rather than specifying the means to those ends. They are generally superior to engineering or design standards because performance standards give the regulated parties the flexibility to achieve regulatory objectives in the most cost-effective way. In general, you should take into account both the cost savings to the regulated parties of the greater flexibility and the costs of assuring compliance through monitoring or some other means.

Market-Oriented Approaches Rather than Direct Controls

Market-oriented approaches that use economic incentives should be explored. These alternatives include fees, penalties, subsidies, marketable permits or offsets, changes in liability or property rights (including policies that alter the incentives of insurers and insured parties), and required bonds, insurance or warranties. One example of a market-oriented approach is a program that allows for averaging, banking, and/or trading (ABT) of credits for achieving additional emission reductions beyond the required air emission standards. ABT programs can be extremely valuable in reducing costs or achieving earlier or greater benefits, particularly when the costs of achieving compliance vary across production lines, facilities, or firms. ABT can be allowed on a plant-wide, firm-wide, or region-wide basis rather than vent by vent, provided this does not produce unacceptable local air quality outcomes (such as "hot spots" from local pollution concentration).

Informational Measures Rather than Regulation

If intervention is contemplated to address a market failure that arises from inadequate or asymmetric information, informational remedies will often be preferred. Measures to improve the availability of information include government establishment of a standardized testing and rating system (the use of which could be mandatory or voluntary), mandatory disclosure requirements (e.g., by advertising, labeling, or enclosures), and government provision of information (e.g., by government publications, telephone hotlines, or public interest broadcast announcements). A regulatory measure to improve the availability of information, particularly about the concealed characteristics of products, provides consumers a greater choice than a mandatory product standard or ban.

Specific informational measures should be evaluated in terms of their benefits and costs. Some effects of informational measures are easily overlooked. The costs of a mandatory disclosure requirement for a consumer product will include not only the cost of gathering and communicating the required information, but also the loss of net benefits of any information displaced by the mandated information. The other costs also may include the effect of providing information that is ignored or misinterpreted, and inefficiencies arising from the incentive that mandatory disclosure may give to overinvest in a particular characteristic of a product or service.

Where information on the benefits and costs of alternative informational measures is insufficient to provide a clear choice between them, you should consider the least intrusive informational alternative sufficient to accomplish the regulatory objective. To correct an informational market failure it may be sufficient for government to establish a standardized testing and rating system without mandating its use, because competing firms that score well according to the system should thereby have an incentive to publicize the fact.

D. Analytical Approaches

Both benefit-cost analysis (BCA) and cost-effectiveness analysis (CEA) provide a systematic framework for identifying and evaluating the likely outcomes of alternative regulatory choices. A major rulemaking should be supported by both types of analysis wherever possible. Specifically, you should prepare a CEA for all major rulemakings for which the primary benefits are improved public health and safety to the extent that a valid effectiveness measure can be developed to represent expected health and safety outcomes. You should also perform a BCA for major health and safety rulemakings to the extent that valid monetary values can be assigned to the primary expected health and safety outcomes. In undertaking these analyses, it is important to keep in mind the larger objective of analytical consistency in estimating benefits and costs across regulations and agencies, subject to statutory limitations. Failure to maintain such consistency may prevent achievement of the most risk reduction for a given level of resource expenditure. For all other major rulemakings, you should carry out a BCA. If some of the primary benefit categories cannot be expressed in monetary units, you should also conduct a CEA. In unusual cases where no quantified information on benefits, costs and effectiveness can be produced, the regulatory analysis should present a qualitative discussion of the issues and evidence.

Benefit-Cost Analysis

A distinctive feature of BCA is that both benefits and costs are expressed in monetary units, which allows you to evaluate different regulatory options with a variety of attributes using a common measure.[4] By measuring incremental benefits and costs of successively more stringent regulatory alternatives, you can identify the alternative that maximizes net benefits.

The size of net benefits, the absolute difference between the projected benefits and costs, indicates whether one policy is more efficient than another. The ratio of benefits to costs is not a meaningful indicator of net

---

[4]Mishan EJ (1994), *Cost-Benefit Analysis*, fourth edition, Routledge, New York.

benefits and should not be used for that purpose. It is well known that considering such ratios alone can yield misleading results.

Even when a benefit or cost cannot be expressed in monetary units, you should still try to measure it in terms of its physical units. If it is not possible to measure the physical units, you should still describe the benefit or cost qualitatively. For more information on describing qualitative information, see the section "*Developing Benefit and Cost Estimates.*"

When important benefits and costs cannot be expressed in monetary units, BCA is less useful, and it can even be misleading, because the calculation of net benefits in such cases does not provide a full evaluation of all relevant benefits and costs.

You should exercise professional judgment in identifying the importance of non-quantified factors and assess as best you can how they might change the ranking of alternatives based on estimated net benefits. If the non-quantified benefits and costs are likely to be important, you should recommend which of the non-quantified factors are of sufficient importance to justify consideration in the regulatory decision. This discussion should also include a clear explanation that support designating these non-quantified factors as important. In this case, you should also consider conducting a threshold analysis to help decision makers and other users of the analysis to understand the potential significance of these factors to the overall analysis.

Cost-Effectiveness Analysis[5]

Cost-effectiveness analysis can provide a rigorous way to identify options that achieve the most effective use of the resources available without requiring monetization of all of relevant benefits or costs. Generally, cost-effectiveness analysis is designed to compare a set of regulatory actions with the same primary outcome (e.g., an increase in the acres of wetlands protected) or multiple outcomes that can be integrated into a single numerical index (e.g., units of health improvement).

Cost-effectiveness results based on averages need to be treated with great care. They suffer from the same drawbacks as benefit–cost ratios. The alternative that exhibits the smallest cost-effectiveness ratio may not be the best option, just as the alternative with the highest benefit–cost ratio is not always the one that maximizes net benefits. Incremental cost-effectiveness

---

[5]For a full discussion of CEA, see Gold, ML, Siegel, JE, Russell, LB, and Weinstein, MC (1996), *Cost Effectiveness in Health and Medicine: The Report of the Panel on Cost-Effectiveness in Health and Medicine*, Oxford University Press, New York.

analysis (discussed below) can help to avoid mistakes that can occur when policy choices are based on average cost-effectiveness.

CEA can also be misleading when the "effectiveness" measure does not appropriately weight the consequences of the alternatives. For example, when effectiveness is measured in tons of reduced pollutant emissions, cost-effectiveness estimates will be misleading unless the reduced emissions of diverse pollutants result in the same health and environmental benefits.

When you have identified a range of alternatives (e.g., different levels of stringency), you should determine the cost-effectiveness of each option compared with the baseline as well as its incremental cost-effectiveness compared with successively more stringent requirements. Ideally, your CEA would present an array of cost-effectiveness estimates that would allow comparison across different alternatives. However, analyzing all possible combinations is not practical when there are many options (including possible interaction effects). In these cases, you should use your judgment to choose reasonable alternatives for careful consideration.

When constructing and comparing incremental cost-effectiveness ratios, you should be careful to determine whether the various alternatives are mutually exclusive or whether they can be combined. If they can be combined, you should consider which might be favored under different regulatory budget constraints (implicit or explicit). You should also make sure that inferior alternatives identified by the principles of strong and weak dominance are eliminated from consideration.[6]

The value of CEA is enhanced when there is consistency in the analysis across a diverse set of possible regulatory actions. To achieve consistency, you need to carefully construct the two key components of any CEA: the cost and the "effectiveness" or performance measures for the alternative policy options.

With regard to measuring costs, you should be sure to include all the relevant costs to society B whether public or private. Rulemakings may also yield cost savings (e.g., energy savings associated with new technologies). The numerator in the cost-effectiveness ratio should reflect net costs, defined as the gross cost incurred to comply with the requirements (sometimes called "total" costs) minus any cost savings. You should be careful to avoid double-counting effects in both the numerator and the denominator of the cost-effectiveness ratios. For example, it would be incorrect to reduce gross

---

[6]Gold ML, Siegel JE, Russell LB, and Weinstein MC (1996), *Cost Effectiveness in Health and Medicine: The Report of the Panel on Cost-Effectiveness in Health and Medicine*, Oxford University Press, New York, pp. 284–285.

costs by an estimated monetary value on life extension if life-years are already used as the effectiveness measure in the denominator.

In constructing measures of "effectiveness", final outcomes, such as lives saved or life-years saved, are preferred to measures of intermediate outputs, such as tons of pollution reduced, crashes avoided, or cases of disease avoided. Where the quality of the measured unit varies (e.g., acres of wetlands vary substantially in terms of their ecological benefits), it is important that the measure capture the variability in the value of the selected "outcome" measure. You should provide an explanation of your choice of effectiveness measure.

Where regulation may yield several different beneficial outcomes, a cost-effectiveness comparison becomes more difficult to interpret because there is more than one measure of effectiveness to incorporate in the analysis. To arrive at a single measure you will need to weight the value of disparate benefit categories, but this computation raises some of the same difficulties you will encounter in BCA. If you can assign a reasonable monetary value to all of the regulation's different benefits, then you should do so. But in this case, you will be doing BCA, not CEA.

When you can estimate the monetary value of some but not all of the ancillary benefits of a regulation, but cannot assign a monetary value to the primary measure of effectiveness, you should subtract the monetary estimate of the ancillary benefits from the gross cost estimate to yield an estimated net cost. (This net cost estimate for the rule may turn out to be negative—that is, the monetized benefits exceed the cost of the rule.) If you are unable to estimate the value of some of the ancillary benefits, the cost-effectiveness ratio will be overstated, and this should be acknowledged in your analysis. CEA does not yield an unambiguous choice when there are benefits or costs that have not been incorporated in the net-cost estimates. You also may use CEA to compare regulatory alternatives in cases where the statute specifies the level of benefits to be achieved.

The Effectiveness Metric for Public Health and Safety Rulemakings

When CEA is applied to public health and safety rulemakings, one or more measures of effectiveness must be selected that permits comparison of regulatory alternatives. Agencies currently use a variety of effectiveness measures.

There are relatively simple measures such as the number of lives saved, cases of cancer reduced, and cases of paraplegia prevented. Sometimes these measures account only for mortality information, such as the number of lives saved and the number of years of life saved. There are also more comprehensive, integrated measures of effectiveness such as the number of "equivalent lives" (ELs) saved and the number of "quality-adjusted life years" (QALYs) saved.

The main advantage of the integrated measures of effectiveness is that they account for a rule's impact on morbidity (nonfatal illness, injury, impairment and quality of life) as well as premature death. The inclusion of morbidity effects is important because (a) some illnesses (e.g., asthma) cause more instances of pain and suffering than they do premature death, (b) some population groups are known to experience elevated rates of morbidity (e.g, the elderly and the poor) and thus have a strong interest in morbidity measurement[7], and (c) some regulatory alternatives may be more effective at preventing morbidity than premature death (e.g., some advanced airbag designs may diminish the nonfatal injuries caused by airbag inflation without changing the frequency of fatal injury prevented by airbags).

However, the main drawback of these integrated measures is that they must meet some restrictive assumptions to represent a valid measure of individual preferences.[8] For example, a QALY measure implicitly assumes that the fraction of remaining lifespan an individual would give up for an improvement in health-related quality of life does not depend on the remaining lifespan. Thus, if an individual is willing to give up 10 years of life among 50 remaining years for a given health improvement, he or she would also be willing to give up 1 year of life among 5 remaining years. To the extent that individual preferences deviate from these assumptions, analytic results from CEA using QALYs could differ from analytic results based on willingness-to-pay-measures.[9] Though willingness to pay is generally the preferred economic method for evaluating preferences, the CEA method, as applied in medicine and health, does not evaluate health changes using individual willingness to pay. When performing CEA, you should consider using at least one integrated measure of effectiveness when a rule creates a significant impact on both mortality and morbidity.

When CEA is performed in specific rulemaking contexts, you should be prepared to make appropriate adjustments to ensure fair treatment of all segments of the population. Fairness is important in the choice and execution of effectiveness measures. For example, if QALYs are used to evaluate a lifesaving rule aimed at a population that happens to experience a high

---

[7]Russell LB and Sisk JE (2000), "Modeling Age Differences in Cost Effectiveness Analysis", *International Journal of Technology Assessment in Health Care*, 16(4), 1158–1167.

[8]Pliskin JS, Shepard DS, and Weinstein MC (1980), "Utility Functions for Life Years and Health Status," *Operations Research*, 28(1), 206–224.

[9]Hammitt JK (2002), "QALYs Versus WTP," *Risk Analysis*, 22(5), pp. 985–1002.

rate of disability (i.e., where the rule is not designed to affect the disability), the number of life years saved should not necessarily be diminished simply because the rule saves the lives of people with life-shortening disabilities. Both analytic simplicity and fairness suggest that the estimated number of life years saved for the disabled population should be based on average life expectancy information for the relevant age cohorts. More generally, when numeric adjustments are made for life expectancy or quality of life, analysts should prefer use of population averages rather than information derived from subgroups dominated by a particular demographic or income group.

OMB does not require agencies to use any specific measure of effectiveness. In fact, OMB encourages agencies to report results with multiple measures of effectiveness that offer different insights and perspectives. The regulatory analysis should explain which measures were selected and why, and how they were implemented.

The analytic discretion provided in choice of effectiveness measure will create some inconsistency in how agencies evaluate the same injuries and diseases, and it will be difficult for OMB and the public to draw meaningful comparisons between rulemakings that employ different effectiveness measures. As a result, agencies should use their web site to provide OMB and the public with the underlying data, including mortality and morbidity data, the age distribution of the affected populations, and the severity and duration of disease conditions and trauma, so that OMB and the public can construct apples-to-apples comparisons between rulemakings that employ different measures.

There are sensitive technical and ethical issues associated with choosing one or more of these integrated measures for use throughout the Federal government. The Institute of Medicine (IOM) may assemble a panel of specialists in cost-effectiveness analysis and bioethics to evaluate the advantages and disadvantages of these different measures and other measures that have been suggested in the academic literature. OMB believes that the IOM guidance will provide Federal agencies and OMB useful insight into how to improve the measurement of effectiveness of public health and safety regulations.

Distributional Effects

Those who bear the costs of a regulation and those who enjoy its benefits often are not the same people. The term "distributional effect" refers to the impact of a regulatory action across the population and economy, divided up in various ways (e.g., income groups, race, sex, industrial sector, geography). Benefits and costs of a regulation may also be distributed unevenly over time, perhaps spanning several generations. Distributional effects may arise through "transfer payments" that stem from a regulatory action as well. For example, the revenue collected through a fee, surcharge in excess of the cost of services provided, or tax is a transfer payment.

Your regulatory analysis should provide a separate description of distributional effects (i.e., how both benefits and costs are distributed among sub-populations of particular concern) so that decision makers can properly consider them along with the effects on economic efficiency. Executive Order 12866 authorizes this approach. Where distributive effects are thought to be important, the effects of various regulatory alternatives should be described quantitatively to the extent possible, including the magnitude, likelihood, and severity of impacts on particular groups. You should be alert for situations in which regulatory alternatives result in significant changes in treatment or outcomes for different groups. Effects on the distribution of income that are transmitted through changes in market prices can be important, albeit sometimes difficult to assess. Your analysis should also present information on the streams of benefits and costs over time in order to provide a basis for assessing intertemporal distributional consequences, particularly where intergenerational effects are concerned.

E. Identifying and Measuring Benefits and Costs

This Section provides guidelines for your preparation of the benefit and cost estimates required by Executive Order 12866 and the "Regulatory Right-to-Know Act." The discussions in previous sections will help you identify a workable number of alternatives for consideration in your analysis and an appropriate analytical approach to use.

General Issues

1. Scope of Analysis

Your analysis should focus on benefits and costs that accrue to citizens and residents of the United States. Where you choose to evaluate a regulation that is likely to have effects beyond the borders of the United States, these effects should be reported separately. The time frame for your analysis should cover a period long enough to encompass all the important benefits and costs likely to result from the rule.

2. Developing a Baseline

You need to measure the benefits and costs of a rule against a baseline. This baseline should be the best assessment of the way the world would look absent the proposed action. The choice of an appropriate baseline may require consideration of a wide range of potential factors, including:

- evolution of the market,
- changes in external factors affecting expected benefits and costs,
- changes in regulations promulgated by the agency or other government entities, and
- the degree of compliance by regulated entities with other regulations.

It may be reasonable to forecast that the world absent the regulation will resemble the present. If this is the case, however, your baseline should reflect the future effect of current government programs and policies. For review of an existing regulation, a baseline assuming "no change" in the regulatory program generally provides an appropriate basis for evaluating regulatory alternatives. When more than one baseline is reasonable and the choice of baseline will significantly affect estimated benefits and costs, you should consider measuring benefits and costs against alternative baselines. In doing so you can analyze the effects on benefits and costs of making different assumptions about other agencies' regulations, or the degree of compliance with your own existing rules. In all cases, you must evaluate benefits and costs against the same baseline. You should also discuss the reasonableness of the baselines used in the sensitivity analyses. For each baseline you use, you should identify the key uncertainties in your forecast.

EPA's 1998 final PCB disposal rule provides a good example of using different baselines. EPA used several alternative baselines, each reflecting a different interpretation of existing regulatory requirements. In particular, one baseline reflected a literal interpretation of EPA's 1979 rule and another the actual implementation of that rule in the year immediately preceding the 1998 revision. The use of multiple baselines illustrated the substantial effect changes in EPA's implementation policy could have on the cost of a regulatory program. In the years after EPA adopted the 1979 PCB disposal rule, changes in EPA policy—especially allowing the disposal of automobile "shredder fluff" in municipal landfills—reduced the cost of the program by more than $500 million per year.

In some cases, substantial portions of a rule may simply restate statutory requirements that would be self-implementing, even in the absence of the regulatory action. In these cases, you should use a pre-statute baseline. If you are able to separate out those areas where the agency has discretion, you may also use a post-statute baseline to evaluate the discretionary elements of the action.

3. Evaluation of Alternatives

You should describe the alternatives available to you and the reasons for choosing one alternative over another. As noted previously, alternatives that rely on incentives and offer increased flexibility are often more cost-effective than more prescriptive approaches. For instance, user fees and information dissemination may be good alternatives to direct command-and-control regulation. Within a command-and-control regulatory program, performance-based standards generally offer advantages over standards specifying design, behavior, or manner of compliance.

You should carefully consider all appropriate alternatives for the key attributes or provisions of the rule. The previous discussion outlines examples of appropriate alternatives. Where there is a "continuum" of alternatives for a standard (such as the level of stringency), you generally should analyze at least three options: the preferred option; a more stringent option that achieves additional benefits (and presumably costs more) beyond those realized by the preferred option; and a less stringent option that costs less (and presumably generates fewer benefits) than the preferred option.

You should choose reasonable alternatives deserving careful consideration. In some cases, a regulatory program will focus on an option that is near or at the limit of technical feasibility. In this case, the analysis would not need to examine a more stringent option. For each of the options analyzed, you should compare the anticipated benefits to the corresponding costs.

It is not adequate simply to report a comparison of the agency's preferred option to the chosen baseline. Whenever you report the benefits and costs of alternative options, you should present both total and incremental benefits and costs. You should present incremental benefits and costs as differences from the corresponding estimates associated with the next less-stringent alternative.[10] It is important to emphasize that incremental effects are simply differences between successively more stringent alternatives.

---

[10]For the least stringent alternative, you should estimate the incremental benefits and costs relative to the baseline. Thus, for this alternative, the incremental effects would be the same as the corresponding totals. For each alternative that is more stringent than the least stringent alternative, you should estimate the incremental benefits and costs relative to the closest less-stringent alternative.

Results involving a comparison to a "next best" alternative may be especially useful.

In some cases, you may decide to analyze a wide array of options. In 1998, DOE analyzed a large number of options in setting new energy efficiency standards for refrigerators and freezers and produced a rich amount of information on their relative effects. This analysis—examining more than 20 alternative performance standards for one class of refrigerators with top-mounted freezers—enabled DOE to select an option that produced $200 more in estimated net benefits per refrigerator than the least attractive option.

You should analyze the benefits and costs of different regulatory provisions separately when a rule includes a number of distinct provisions. If the existence of one provision affects the benefits or costs arising from another provision, the analysis becomes more complicated, but the need to examine provisions separately remains. In this case, you should evaluate each specific provision by determining the net benefits of the proposed regulation with and without it.

Analyzing all possible combinations of provisions is impractical if the number is large and interaction effects are widespread. You need to use judgment to select the most significant or relevant provisions for such analysis. You are expected to document all of the alternatives that were considered in a list or table and which were selected for emphasis in the main analysis.

You should also discuss the statutory requirements that affect the selection of regulatory approaches. If legal constraints prevent the selection of a regulatory action that best satisfies the philosophy and principles of Executive Order 12866, you should identify these constraints and estimate their opportunity cost. Such information may be useful to Congress under the Regulatory Right-to-Know Act.

4.   Transparency and Reproducibility of Results

Because of its influential nature and its special role in the rulemaking process, it is appropriate to set minimum quality standards for regulatory analysis. You should provide documentation that the analysis is based on the best reasonably obtainable scientific, technical, and economic information available. To achieve this, you should rely on peer-reviewed literature, where available, and provide the source for all original information.

A good analysis should be transparent and your results must be reproducible. You should clearly set out the basic assumptions, methods, and data underlying the analysis and discuss the uncertainties associated with the estimates. A qualified third party reading the analysis should be able to understand the basic elements of your analysis and the way in which you developed your estimates.

To provide greater access to your analysis, you should generally post it, with all the supporting documents, on the internet so the public can review the findings. You should also disclose the use of outside consultants, their qualifications, and history of contracts and employment with the agency (e.g., in a preface to the RIA). Where other compelling interests (such as privacy, intellectual property, trade secrets, etc.) prevent the public release of data or key elements of the analysis, you should apply especially rigorous robustness checks to analytic results and document the analytical checks used.

Finally, you should assure compliance with the Information Quality Guidelines for your agency and OMB's "Guidelines for Ensuring and Maximizing the Quality, Objectivity, Utility, and Integrity of Information Disseminated by Federal Agencies" ("data quality guidelines") http://www.whitehouse.gov/omb/fedreg/reproducible.html.

Developing Benefit and Cost Estimates

1. Some General Considerations

The analysis document should discuss the expected benefits and costs of the selected regulatory option and any reasonable alternatives. How is the proposed action expected to provide the anticipated benefits and costs? What are the monetized values of the potential real incremental benefits and costs to society? To present your results, you should:

- include separate schedules of the monetized benefits and costs that show the type and timing of benefits and costs, and express the estimates in this table in constant, undiscounted dollars (for more on discounting see "Discount Rates" below);
- list the benefits and costs you can quantify, but cannot monetize, including their timing;
- describe benefits and costs you cannot quantify; and
- identify or cross-reference the data or studies on which you base the benefit and cost estimates.

When benefit and cost estimates are uncertain (for more on this see "*Treatment of Uncertainty*" below), you should report benefit and cost estimates (including benefits of risk reductions) that reflect the full probability distribution of potential consequences. Where possible, present probability distributions of benefits and costs and include the upper and lower bound estimates as complements to central tendency and other estimates.

If fundamental scientific disagreement or lack of knowledge prevents construction of a scientifically defensible probability distribution, you should describe benefits or costs under plausible scenarios and characterize the evidence and assumptions underlying each alternative scenario.

2. The Key Concepts Needed to Estimate Benefits and Costs

"Opportunity cost" is the appropriate concept for valuing both benefits and costs. The principle of "willingness-to-pay" (WTP) captures the notion of opportunity cost by measuring what individuals are willing to forgo to enjoy a particular benefit. In general, economists tend to view WTP as the most appropriate measure of opportunity cost, but an individual's "willingness-to-accept" (WTA) compensation for not receiving the improvement can also provide a valid measure of opportunity cost.

WTP and WTA are comparable measures under special circumstances. WTP and WTA measures may be comparable in the following situations: if a regulation affects a price change rather than a quantity change; the change being evaluated is small; there are reasonably close substitutes available; and the income effect is small.[11] However, empirical evidence from experimental economics and psychology shows that even when income/wealth effects are "small", the measured differences between WTP and WTA can be large.[12] WTP is generally considered to be more readily measurable. Adoption of WTP as the measure of value implies that individual preferences of the affected population should be a guiding factor in the regulatory analysis.

Market prices provide rich data for estimating benefits and costs based on willingness-to-pay if the goods and services affected by the regulation are traded in well-functioning competitive markets. The opportunity cost of an alternative includes the value of the benefits forgone as a result of choosing that alternative. The opportunity cost of banning a product—a drug, food additive, or hazardous chemical—is the forgone net benefit (i.e.,

---

[11]See Hanemann WM (1991), *American Economic Review*, 81(3), 635–647.

[12]See Kahneman D, Knetsch JL, and Thaler RH (1991), "Anomalies: The Endowment Effect, Loss Aversion, and Status Quo Bias," *Journal of Economic Perspectives* 3(1), 192–206.

lost consumer and producer surplus[13]) of that product, taking into account the mitigating effects of potential substitutes.

The use of any resource has an opportunity cost regardless of whether the resource is already owned or has to be purchased. That opportunity cost is equal to the net benefit the resource would have provided in the absence of the requirement. For example, if regulation of an industrial plant affects the use of additional land or buildings within the existing plant boundary, the cost analysis should include the opportunity cost of using the additional land or facilities.

To the extent possible, you should monetize any such forgone benefits and add them to the other costs of that alternative. You should also try to monetize any cost savings as a result of an alternative and either add it to the benefits or subtract it from the costs of that alternative. However, you should not assume that the "avoided" costs of not doing another regulatory alternative represent the benefits of a regulatory action where there is no direct, necessary relationship between the two. You should also be careful when the costs avoided are attributable to an existing regulation. Even when there is a direct relationship between the two regulatory actions, the use of avoided costs is problematic because the existing regulation may not maximize net benefits and thus may itself be questionable policy. (See the section, "Direct Use of Market Data," for more detail.)

Estimating benefits and costs when market prices are hard to measure or markets do not exist is more difficult. In these cases, you need to develop appropriate proxies that simulate market exchange. Estimates of willingness-to-pay based on revealed preference methods can be quite useful. As one example, analysts sometimes use "hedonic price equations" based on multiple regression analysis of market behavior to simulate market prices for the commodity of interest. The hedonic technique allows analysts to develop an estimate of the price for specific attributes associated with a product. For instance, a house is a product characterized by a variety of attributes including the number of rooms, total floor area, and type of heating and cooling. If there are enough data on transactions in the housing

---

[13]Consumer surplus is the difference between what a consumer pays for a unit of a good and the maximum amount the consumer would be willing to pay for that unit. It is measured by the area between the price and the demand curve for that unit. Producer surplus is the difference between the amount a producer is paid for a unit of a good and the minimum amount the producer would accept to supply that unit. It is measured by the area between the price and the supply curve for that unit.

market, it is possible to develop an estimate of the implicit price for specific attributes, such as the implicit price of an additional bathroom or for central air conditioning. This technique can be extended, as well, to develop an estimate for the implicit price of public goods that are not directly traded in markets. An analyst can develop implicit price estimates for public goods like air quality and access to public parks by assessing the effects of these goods on the housing market. Going through the analytical process of deriving benefit estimates by simulating markets may also suggest alternative regulatory strategies that create such markets.

You need to guard against double-counting, since some attributes are embedded in other broader measures. To illustrate, when a regulation improves the quality of the environment in a community, the value of real estate in the community generally rises to reflect the greater attractiveness of living in a better environment. Simply adding the increase in property values to the estimated value of improved public health would be double counting if the increase in property values reflects the improvement in public health. To avoid this problem you should separate the embedded effects on the value of property arising from improved public health. At the same time, an analysis that fails to incorporate the consequence of land use changes when accounting for costs will not capture the full effects of regulation.

3.   Revealed Preference Methods

Revealed preference methods develop estimates of the value of goods and services—or attributes of those goods and services—based on actual market decisions by consumers, workers and other market participants. If the market participant is well informed and confronted with a real choice, it may be feasible to determine accurately and precisely the monetary value needed for a rulemaking. There is a large and well-developed literature on revealed preference in the peer-reviewed, applied economics literature.

Although these methods are well grounded in economic theory, they are sometimes difficult to implement given the complexity of market transactions and the paucity of relevant data. When designing or evaluating a revealed preference study, the following principles should be considered:

- the market should be competitive. If the market isn't competitive (e.g., monopoly, oligopoly), then you should consider making adjustments such that the price reflects the true value to society (often called the "shadow price");
- the market should not exhibit a significant information gap or asymmetric information problem. If the market suffers from information problems, then you should discuss the divergence of the price from

the underlying shadow price and consider possible adjustments to reflect the underlying shadow price;

- the market should not exhibit an externality. In this case, you should discuss the divergence of the price from the underlying shadow price and consider possible adjustments to reflect the underlying shadow price;
- the specific market participants being studied should be representative of the target populations to be affected by the rulemaking under consideration;
- a valid research design and framework for analysis should be adopted. Examples include using data and/or model specifications that include the markets for substitute and complementary goods and services and using reasonably unrestricted functional forms. When specifying substitute and complementary goods, the analysis should preferably be based on data about the range of alternatives perceived by market participants. If such data are not available, you should adopt plausible assumptions and describe the limitations of the analysis.
- the statistical and econometric models employed should be appropriate for the application and the resulting estimates should be robust in response to plausible changes in model specification and estimation technique; and
- the results should be consistent with economic theory.

You should also determine whether there are multiple revealed-preference studies of the same good or service and whether anything can be learned by comparing the methods, data and findings from different studies. Professional judgment is required to determine whether a particular study is of sufficient quality to justify use in regulatory analysis. When studies are used in regulatory analysis despite their technical weaknesses (e.g., due to the absence of other evidence), the regulatory analysis should discuss any biases or uncertainties that are likely to arise due to those weaknesses. If a study has major weaknesses, the study should not be used in regulatory analysis.

a. Direct Uses of Market Data

Economists ordinarily consider market prices as the most accurate measure of the marginal value of goods and services to society. In some instances, however, market prices may not reflect the true value of goods and services due to market imperfections or government intervention. If a regulation involves changes to goods or services where the market price is not a good measure of the value to society, you should use an estimate that reflects the shadow price. Suppose a particular air pollutant damages crops.

One of the benefits of controlling that pollutant is the value of the crop yield increase as a result of the controls. That value is typically measured by the price of the crop. However, if the price is held above the market price by a government program that affects supply, a value estimate based on this price may not reflect the true benefits of controlling the pollutant. In this case, you should calculate the value to society of the increase in crop yields by estimating the shadow price, which reflects the value to society of the marginal use of the crop. If the marginal use is for exports, you should use the world price. If the marginal use is to add to very large surplus stockpiles, you should use the value of the last units released from storage minus storage cost. If stockpiles are large and growing, the shadow price may be low or even negative.

Other goods whose market prices may not reflect their true value include those whose production or consumption results in substantial (1) positive or negative external effects or (2) transfer payments. For example, the observed market price of gasoline may not reflect marginal social value due to the inclusion of taxes, other government interventions, and negative externalities (e.g., pollution). This shadow price may also be needed for goods whose market price is substantially affected by existing regulations that do not maximize net benefits.

b. Indirect Uses of Market Data

Many goods or attributes of goods that are affected by regulation—such as preserving environmental or cultural amenities—are not traded directly in markets. The value for these goods or attributes arise both from use and non-use. Estimation of these values is difficult because of the absence of an organized market. However, overlooking or ignoring these values in your regulatory analysis may significantly understate the benefits and/or costs of regulatory action.

"Use values" arise where an individual derives satisfaction from using the resource, either now or in the future. Use values are associated with activities such as swimming, hunting, and hiking where the individual makes use of the natural environment.

"Non-use values" arise where an individual places value on a resource, good or service even though the individual will not use the resource, now or in the future. Non-use value includes bequest and existence values.

General altruism for the health and welfare of others is a closely related concept but may not be strictly considered a "non-use" value.[14] A general

---

[14]See McConnell KE (1997), *Journal of Environmental Economics and Management*, 32, 22–37.

concern for the welfare of others should supplement benefits and costs equally; hence, it is not necessary to measure the size of general altruism in regulatory analysis. If there is evidence of selective altruism, it needs to be considered specifically in both benefits and costs.

Some goods and services are indirectly traded in markets, which means that their value is reflected in the prices of related goods and services that are directly traded in markets. Their use values are typically estimated through revealed preference methods. Examples include estimates of the values of environmental amenities derived from travel-cost studies, and hedonic price models that measure differences or changes in the value of real estate. It is important that you utilize revealed preference models that adhere to economic criteria that are consistent with utility maximizing behavior. Also, you should take particular care in designing protocols for reliably estimating the values of these attributes.

4. Stated Preference Methods

Stated Preference Methods (SPM) have been developed and used in the peer-reviewed literature to estimate both "use" and "non-use" values of goods and services. They have also been widely used in regulatory analyses by Federal agencies, in part, because these methods can be creatively employed to address a wide variety of goods and services that are not easy to study through revealed preference methods.

The distinguishing feature of these methods is that hypothetical questions about use or non-use values are posed to survey respondents in order to obtain willingness-to-pay estimates relevant to benefit or cost estimation. Some examples of SPM include contingent valuation, conjoint analysis and risk-tradeoff analysis. The surveys used to obtain the health-utility values used in CEA are similar to stated-preference surveys but do not entail monetary measurement of value. Nevertheless, the principles governing quality stated-preference research, with some obvious exceptions involving monetization, are also relevant in designing quality health-utility research.

When you are designing or evaluating a stated-preference study, the following principles should be considered:

- the good or service being evaluated should be explained to the respondent in a clear, complete and objective fashion, and the survey instrument should be pre-tested;
- willingness-to-pay questions should be designed to focus the respondent on the reality of budgetary limitations and alerted to the availability of substitute goods and alternative expenditure options;
- the survey instrument should be designed to probe beyond general attitudes (e.g., a "warm glow" effect for a particular use or non-use

value) and focus on the magnitude of the respondent's economic valuation;

- the analytic results should be consistent with economic theory using both "internal" (within respondent) and "external" (between respondent) scope tests such as the willingness to pay is larger (smaller) when more (less) of a good is provided;
- the subjects being interviewed should be selected/sampled in a statistically appropriate manner. The sample frame should adequately cover the target population. The sample should be drawn using probability methods in order to generalize the results to the target population;
- response rates should be as high as reasonably possible. Best survey practices should be followed to achieve high response rates. Low response rates increase the potential for bias and raise concerns about the generalizability of the results. If response rates are not adequate, you should conduct an analysis of non-response bias or further study. Caution should be used in assessing the representativeness of the sample based solely on demographic profiles. Statistical adjustments to reduce non-response bias should be undertaken whenever feasible and appropriate;
- the mode of administration of surveys (in-person, phone, mail, computer, internet or multiple modes) should be appropriate in light of the nature of the questions being posed to respondents and the length and complexity of the instrument;
- documentation should be provided about the target population, the sampling frame used and its coverage of the target population, the design of the sample including any stratification or clustering, the cumulative response rate (including response rate at each stage of selection if applicable); the item non-response rate for critical questions; the exact wording and sequence of questions and other information provided to respondents; and the training of interviewers and techniques they employed (as appropriate);
- the statistical and econometric methods used to analyze the collected data should be transparent, well suited for the analysis, and applied with rigor and care.

Professional judgment is necessary to apply these criteria to one or more studies, and thus there is no mechanical formula that can be used to determine whether a particular study is of sufficient quality to justify use in regulatory analysis. When studies are used despite having weaknesses on one or more of these criteria, those weaknesses should be acknowledged in the regulatory analysis, including any resulting biases or uncertainties that are likely to result. If a study has too many weaknesses with unknown consequences for the quality of the data, the study should not be used.

The challenge in designing quality stated-preference studies is arguably greater for non-use values and unfamiliar use values than for familiar goods or services that are traded (directly or indirectly) in market transactions. The good being valued may have little meaning to respondents, and respondents may be forming their valuations for the first time in response to the questions posed. Since these values are effectively constructed by the respondent during the elicitation, the instrument and mode of administration should be rigorously pre-tested to make sure that responses are not simply an artifact of specific features of instrument design and/or mode of administration.

Since SPM generate data from respondents in a hypothetical setting, often on complex and unfamiliar goods, special care is demanded in the design and execution of surveys, analysis of the results, and characterization of the uncertainties. A stated-preference study may be the only way to obtain quantitative information about non-use values, though a number based on a poor quality study is not necessarily superior to no number at all. Non-use values that are not quantified should be presented as an "intangible" benefit or cost.

If both revealed-preference and stated-preference studies that are directly applicable to regulatory analysis are available, you should consider both kinds of evidence and compare the findings. If the results diverge significantly, you should compare the overall size and quality of the two bodies of evidence. Other things equal, you should prefer revealed preference data over stated preference data because revealed preference data are based on actual decisions, where market participants enjoy or suffer the consequences of their decisions. This is not generally the case for respondents in stated preference surveys, where respondents may not have sufficient incentives to offer thoughtful responses that are more consistent with their preferences or may be inclined to bias their responses for one reason or another.

5. Benefit-Transfer Methods

It is often preferable to collect original data on revealed preference or stated preference to support regulatory analysis. Yet conducting an original study may not be feasible due to the time and expense involved. One alternative to conducting an original study is the use of "benefit transfer" methods. (The transfer may involve cost determination as well). The practice of "benefit transfer" began with transferring existing estimates obtained from indirect market and stated preference studies to new contexts (i.e., the context posed by the rulemaking). The principles that guide transferring estimates from indirect market and stated preference studies should apply to direct market studies as well.

Although benefit-transfer can provide a quick, low-cost approach for obtaining desired monetary values, the methods are often associated with uncertainties and potential biases of unknown magnitude. It should therefore be treated as a last-resort option and not used without explicit justification.

In conducting benefit transfer, the first step is to specify the value to be estimated for the rulemaking. You should identify the relevant measure of the policy change at this initial stage. For instance, you can derive the relevant willingness-to-pay measure by specifying an indirect utility function. This identification allows you to "zero in" on key aspects of the benefit transfer.

The next step is to identify appropriate studies to conduct benefit transfer. In selecting transfer studies for either point transfers or function transfers, you should base your choices on the following criteria:

- The selected studies should be based on adequate data, sound and defensible empirical methods and techniques.
- The selected studies should document parameter estimates of the valuation function.
- The study context and policy context should have similar populations (e.g., demographic characteristics). The market size (e.g., target population) between the study site and the policy site should be similar. For example, a study valuing water quality improvement in Rhode Island should not be used to value policy that will affect water quality throughout the United States.
- The good, and the magnitude of change in that good, should be similar in the study and policy contexts.
- The relevant characteristics of the study and the policy contexts should be similar. For example, the effects examined in the original study should be "reversible" or "irreversible" to a degree that is similar to the regulatory actions under consideration.
- The distribution of property rights should be similar so that the analysis uses the same welfare measure. If the property rights in the study context support the use of WTA measures while the rights in the rulemaking context support the use of WTP measures, benefit transfer is not appropriate.
- The availability of substitutes across study and policy contexts should be similar.

If you can choose between transferring a function or a point estimate, you should transfer the entire demand function (referred to as benefit function transfer) rather than adopting a single point estimate (referred to as benefit point transfer).[15]

Finally, you should not use benefit transfer in estimating benefits if:

- resources are unique or have unique attributes. For example, if a policy change affects snowmobile use in Yellowstone National Park, then a study valuing snowmobile use in the state of Michigan should not be used to value changes in snowmobile use in the Yellowstone National Park.
- If the study examines a resource that is unique or has unique attributes, you should not transfer benefit estimates or benefit functions to value a different resource and vice versa. For example, if a study values visibility improvements at the Grand Canyon, these results should not be used to value visibility improvements in urban areas.
- There are significant problems with applying an "*ex ante*" valuation estimate to an "ex post" policy context. If a policy yields a significant change in the attributes of the good, you should not use the study estimates to value the change using a benefit transfer approach.
- You also should not use a value developed from a study involving, small marginal changes in a policy context involving large changes in the quantity of the good.

Clearly, all of these criteria are difficult to meet. However, you should attempt to satisfy as many as possible when choosing studies from the existing economic literature. Professional judgment is required in determining whether a particular transfer is too speculative to use in regulatory analysis.

6. Ancillary Benefits and Countervailing Risks

Your analysis should look beyond the direct benefits and direct costs of your rulemaking and consider any important ancillary benefits and countervailing risks. An ancillary benefit is a favorable impact of the rule that is typically unrelated or secondary to the statutory purpose of the rulemaking (e.g., reduced refinery emissions due to more stringent fuel economy standards for light trucks) while a countervailing risk is an adverse economic,

---

[15]See Loomis JB (1992), *Water Resources Research*, 28(3), 701–705 and Kirchoff, S, Colby, BG, and LaFrance, JT (1997), *Journal of Environmental Economics and Management*, 33, 75–93.

health, safety, or environmental consequence that occurs due to a rule and is not already accounted for in the direct cost of the rule (e.g., adverse safety impacts from more stringent fuel-economy standards for light trucks).

You should begin by considering and perhaps listing the possible ancillary benefits and countervailing risks. However, highly speculative or minor consequences may not be worth further formal analysis. Analytic priority should be given to those ancillary benefits and countervailing risks that are important enough to potentially change the rank ordering of the main alternatives in the analysis. In some cases the mere consideration of these secondary effects may help in the generation of a superior regulatory alternative with strong ancillary benefits and fewer countervailing risks. For instance, a recent study suggested that weight-based, fuel-economy standards could achieve energy savings with fewer safety risks and employment losses than would occur under the current regulatory structure.

Like other benefits and costs, an effort should be made to quantify and monetize ancillary benefits and countervailing risks. If monetization is not feasible, quantification should be attempted through use of informative physical units. If both monetization and quantification are not feasible, then these issues should be presented as non-quantified benefits and costs. The same standards of information and analysis quality that apply to direct benefits and costs should be applied to ancillary benefits and countervailing risks.

One way to combine ancillary benefits and countervailing risks is to evaluate these effects separately and then put both of these effects on the benefits side, not on the cost side. Although it is theoretically appropriate to include disbenefits on the cost side, legal and programmatic considerations generally support subtracting the disbenefits from direct benefits.

7. Methods for Treating Non-Monetized Benefits and Costs

Sound quantitative estimates of benefits and costs, where feasible, are preferable to qualitative descriptions of benefits and costs because they help decision makers understand the magnitudes of the effects of alternative actions. However, some important benefits and costs (e.g., privacy protection) may be inherently too difficult to quantify or monetize given current data and methods. You should carry out a careful evaluation of non-quantified benefits and costs. Some authorities[16] refer to these non-monetized and non-quantified effects as "intangible".

---

[16]Mishan EJ (1994), *Cost-Benefit Analysis*, fourth edition, Routledge, New York.

a. Benefits and Costs that are Difficult to Monetize

You should monetize quantitative estimates whenever possible. Use sound and defensible values or procedures to monetize benefits and costs, and ensure that key analytical assumptions are defensible. If monetization is impossible, explain why and present all available quantitative information. For example, if you can quantify but cannot monetize increases in water quality and fish populations resulting from water quality regulation, you can describe benefits in terms of stream miles of improved water quality for boaters and increases in game fish populations for anglers. You should describe the timing and likelihood of such effects and avoid double-counting of benefits when estimates of monetized and physical effects are mixed in the same analysis.

b. Benefits and Costs that are Difficult to Quantify

If you are not able to quantify the effects, you should present any relevant quantitative information along with a description of the unquantified effects, such as ecological gains, improvements in quality of life, and aesthetic beauty. You should provide a discussion of the strengths and limitations of the qualitative information. This should include information on the key reason(s) why they cannot be quantified. In one instance, you may know with certainty the magnitude of a risk to which a substantial, but unknown, number of individuals are exposed. In another instance, the existence of a risk may be based on highly speculative assumptions, and the magnitude of the risk may be unknown.

For cases in which the unquantified benefits or costs affect a policy choice, you should provide a clear explanation of the rationale behind the choice. Such an explanation could include detailed information on the nature, timing, likelihood, location, and distribution of the unquantified benefits and costs. Also, please include a summary table that lists all the unquantified benefits and costs, and use your professional judgment to highlight (e.g., with categories or rank ordering) those that you believe are most important (e.g., by considering factors such as the degree of certainty, expected magnitude, and reversibility of effects).

While the focus is often placed on difficult to quantify benefits of regulatory action, some costs are difficult to quantify as well. Certain permitting requirements (e.g., EPA's New Source Review program) restrict the decisions of production facilities to shift to new products and adopt innovative methods of production. While these programs may impose substantial costs on the economy, it is very difficult to quantify and monetize these effects. Similarly, regulations that establish emission standards for recreational vehicles, like motor bikes, may adversely affect the performance of the vehicles in terms of driveability and 0 to 60 miles per hour acceleration. Again, the cost associated with the loss of these attributes may be difficult to quantify and monetize. They need to be analyzed qualitatively.

8. Monetizing Health and Safety Benefits and Costs

We expect you to provide a benefit-cost analysis of major health and safety rulemakings in addition to a CEA. The BCA provides additional insight because (a) it provides some indication of what the public is willing to pay for improvements in health and safety and (b) it offers additional information on preferences for health using a different research design than is used in CEA. Since the health-preference methods used to support CEA and BCA have some different strengths and drawbacks, it is important that you provide decision makers with both perspectives.

In monetizing health benefits, a WTP measure is the conceptually appropriate measure as compared to other alternatives (e.g., cost of illness or lifetime earnings), in part because it attempts to capture pain and suffering and other quality-of-life effects. Using the WTP measure for health and safety allows you to directly compare your results to the other benefits and costs in your analysis, which will typically be based on WTP.

If well-conducted revealed-preference studies of relevant health and safety risks are available, you should consider using them in developing your monetary estimates. If appropriate revealed-preference data are not available, you should use valid and relevant data from stated-preference studies. You will need to use your professional judgment when you are faced with limited information on revealed preference studies and substantial information based on stated preference studies.

A key advantage of stated-preference and health-utility methods compared to revealed preference methods is that they can be tailored to address the ranges of probabilities, types of health risks and specific populations affected by your rule. In many rulemakings there will be no relevant information from revealed-preference studies. In this situation you should consider commissioning a stated-preference study or using values from published stated-preference studies. For the reasons discussed previously, you should be cautious about using values from stated-preference studies and describe in the analysis the drawbacks of this approach.

a. Nonfatal Health and Safety Risks

With regard to nonfatal health and safety risks, there is enormous diversity in the nature and severity of impaired health states. A traumatic injury that can be treated effectively in the emergency room without hospitalization or long-term care is different from a traumatic injury resulting in paraplegia. Severity differences are also important in evaluation of chronic diseases. A severe bout of bronchitis, though perhaps less frequent, is far more painful and debilitating than the more frequent bouts of mild bronchitis. The duration of an impaired health state, which can range from a day or two to several years or even a lifetime (e.g., birth defects inducing mental retardation), need to be considered carefully. Information on both the severity and duration of an impaired health state is necessary before the task of monetization can be performed.

When monetizing nonfatal health effects, it is important to consider two components: (1) the private demand for prevention of the nonfatal health effect, to be represented by the preferences of the target population at risk, and (2) the net financial externalities associated with poor health such as net changes in public medical costs and any net changes in economic production that are not experienced by the target population. Revealed-preference or stated-preference studies are necessary to estimate the private demand; health economics data from published sources can typically be used to estimate the financial externalities caused by changes in health status. If you use literature values to monetize nonfatal health and safety risks, it is important to make sure that the values you have selected are appropriate for the severity and duration of health effects to be addressed by your rule.

If data are not available to support monetization, you might consider an alternative approach that makes use of health-utility studies. Although the economics literature on the monetary valuation of impaired health states is growing, there is a much larger clinical literature on how patients, providers and community residents value diverse health states. This literature typically measures health utilities based on the standard gamble, the time tradeoff or the rating scale methods. This health utility information may be combined with known monetary values for well-defined health states to estimate monetary values for a wide range of health states of different severity and duration. If you use this approach, you should be careful to acknowledge your assumptions and the limitations of your estimates.

b. Fatality Risks

Since agencies often design health and safety regulation to reduce risks to life, evaluation of these benefits can be the key part of the analysis. A good analysis must present these benefits clearly and show their importance. Agencies may choose to monetize these benefits. The willingness-to-pay approach is the best methodology to use if reductions in fatality risk are monetized.

Some describe the monetized value of small changes in fatality risk as the "value of statistical life" (VSL) or, less precisely, the "value of a life." The latter phrase can be misleading because it suggests erroneously that the monetization exercise tries to place a "value" on individual lives. You should make clear that these terms refer to the measurement of willingness to pay for reductions in only small risks of premature death. They have no application to an identifiable individual or to very large reductions in individual risks. They do not suggest that any individual's life can be expressed in monetary terms. Their sole purpose is to help describe better the likely benefits of a regulatory action.

Confusion about the term "statistical life" is also widespread. This term refers to the sum of risk reductions expected in a population. For example, if the annual risk of death is reduced by one in a million for each of two million people, that is said to represent two "statistical lives" extended per year (2 million people x 1/1,000,000 = 2). If the annual risk of death is reduced by one in 10 million for each of 20 million people, that also represents two statistical lives extended.

The adoption of a value for the projected reduction in the risk of premature mortality is the subject of continuing discussion within the economic and public policy analysis community. A considerable body of academic literature is available on this subject. This literature involves either explicit or implicit valuation of fatality risks, and generally involves the use of estimates of VSL from studies on wage compensation for occupational hazards (which generally are in the range of 10^{-4} annually), on consumer product purchase and use decisions, or from an emerging literature using stated preference approaches. A substantial majority of the resulting estimates of VSL vary from roughly $1 million to $10 million per statistical life.[17]

There is a continuing debate within the economic and public policy analysis community on the merits of using a single VSL for all situations versus adjusting the VSL estimates to reflect the specific rule context. A variety of factors have been identified, including whether the mortality risk involves sudden death, the fear of cancer, and the extent to which the risk is voluntarily incurred.[18] The consensus of EPA's recent Science Advisory

[17]See Viscusi WK and Aldy JE, *Journal of Risk and Uncertainty* (forthcoming) and Mrozek JR and Taylor LO (2002), *Journal of Policy Analysis and Management*, 21(2), 253–270.

[18]Distinctions between "voluntary" and "involuntary" should be treated with care. Risks are best considered to fall within a continuum from "voluntary" to "involuntary" with very few risks at either end of this range. These terms are also related to differences in the cost of avoiding risks.

Board (SAB) review of this issue was that the available literature does not support adjustments of VSL for most of these factors. The panel did conclude that it was appropriate to adjust VSL to reflect changes in income and any time lag in the occurrence of adverse health effects.

The age of the affected population has also been identified as an important factor in the theoretical literature. However, the empirical evidence on age and VSL is mixed. In light of the continuing questions over the effect of age on VSL estimates, you should not use an age-adjustment factor in an analysis using VSL estimates.[19]

Another way that has been used to express reductions in fatality risks is to use the life expectancy method, the "value of statistical life-years (VSLY) extended." If a regulation protects individuals whose average remaining life expectancy is 40 years, a risk reduction of one fatality is expressed as "40 life-years extended." Those who favor this alternative approach emphasize that the value of a statistical life is not a single number relevant for all situations. In particular, when there are significant differences between the effect on life expectancy for the population affected by a particular health risk and the populations studied in the labor market studies, they prefer to adopt a VSLY approach to reflect those differences. You should consider providing estimates of both VSL and VSLY, while recognizing the developing state of knowledge in this area.

Longevity may be only one of a number of relevant considerations pertaining to the rule. You should keep in mind that regulations with greater numbers of life-years extended are not necessarily better than regulations with fewer numbers of life-years extended. In any event, when you present estimates based on the VSLY method, you should adopt a larger VSLY estimate for senior citizens because senior citizens face larger overall health risks from all causes and they may have accumulated savings to spend on their health and safety.[20]

The valuation of fatality risk reduction is an evolving area in both results and methodology. Hence, you should utilize valuation methods that you consider appropriate for the regulatory circumstances. Since the literature-based VSL estimates may not be entirely appropriate for the risk being evaluated (e.g., the use of occupational risk premia to value reductions

---

[19]Graham JD (2003), Memorandum to the President's Management Council, Benefit-Cost Methods and Lifesaving Rules. This memorandum can be found at http://www.whitehouse. gov/omb/inforeg/pmc_benefit_cost_memo.pdf

[20]Office of Information and Regulatory Affairs, OMB, Memorandum to the President's Management Council, ibid.

in risks from environmental hazards), you should explain your selection of estimates and any adjustments of the estimates to reflect the nature of the risk being evaluated. You should present estimates based on alternative approaches, and if you monetize mortality risk reduction, you should do so on a consistent basis to the extent feasible. You should clearly indicate the methodology used and document your choice of a particular methodology. You should explain any significant deviations from the prevailing state of knowledge. If you use different methodologies in different rules, you should clearly disclose the fact and explain your choices.

c.   Valuation of Reductions in Health and Safety Risks to Children

The valuation of health outcomes for children and infants poses special challenges. It is rarely feasible to measure a child's willingness to pay for health improvement and an adult's concern for his or her own health is not necessarily relevant to valuation of child health. For example, the wage premiums demanded by workers to accept hazardous jobs are not readily transferred to rules that accomplish health gains for children.

There are a few studies that examine parental willingness to pay to invest in health and safety for their children. Some of these studies suggest that parents may value children's health more strongly than their own health. Although this parental perspective is a promising research strategy, it may need to be expanded to include a societal interest in child health and safety.

Where the primary objective of a rule is to reduce the risk of injury, disease or mortality among children, you should conduct a cost-effectiveness analysis of the rule. You may also develop a benefit-cost analysis to the extent that valid monetary values can be assigned to the primary expected health outcomes. For rules where health gains are expected among both children and adults and you decide to perform a benefit-cost analysis, the monetary values for children should be at least as large as the values for adults (for the same probabilities and outcomes) unless there is specific and compelling evidence to suggest otherwise.[21]

Discount Rates

Benefits and costs do not always take place in the same time period. When they do not, it is incorrect simply to add all of the expected net benefits or costs without taking account of when the actually occur. If

---

[21]For more information, see Dockins C., Jenkins RR, Owens N, Simon NB, and Wiggins LB (2002), *Risk Analysis*, 22(2), 335–346.

benefits or costs are delayed or otherwise separated in time from each other, the difference in timing should be reflected in your analysis.

As a first step, you should present the annual time stream of benefits and costs expected to result from the rule, clearly identifying when the benefits and costs are expected to occur. The beginning point for your stream of estimates should be the year in which the final rule will begin to have effects, even if that is expected to be some time in the future. The ending point should be far enough in the future to encompass all the significant benefits and costs likely to result from the rule.

In presenting the stream of benefits and costs, it is important to measure them in constant dollars to avoid the misleading effects of inflation in your estimates. If the benefits and costs are initially measured in prices reflecting expected future inflation, you can convert them to constant dollars by dividing through by an appropriate inflation index, one that corresponds to the inflation rate underlying the initial estimates of benefits or costs.

1. The Rationale for Discounting

Once these preliminaries are out of the way, you can begin to adjust your estimates for differences in timing. (This is a separate calculation from the adjustment needed to remove the effects of future inflation.) Benefits or costs that occur sooner are generally more valuable. The main rationales for the discounting of future impacts are:

a) Resources that are invested will normally earn a positive return, so current consumption is more expensive than future consumption, since you are giving up that expected return on investment when you consume today.

b) Postponed benefits also have a cost because people generally prefer present to future consumption. They are said to have positive time preference.

c) Also, if consumption continues to increase over time, as it has for most of U.S. history, an increment of consumption will be less valuable in the future than it would be today, because the principle of diminishing marginal utility implies that as total consumption increases, the value of a marginal unit of consumption tends to decline.

There is wide agreement with point (a). Capital investment is productive, but that point is not sufficient by itself to explain positive interest rates and observed saving behavior. To understand these phenomena, points (b) and (c) are also necessary. If people are really indifferent between consumption now and later, then they should be willing to forgo current consumption in order to consume an equal or slightly greater amount in the future. That would cause saving rates and investment to rise until interest rates were driven to zero and capital was no longer productive. As long as we observe positive interest rates and saving rates below 100 percent, people must be placing a higher value on current consumption than on future consumption.

To reflect this preference, a discount factor should be used to adjust the estimated benefits and costs for differences in timing. The further in the future the benefits and costs are expected to occur, the more they should be discounted. The discount factor can be calculated given a discount rate. The formula is $1/(1+ \text{the discount rate})^t$ where "t" measures the number of years in the future that the benefits or costs are expected to occur. Benefits or costs that have been adjusted in this way are called "discounted present values" or simply "present values". When, and only when, the estimated benefits and costs have been discounted, they can be added to determine the overall value of net benefits.

2.   Real Discount Rates of 3 percent and 7 percent

OMB's basic guidance on the discount rate is provided in OMB Circular A-94 (http://www.whitehouse.gov/omb/circulars/index.html). This Circular points out that the analytically preferred method of handling temporal differences between benefits and costs is to adjust all the benefits and costs to reflect their value in equivalent units of consumption and to discount them at the rate consumers and savers would normally use in discounting future consumption benefits. This is sometimes called the "shadow price" approach to discounting because doing such calculations requires you to value benefits and costs using shadow prices, especially for capital goods, to correct for market distortions. These shadow prices are not well established for the United States. Furthermore, the distribution of impacts from regulations on capital and consumption are not always well known. Consequently, any agency that wishes to tackle this challenging analytical task should check with OMB before proceeding.

As a default position, OMB Circular A-94 states that a real discount rate of 7 percent should be used as a base-case for regulatory analysis. The 7 percent rate is an estimate of the average before-tax rate of return to private capital in the U.S. economy. It is a broad measure that reflects the returns to real estate and small business capital as well as corporate capital. It approximates the opportunity cost of capital, and it is the appropriate discount rate whenever the main effect of a regulation is to displace or alter the use of capital in the private sector. OMB revised Circular A-94 in 1992 after extensive internal review and public comment. In a recent analysis, OMB found that the average rate of return to capital remains near the

7 percent rate estimated in 1992. Circular A-94 also recommends using other discount rates to show the sensitivity of the estimates to the discount rate assumption.

Economic distortions, including taxes on capital, create a divergence between the rate of return that savers earn and the private rate of return to capital. This divergence persists despite the tendency for capital to flow to where it can earn the highest rate of return. Although market forces will push after-tax rates of return in different sectors of the economy toward equality, that process will not equate pre-tax rates of return when there are differences in the tax treatment of investment. Corporate capital, in particular, pays an additional layer of taxation, the corporate income tax, which requires it to earn a higher pre-tax rate of return in order to provide investors with similar after-tax rates of return compared with non-corporate investments. The pre-tax rates of return better measure society's gains from investment. Since the rates of return on capital are higher in some sectors of the economy than others, the government needs to be sensitive to possible impacts of regulatory policy on capital allocation.

The effects of regulation do not always fall exclusively or primarily on the allocation of capital. When regulation primarily and directly affects private consumption (e.g., through higher consumer prices for goods and services), a lower discount rate is appropriate. The alternative most often used is sometimes called the "social rate of time preference." This simply means the rate at which "society" discounts future consumption flows to their present value. If we take the rate that the average saver uses to discount future consumption as our measure of the social rate of time preference, then the real rate of return on long-term government debt may provide a fair approximation. Over the last thirty years, this rate has averaged around 3 percent in real terms on a pre-tax basis. For example, the yield on 10-year Treasury notes has averaged 8.1 percent since 1973 while the average annual rate of change in the CPI over this period has been 5.0 percent, implying a real 10-year rate of 3.1 percent.

For regulatory analysis, you should provide estimates of net benefits using both 3 percent and 7 percent. An example of this approach is EPA's analysis of its 1998 rule setting both effluent limits for wastewater discharges and air toxic emission limits for pulp and paper mills. In this analysis, EPA developed its present-value estimates using real discount rates of 3 and 7 percent applied to benefit and cost streams that extended forward for 30 years. You should present a similar analysis in your own work.

In some instances, if there is reason to expect that the regulation will cause resources to be reallocated away from private investment in the corporate sector, then the opportunity cost may lie outside the range of 3 to

7 percent. For example, the average real rate of return on corporate capital in the United States was approximately 10 percent in the 1990s, returning to the same level observed in the 1950s and 1960s. If you are uncertain about the nature of the opportunity cost, then you should present benefit and cost estimates using a higher discount rate as a further sensitivity analysis as well as using the 3 and 7 percent rates.

3.   Time Preference for Health-Related Benefits and Costs

When future benefits or costs are health-related, some have questioned whether discounting is appropriate, since the rationale for discounting money may not appear to apply to health. It is true that lives saved today cannot be invested in a bank to save more lives in the future. But the resources that would have been used to save those lives can be invested to earn a higher payoff in future lives saved. People have been observed to prefer health gains that occur immediately to identical health gains that occur in the future. Also, if future health gains are not discounted while future costs are, then the following perverse result occurs: an attractive investment today in future health improvement can always be made more attractive by delaying the investment. For such reasons, there is a professional consensus that future health effects, including both benefits and costs, should be discounted at the same rate. This consensus applies to both BCA and CEA.

A common challenge in health-related analysis is to quantify the time lag between when a rule takes effect and when the resulting physical improvements in health status will be observed in the target population. In such situations, you must carefully consider the timing of health benefits before performing present-value calculations. It is not reasonable to assume that all of the benefits of reducing chronic diseases such as cancer and cardiovascular disease will occur immediately when the rule takes effect. For rules addressing traumatic injury, this lag period may be short. For chronic diseases it may take years or even decades for a rule to induce its full beneficial effects in the target population.

When a delay period between exposure to a toxin and increased probability of disease is likely (a so-called latency period), a lag between exposure reduction and reduced probability of disease is also likely. This latter period has sometimes been referred to as a "cessation lag," and it may or may not be of the same duration as the latency period. As a general matter, cessation lags will only apply to populations with at least some high-level exposure (e.g., before the rule takes effect). For populations with no such prior exposure, such as those born after the rule takes effect, only the latency period will be relevant.

Ideally, your exposure-risk model would allow calculation of reduced risk for each year following exposure cessation, accounting for total cumulative exposure and age at the time of exposure reduction. The present-value benefits estimate could then reflect an appropriate discount factor for each year's risk reduction. Recent analyses of the cancer benefits stemming from reduction in public exposure to radon in drinking water have adopted this approach. They were supported by formal risk-assessment models that allowed estimates of the timing of lung cancer incidence and mortality to vary in response to different radon exposure levels.[22]

In many cases, you will not have the benefit of such detailed risk assessment modeling. You will need to use your professional judgment as to the average cessation lag for the chronic diseases affected by your rule. In situations where information exists on latency but not on cessation lags, it may be reasonable to use latency as a proxy for the cessation lag, unless there is reason to believe that the two are different. When the average lag time between exposures and disease is unknown, a range of plausible alternative values for the time lag should be used in your analysis.

4.   Intergenerational Discounting

Special ethical considerations arise when comparing benefits and costs across generations. Although most people demonstrate time preference in their own consumption behavior, it may not be appropriate for society to demonstrate a similar preference when deciding between the well-being of current and future generations. Future citizens who are affected by such choices cannot take part in making them, and today's society must act with some consideration of their interest.

One way to do this would be to follow the same discounting techniques described above and supplement the analysis with an explicit discussion of the intergenerational concerns (how future generations will be affected by the regulatory decision). Policymakers would be provided with this additional information without changing the general approach to discounting.

Using the same discount rate across generations has the advantage of preventing time-inconsistency problems. For example, if one uses a lower discount rate for future generations, then the evaluation of a rule that has short-term costs and long-term benefits would become more favorable merely by waiting a year to do the analysis. Further, using the same dis-

---

[22]Committee on Risk Assessment of Exposure to Radon in Drinking Water, Board on Radiation Effects Research, Commission on Life Sciences (1996), *Risk Assessment of Radon in Drinking Water*, National Research Council, National Academy Press, Washington, DC.

count rate across generations is attractive from an ethical standpoint. If one expects future generations to be better off, then giving them the advantage of a lower discount rate would in effect transfer resources from poorer people today to richer people tomorrow.

Some believe, however, that it is ethically impermissible to discount the utility of future generations. That is, government should treat all generations equally. Even under this approach, it would still be correct to discount future costs and consumption benefits generally (perhaps at a lower rate than for intragenerational analysis), due to the expectation that future generations will be wealthier and thus will value a marginal dollar of benefits or costs by less than those alive today. Therefore, it is appropriate to discount future benefits and costs relative to current benefits and costs, even if the welfare of future generations is not being discounted. Estimates of the appropriate discount rate appropriate in this case, from the 1990s, ranged from 1 to 3 percent per annum.[23]

A second reason for discounting the benefits and costs accruing to future generations at a lower rate is increased uncertainty about the appropriate value of the discount rate, the longer the horizon for the analysis. Private market rates provide a reliable reference for determining how society values time within a generation, but for extremely long time periods no comparable private rates exist. As explained by Martin Weitzman[24], in the limit for the deep future, the properly averaged certainty-equivalent discount factor (i.e., $1/[1+r]^t$) corresponds to the minimum discount rate having any substantial positive probability. From today's perspective, the only relevant limiting scenario is the one with the lowest discount rate—all of the other states at the far-distant time are relatively much less important because their expected present value is so severely reduced by the power of compounding at a higher rate.

If your rule will have important intergenerational benefits or costs you might consider a further sensitivity analysis using a lower but positive discount rate in addition to calculating net benefits using discount rates of 3 and 7 percent.

5. Time Preference for Non-Monetized Benefits and Costs

Differences in timing should be considered even for benefits and costs that are not expressed in monetary units, including health benefits. The

---

[23]Portney PR and Weyant JP, eds. (1999), *Discounting and Intergenerational Equity*, Resources for the Future, Washington, DC.

[24]Weitzman ML In Portney PR and Weyant JP, eds. (1999), *Discounting and Intergenerational Equity*, Resources for the Future, Washington, DC.

timing differences can be handled through discounting. EPA estimated cost-effectiveness in its 1998 rule, "Control of Emissions from Nonroad Diesel Engines," by discounting both the monetary costs and the non-monetized emission reduction benefits over the expected useful life of the engines at the 7 percent real rate recommended in OMB Circular A-94.

Alternatively, it may be possible in some cases to avoid discounting non-monetized benefits. If the expected flow of benefits begins as soon as the cost is incurred and is expected to be constant over time, then annualizing the cost stream is sufficient, and further discounting of benefits is unnecessary. Such an analysis might produce an estimate of the annualized cost per ton of reduced emissions of a pollutant.

6.   The Internal Rate of Return

The internal rate of return is the discount rate that sets the net present value of the discounted benefits and costs equal to zero. The internal rate of return does not generally provide an acceptable decision criterion, and regulations with the highest internal rate of return are not necessarily the most beneficial. Nevertheless, it does provide useful information and for many it will offer a meaningful indication of regulation's impact. You should consider including the internal rate of return implied by your regulatory analysis along with other information about discounted net present values.

Other Key Considerations

1.   Other Benefit and Cost Considerations

You should include these effects in your analysis and provide estimates of their monetary values when they are significant:

- Private-sector compliance costs and savings;
- Government administrative costs and savings;
- Gains or losses in consumers' or producers' surpluses;
- Discomfort or inconvenience costs and benefits; and
- Gains or losses of time in work, leisure and/or commuting/travel settings.

Estimates of benefits and costs should be based on credible changes in technology over time. For example, retrospective studies may provide evidence that "learning" will likely reduce the cost of regulation in future years. The weight you give to a study of past rates of cost savings resulting from innovation (including "learning curve" effects) should depend on both its timeliness and direct relevance to the processes affected by the regulatory alternative under consideration. In addition, you should take into account cost-saving innovations that result from a shift to regulatory performance standards and incentive-based policies. On the other hand, significant costs may result from a slowing in the rate of innovation or of adoption of new technology due to delays in the regulatory approval process or the setting of more stringent standards for new facilities than existing ones. In some cases agencies are limited under statute to consider only technologies that have been demonstrated to be feasible. In these situations, it may be useful to estimate costs and cost savings assuming a wider range of technical possibilities.

When characterizing technology changes over time, you should assess the likely technology changes that would have occurred in the absence of the regulatory action (technology baseline). Technologies change over time in both reasonably functioning markets and imperfect markets. If you assume that technology will remain unchanged in the absence of regulation when technology changes are likely, then your analysis will over-state both the benefits and costs attributable to the regulation.

Occasionally, cost savings or other forms of benefits accrue to parties affected by a rule who also bear its costs. For example, a requirement that engine manufacturers reduce emissions from engines may lead to technologies that improve fuel economy. These fuel savings will normally accrue to the engine purchasers, who also bear the costs of the technologies. There is no apparent market failure with regard to the market value of fuel saved because one would expect that consumers would be willing to pay for increased fuel economy that exceeded the cost of providing it. When these cost savings are substantial, and particularly when you estimate them to be greater than the cost associated with achieving them, you should examine and discuss why market forces would not accomplish these gains in the absence of regulation. As a general matter, any direct costs that are averted as a result of a regulatory action should be monetized wherever possible and either added to the benefits or subtracted from the costs of that alternative.

2. The Difference between Costs (or Benefits) and Transfer Payments

Distinguishing between real costs and transfer payments is an important, but sometimes difficult, problem in cost estimation. Benefit and cost estimates should reflect real resource use. Transfer payments are monetary payments from one group to another that do not affect total resources available to society. A regulation that restricts the supply of a good, causing its price to rise, produces a transfer from buyers to sellers. The net reduction in the total surplus (consumer plus producer) is a real cost to society, but the transfer from buyers to sellers resulting from a higher price is not a real cost since the net reduction automatically accounts for the transfer from buyers to sellers. However, transfers from the United States to other nations *should* be included as costs, and transfers from other nations to the United States as benefits, as long as the analysis is conducted from the United States perspective.

You should not include transfers in the estimates of the benefits and costs of a regulation. Instead, address them in a separate discussion of the regulation's distributional effects. Examples of transfer payments include the following:

- Scarcity rents and monopoly profits
- Insurance payments
- Indirect taxes and subsidies

Treatment of Uncertainty

The precise consequences (benefits and costs) of regulatory options are not always known for certain, but the probability of their occurrence can often be developed. The important uncertainties connected with your regulatory decisions need to be analyzed and presented as part of the overall regulatory analysis. You should begin your analysis of uncertainty at the earliest possible stage in developing your analysis. You should consider both the statistical variability of key elements underlying the estimates of benefits and costs (for example, the expected change in the distribution of automobile accidents that might result from a change in automobile safety standards) and the incomplete knowledge about the relevant relationships (for example, the uncertain knowledge of how some economic activities might affect future climate change).[25] By assessing the sources of uncertainty and the way in which benefit and cost estimates may be affected under plausible assumptions, you can shape your analysis to inform decision makers and the public about the effects and the uncertainties of alternative regulatory actions.

The treatment of uncertainty must be guided by the same principles of full disclosure and transparency that apply to other elements of your regulatory analysis. Your analysis should be credible, objective, realistic, and scientifically balanced.[26] Any data and models that you use to analyze

---

[25]In some contexts, the word "variability" is used as a synonym for statistical variation that can be described by a theoretically valid distribution function, whereas "uncertainty" refers to a more fundamental lack of knowledge. Throughout this discussion, we use the term "uncertainty" to refer to both concepts.

[26]When disseminating information, agencies should follow their own information quality guidelines, issued in conformance with the OMB government-wide guidelines (67 FR 8452, February 22, 2002).

uncertainty should be fully identified. You should also discuss the quality of the available data used. Inferences and assumptions used in your analysis should be identified, and your analytical choices should be explicitly evaluated and adequately justified. In your presentation, you should delineate the strengths of your analysis along with any uncertainties about its conclusions. Your presentation should also explain how your analytical choices have affected your results.

In some cases, the level of scientific uncertainty may be so large that you can only present discrete alternative scenarios without assessing the relative likelihood of each scenario quantitatively. For instance, in assessing the potential outcomes of an environmental effect, there may be a limited number of scientific studies with strongly divergent results. In such cases, you might present results from a range of plausible scenarios, together with any available information that might help in qualitatively determining which scenario is most likely to occur.

When uncertainty has significant effects on the final conclusion about net benefits, your agency should consider additional research prior to rulemaking. The costs of being wrong may outweigh the benefits of a faster decision. This is true especially for cases with irreversible or large upfront investments. If your agency decides to proceed with rulemaking, you should explain why the costs of developing additional information—including any harm from delay in public protection—exceed the value of that information.

For example, when the uncertainty is due to a lack of data, you might consider deferring the decision, as an explicit regulatory alternative, pending further study to obtain sufficient data[27]. Delaying a decision will also have costs, as will further efforts at data gathering and analysis. You will need to weigh the benefits of delay against these costs in making your decision. Formal tools for assessing the value of additional information are now well developed in the applied decision sciences and can be used to help resolve this type of complex regulatory question.

"Real options" methods have also formalized the valuation of the added flexibility inherent in delaying a decision. As long as taking time will lower uncertainty, either passively or actively through an investment in information gathering, and some costs are irreversible, such as the potential costs of a sunk investment, a benefit can be assigned to the option to delay a decision. That benefit should be considered a cost of taking immediate

---

[27]Clemen RT (1996), Making Hard Decisions: *An Introduction to Decision Analysis*, second edition, Duxbury Press, Pacific Grove.

action versus the alternative of delaying that action pending more information. However, the burdens of delay—including any harm to public health, safety, and the environment—need to be analyzed carefully.

1.   Quantitative Analysis of Uncertainty

Examples of quantitative analysis, broadly defined, would include formal estimates of the probabilities of environmental damage to soil or water, the possible loss of habitat, or risks to endangered species as well as probabilities of harm to human health and safety. There are also uncertainties associated with estimates of economic benefits and costs, such as the cost savings associated with increased energy efficiency. Thus, your analysis should include two fundamental components: a quantitative analysis characterizing the probabilities of the relevant outcomes and an assignment of economic value to the projected outcomes. It is essential that both parts be conceptually consistent. In particular, the quantitative analysis should be conducted in a way that permits it to be applied within a more general analytical framework, such as benefit-cost analysis. Similarly, the general framework needs to be flexible enough to incorporate the quantitative analysis without oversimplifying the results. For example, you should address explicitly the implications for benefits and costs of any probability distributions developed in your analysis.

As with other elements of regulatory analysis, you will need to balance thoroughness with the practical limits on your analytical capabilities. Your analysis does not have to be exhaustive, nor is it necessary to evaluate each alternative at every step. Attention should be devoted to first resolving or studying the uncertainties that have the largest potential effect on decision making. Many times these will be the largest sources of uncertainties. In the absence of adequate data, you will need to make assumptions. These should be clearly identified and consistent with the relevant science. Your analysis should provide sufficient information for decision makers to grasp the degree of scientific uncertainty and the robustness of estimated probabilities, benefits, and costs to changes in key assumptions.

For major rules involving annual economic effects of $1 billion or more, you should present a formal quantitative analysis of the relevant uncertainties about benefits and costs. In other words, you should try to provide some estimate of the probability distribution of regulatory benefits and costs. In summarizing the probability distributions, you should provide some estimates of the central tendency (e.g., mean and median) along with any other information you think will be useful such as ranges, variances, specified low-end and high-end percentile estimates, and other characteristics of the distribution.

Your estimates cannot be more precise than their most uncertain component. Thus, your analysis should report estimates in a way that reflects the degree of uncertainty and not create a false sense of precision. Worst-case or conservative analyses are not usually adequate because they do not convey the complete probability distribution of outcomes, and they do not permit calculation of an expected value of net benefits. In many health and safety rules, economists conducting benefit-cost analyses must rely on formal risk assessments that address a variety of risk management questions such as the baseline risk for the affected population, the safe level of exposure or, the amount of risk to be reduced by various interventions. Because the answers to some of these questions are directly used in benefits analyses, the risk assessment methodology must allow for the determination of expected benefits in order to be comparable to expected costs. This means that conservative assumptions and defaults (whether motivated by science policy or by precautionary instincts), will be incompatible with benefit analyses as they will result in benefit estimates that exceed the expected value. Whenever it is possible to characterize quantitatively the probability distributions, some estimates of expected value (e.g., mean and median) must be provided in addition to ranges, variances, specified low-end and high-end percentile estimates, and other characteristics of the distribution.

Whenever possible, you should use appropriate statistical techniques to determine a probability distribution of the relevant outcomes. For rules that exceed the $1 billion annual threshold, a formal quantitative analysis of uncertainty is required. For rules with annual benefits and/or costs in the range from 100 million to $1 billion, you should seek to use more rigorous approaches with higher consequence rules. This is especially the case where net benefits are close to zero. More rigorous uncertainty analysis may not be necessary for rules in this category if simpler techniques are sufficient to show robustness. You may consider the following analytical approaches that entail increasing levels of complexity:

- Disclose qualitatively the main uncertainties in each important input to the calculation of benefits and costs. These disclosures should address the uncertainties in the data as well as in the analytical results. However, major rules above the $1 billion annual threshold require a formal treatment.
- Use a numerical sensitivity analysis to examine how the results of your analysis vary with plausible changes in assumptions, choices of input data, and alternative analytical approaches. Sensitivity analysis is especially valuable when the information is lacking to carry out a formal probabilistic simulation. Sensitivity analysis can be used to find "switch points"—critical parameter values at which estimated net benefits change sign or the low cost alternative switches. Sensitiv-

ity analysis usually proceeds by changing one variable or assumption at a time, but it can also be done by varying a combination of variables simultaneously to learn more about the robustness of your results to widespread changes. Again, however, major rules above the $1 billion annual threshold require a formal treatment.

- Apply a formal probabilistic analysis of the relevant uncertainties B possibly using simulation models and/or expert judgment as revealed, for example, through Delphi methods.[28] Such a formal analytical approach is appropriate for complex rules where there are large, multiple uncertainties whose analysis raises technical challenges, or where the effects cascade; it is required for rules that exceed the $1 billion annual threshold. For example, in the analysis of regulations addressing air pollution, there is uncertainty about the effects of the rule on future emissions, uncertainty about how the change in emissions will affect air quality, uncertainty about how changes in air quality will affect health, and finally uncertainty about the economic and social value of the change in health outcomes. In formal probabilistic assessments, expert solicitation is a useful way to fill key gaps in your ability to assess uncertainty.[29] In general, experts can be used to quantify the probability distributions of key parameters and relationships. These solicitations, combined with other sources of data, can be combined in Monte Carlo simulations to derive a probability distribution of benefits and costs. You should pay attention to correlated inputs. Often times, the standard defaults in Monte Carlo and other similar simulation packages assume independence across distributions. Failing to correctly account for correlated distributions of inputs can cause the resultant output uncertainty intervals to be too large, although in many cases the overall effect is ambiguous. You should make a special effort to portray the probabilistic results—in graphs and/or tables—clearly and meaningfully.

New methods may become available in the future. This document is not intended to discourage or inhibit their use, but rather to encourage and stimulate their development.

---

[28]The purpose of Delphi methods is to generate suitable information for decision making by eliciting expect judgment. The elicitation is conducted through a survey process which eliminates the interactions between experts. See Morgan MG and Henrion M (1990), *Uncertainty: A Guide to Dealing with Uncertainty in Quantitative Riskand Policy Analysis*, Cambridge University Press.

[29]Cooke RM (1991), *Experts in Uncertainty: Opinion and Subjective Probability in Science*, Oxford University Press.

2. Economic Values of Uncertain Outcomes

In developing benefit and cost estimates, you may find that there are probability distributions of values as well for each of the outcomes. Where this is the case, you will need to combine these probability distributions to provide estimated benefits and costs.

Where there is a distribution of outcomes, you will often find it useful to emphasize summary statistics or figures that can be readily understood and compared to achieve the broadest public understanding of your findings. It is a common practice to compare the "best estimates" of both benefits and costs with those of competing alternatives. These "best estimates" are usually the average or the expected value of benefits and costs. Emphasis on these expected values is appropriate as long as society is "risk neutral" with respect to the regulatory alternatives. While this may not always be the case, you should in general assume "risk neutrality" in your analysis. If you adopt a different assumption on risk preference, you should explain your reasons for doing so.

3. Alternative Assumptions

If benefit or cost estimates depend heavily on certain assumptions, you should make those assumptions explicit and carry out sensitivity analyses using plausible alternative assumptions. If the value of net benefits changes from positive to negative (or vice versa) or if the relative ranking of regulatory options changes with alternative plausible assumptions, you should conduct further analysis to determine which of the alternative assumptions is more appropriate. Because different estimation methods may have hidden assumptions, you should analyze estimation methods carefully to make any hidden assumptions explicit.

F. Specialized Analytical Requirements

In preparing analytical support for your rulemaking, you should be aware that there are a number of analytic requirements imposed by law and Executive Order. In addition to the regulatory analysis requirements of Executive Order 12866, you should also consider whether your rule will need specialized analysis of any of the following issues.

Impact on Small Businesses and Other Small Entities

Under the Regulatory Flexibility Act (5 U.S.C. chapter 6), agencies must prepare a proposed and final "regulatory flexibility analysis" (RFA) if the rulemaking could "have a significant impact on a substantial number of small entities." You should consider posting your RFA on the internet so the public can review your findings.

Your agency should have guidelines on how to prepare an RFA and you are encouraged to consult with the Chief Counsel for Advocacy of the Small Business Administration on expectations concerning what is an adequate RFA. Executive Order 13272 (67 FR 53461, August 16, 2002) requires you to notify the Chief Counsel for Advocacy of any draft rules that might have a significant economic impact on a substantial number of small entities. Executive Order 13272 also directs agencies to give every appropriate consideration to any comments provided by the Advocacy Office. Under SBREFA, EPA and OSHA are required to consult with small business prior to developing a proposed rule that would have a significant effect on small businesses. OMB encourages other agencies to do so as well.

Analysis of Unfunded Mandates

Under the Unfunded Mandates Act (2 U.S.C. 1532), you must prepare a written statement about benefits and costs prior to issuing a proposed or final rule (for which your agency published a proposed rule) that may result in aggregate expenditure by State, local, and tribal governments, or by the private sector, of $100,000,000 or more in any one year (adjusted annually for inflation). Your analytical requirements under Executive Order 12866 are similar to the analytical requirements under this Act, and thus the same analysis may permit you to comply with both analytical requirements.

Information Collection, Paperwork, and Recordkeeping Burdens

Under the Paperwork Reduction Act (44 U.S.C. chapter 35), you will need to consider whether your rulemaking (or other actions) will create any additional information collection, paperwork or recordkeeping burdens. These burdens are permissible only if you can justify the practical utility of the information for the implementation of your rule. OMB approval will be required of any new requirements for a collection of information imposed on 10 or more persons and a valid OMB control number must be obtained for any covered paperwork. Your agency's CIO should be able to assist you in complying with the Paperwork Reduction Act.

Information Quality Guidelines

Under the Information Quality Law, agency guidelines, in conformance with the OMB government-wide guidelines (67 FR 8452, February 22, 2002), have established basic quality performance goals for all information disseminated by agencies, including information disseminated in support of proposed and final rules. The data and analysis that you use to support your rule must meet these agency and OMB quality standards. Your agency's CIO should be able to assist you in assessing information quality. The Statistical and Science Policy Branch of OMB's Office of Information and Regulatory Affairs can provide you assistance. This circular defines OMB's minimum quality standards for regulatory analysis.

Environmental Impact Statements

The National Environmental Policy Act (42 U.S.C. 4321–4347) and related statutes and executive orders require agencies to consider the environmental impacts of agency decisions, including rulemakings. An environmental impact statement must be prepared for "major Federal actions significantly affecting the quality of the human environment." You must complete NEPA documentation before issuing a final rule. The White House Council on Environmental Quality has issued regulations (40 C.F.R. 1500–1508) and associated guidance for implementation of NEPA, available through CEQ's website (http://www.whitehouse.gov/ceq/).

Impacts on Children

Under Executive Order 13045, "Protection of Children from Environmental Health Risks and Safety Risks," each agency must, with respect to its rules, "to the extent permitted by law and appropriate, and consistent with the agency's mission," "address disproportionate risks to children that result from environmental health risks or safety risks." For any substantive rulemaking action that "is likely to result in" an economically significant rule that concerns "an environmental health risk or safety risk that an agency has reason to believe may disproportionately affect children," the agency must provide OMB/OIRA "an evaluation of the environmental health or safety effects of the planned regulation on children," as well as "an explanation of why the planned regulation is preferable to other potentially and reasonably feasible alternatives considered by the agency."

Energy Impacts

Under Executive Order 13211 (66 FR 28355, May 22, 2001), agencies are required to prepare and submit to OMB a Statement of Energy Effects for significant energy actions, to the extent permitted by law. This Statement is to include a detailed statement of "any adverse effects on energy supply, distribution, or use (including a shortfall in supply, price increases, and increased use of foreign supplies)" for the action and reasonable alternatives and their effects. You need to publish the Statement or a summary in the related NPRM and final rule. For further guidance, see OMB Memorandum 01-27 ("Guidance on Implementing Executive Order 13211", July 13, 2001), available on OMB's website.

G. Accounting Statement

You need to provide an accounting statement with tables reporting benefit and cost estimates for each major final rule for your agency. You should use the guidance outlined above to report these estimates. We have included a suggested format for your consideration.

Categories of Benefits and Costs

To the extent feasible, you should quantify all potential incremental benefits and costs. You should report benefit and cost estimates within the following three categories: monetized quantified, but not monetized; and qualitative, but not quantified or monetized.

These categories are mutually exclusive and exhaustive. Throughout the process of listing preliminary estimates of benefits and costs, agencies should avoid double-counting. This problem may arise if more than one way exists to express the same change in social welfare.

Quantifying and Monetizing Benefits and Costs

You should develop quantitative estimates and convert them to dollar amounts if possible. In many cases, quantified estimates are readily convertible, with a little effort, into dollar equivalents.

Qualitative Benefits and Costs

You should categorize or rank the qualitative effects in terms of their importance (e.g., certainty, likely magnitude, and reversibility). You should distinguish the effects that are likely to be significant enough to warrant serious consideration by decision makers from those that are likely to be minor.

Treatment of Benefits and Costs over Time

You should present undiscounted streams of benefit and cost estimates (monetized and net) for each year of the analytic time horizon. You should present annualized benefits and costs using real discount rates of 3 and

7 percent. The stream of annualized estimates should begin in the year in which the final rule will begin to have effects, even if the rule does not take effect immediately. Please report all monetized effects in 2001 dollars. You should convert dollars expressed in different years to 2001 dollars using the GDP deflator.

Treatment of Risk and Uncertainty

You should provide expected-value estimates as well as distributions about the estimates, where such information exists. When you provide only upper and lower bounds (in addition to best estimates), you should, if possible, use the 95 and 5 percent confidence bounds. Although we encourage you to develop estimates that capture the *distribution* of plausible outcomes for a particular alternative, detailed reporting of such distributions is not required, but should be available upon request.

The principles of full disclosure and transparency apply to the treatment of uncertainty. Where there is significant uncertainty and the resulting inferences and/or assumptions have a critical effect on the benefit and cost estimates, you should describe the benefits and costs under plausible alternative assumptions. You may add footnotes to the table as needed to provide documentation and references, or to express important warnings.

In a previous section, we identified some of the issues associated with developing estimates of the value of reductions in premature mortality risk. Based on this discussion, you should present alternative primary estimates where you use different estimates for valuing reductions in premature mortality risk.

Precision of Estimates

Reported estimates should reflect, to the extent feasible, the precision in the analysis. For example, an estimate of $220 million implies rounding to the nearest $10 million and thus a precision of +/-$5 million; similarly, an estimate of $222 million implies rounding to the nearest $1 million and thus, a precision of +/-$0.5 million.

Separate Reporting of Transfers

You should report transfers separately and avoid the misclassification of transfer payments as benefits or costs. Transfers occur when wealth or income is redistributed without any direct change in aggregate social welfare. To the extent that regulatory outputs reflect transfers rather than net welfare gains to society, you should identify them as transfers rather than benefits or costs. You should also distinguish transfers caused by Federal budget actions—such as those stemming from a rule affecting Social Security payments—from those that involve transfers between non-governmental parties—such as monopoly rents a rule may confer on a private party. You should use as many categories as necessary to describe the major redistributive effects of a regulatory action. If transfers have significant efficiency effects in addition to distributional effects, you should report them.

Effects on State, Local, and Tribal Governments, Small Business, Wages and Economic Growth

You need to identity the portions of benefits, costs, and transfers received by State, local, and tribal governments. To the extent feasible, you also should identify the effects of the rule or program on small businesses, wages, and economic growth.[30] Note that rules with annual costs that are less than one billion dollars are likely to have a minimal effect on economic growth.

H. Effective Date

The effective date of this Circular is January 1, 2004 for regulatory analyses received by OMB in support of proposed rules, and January 1, 2005 for regulatory analyses received by OMB in support of final rules. In other words, this Circular applies to the regulatory analyses for draft proposed rules that are formally submitted to OIRA after December 31, 2003, and for draft final rules that are formally submitted to OIRA after December 31, 2004. (However, if the draft proposed rule is subject to the Circular, then the draft final rule will also be subject to the Circular, even if it is submitted prior to January 1, 2005.) To the extent practicable, agencies should comply earlier than these effective dates. Agencies may, on a case-by-case basis, seek a waiver from OMB if these effective dates are impractical.

---

[30]The Regulatory Flexibility Act (5 U.S.C. 603(c), 604).

D
Acronyms and Glossary

ACRONYMS

ADL	Activities of daily living
AIS	Abbreviated Injury Scale
BCA	Benefit–cost analysis (same as CBA)
CDC	Centers for Disease Control and Prevention
CEA	Cost-effectiveness analysis
CFR	*Code of Federal Regulations*
COI	Cost of illness
CPSC	Consumer Product Safety Commission
CR	Category rating
CUA	Cost-utility analysis
DALY	Disability-adjusted life year
DOT	Department of Transportation
ELS	Equivalent lives saved
EOP	Executive Office of the President
EPA	Environmental Protection Agency
EQ-5D	EuroQoL-5D
FMCSA	Federal Motor Carrier Safety Administration
FSIS	Food Safety and Inspection Service

HALex	Health and Limitations Index
HALY	Health-adjusted life year
HRQL	Health-related quality of life
HSPH	Harvard School of Public Health
HUI	Health Utilities Index
HYE	Healthy year equivalent
MAIS	Maximum Abbreviated Injury Scale
MILY	Morbidity-Inclusive Life Year
NASS	National Accident Sampling System
NHTSA	National Highway Traffic Safety Administration
NOAA	National Oceanic and Atmospheric Administration
OIRA	Office of Information and Regulatory Affairs
OMB	Office of Management and Budget
OSHA	Occupational Safety and Health Administration
PCEHM	Panel on Cost-Effectiveness in Health and Medicine
PTO	Person trade-off
QALD	Quality-adjusted life day
QALY	Quality-adjusted life year
QWB	Quality of Well-Being Scale
RS	Rating scale
SAVE	Saved young life equivalent
SDWA	Safe Drinking Water Act
SG	Standard gamble
TSCA	Toxic Substances Control Act
TTO	Time trade-off
USC	United States Code
VAS	Visual analogue scale
VSL	Value of a statistical life
VSLY	Value of a statistical life year
WTP	Willingness to pay
YHL	Years of healthy life

GLOSSARY

Activities of Daily Living (ADL): The measurement of independence that is based on the following five personal care activities: bathing, dressing, using the toilet, getting in or out of bed or chair, and eating.

Attribute, Health: A state, behavior, or perception that is part of an operational definition of health-related quality of life.

Bayesian Methods: Statistical techniques for synthesizing data from different studies using empirical data and subjective probability. Used in benefits transfer to combine such data with information on the regulatory scenario.

Benefit: Generally used to indicate a positive or desirable outcome. See Chapter 5 for specific definitions relevant to the calculation of cost-effectiveness ratios.

Benefit–Cost Analysis (BCA): Also referred to as cost-benefit analysis (CBA). A type of economic analysis that compares the monetary value of improvements and harms to determine the option that provides the largest net benefits to society.

Benefit Transfer: The practice of applying estimates developed in an existing research study (the "study scenario") to another context, such as a regulatory analysis (the "regulatory scenario"). Generally involves using studies that differ somewhat from the regulatory context in terms of the characteristics of the risks or of the affected population.

Concurrent Validity: A type of validity based on a comparison of scores on a measurement to those obtained by applying alternative, equivalent measurements at the same time.

Construct: A concept or model developed or constructed through informed scientific theory.

Construct Validity: A type of validity that compares results of several contrasting tests of validity (e.g., convergent and divergent validation tests) with predictions from a model.

Content Validity: The extent to which a measurement covers all aspects of the topic being assessed.

Contingent Valuation: A stated preference method that uses surveys to directly elicit estimates of individual willingness to pay. These values are "contingent" on the realization of the scenarios described in the study.

Convergent Validity: The extent to which two or more measuring instruments for the same topic are in accord.

Correlation: A measure of association that conveys the degree to which two or more sets of observations fit a linear relationship.

Cost: Generally used to indicate a measure of the resources that are used or exchanged to obtain or produce a good or service. See Chapter 5 for specific definitions relevant to the calculation of cost-effectiveness ratios.

Cost-Effectiveness Analysis (CEA): An economic analysis in which all costs are related to one common measure of effectiveness. Results are usually presented as a ratio of the increase in costs associated with an increase in effectiveness.

Cost of Illness (COI): The direct medical costs associated with illness, including, for example, resources expended for doctor visits, medication, and hospital stays. May also include indirect costs associated with lost productivity due to morbidity or preventable mortality.

Cost-Utility Analysis: A type of cost-effectiveness analysis that uses a form of health-adjusted life year weighted by a measure of individual preferences or utility as the effectiveness metric. (This report does not use the term because the Committee does not interpret health-adjusted life years as actual measures of utilities.)

Criterion Validity: Validity based on a comparison of results obtained using a measurement scale believed to indicate the true situation.

Decision Analysis: An explicit, quantitative, systematic approach to decision making under uncertain conditions.

Delphi Process: An iterative process for reaching consensus among experts where opinions are exchanged anonymously.

Disability: The temporary or long-term reduction in an individual's functional capacity.

Disability-Adjusted Life Year (DALY): A summary measure of population health status originally used to quantify the global burden of diseases. DALYs are calculated as disability weights, inverse to quality-adjusted life-year weights, assigned to each of 107 categories of health status.

Discounting: The process of converting future cost and benefits to a present value under the assumption that individuals generally prefer to receive desirable benefits soon and to defer costs, using a rate that reflects the opportunity cost associated with these time preferences. The formula is $1/(1+r)^t$ where r equals the discount rate and t measures the number of years into the future when the cost or benefit accrues.

Domains: Components of a health state; categories of function, perception, or experience within a health-related quality-of-life survey instrument.

Economic Efficiency: A criterion for identifying the preferred allocation of scarce resources based on determining the option that generates the largest net benefits to society, ignoring the distribution of the impacts.

Expected Utility: A quantity representing the relative desirability of a given action that has uncertain outcomes. Each possible outcome has a utility or preference rank and a probability of occurrence. The expected utility is the value of a particular outcome multiplied by the probability that outcome will occur, summed over all possible outcomes.

Expected Utility Theory: The dominant theory of individual behavior under conditions of uncertainty. The theory assumes that, under different alternatives, the individual will choose the alternative that has the highest expected utility.

Functional Status: The effective performance or ability of an individual to perform certain activities, roles, and tasks, such as going to work, riding a bicycle, maintaining the house.

Generic Index: Multiattribute health state classification system with predetermined index values, usually anchored by death (0) and perfect or optimal health (1.0). Index values for health states that are described generically in terms of functional (e.g., mobility) and experiential (e.g., pain) attributes or domains are usually established by community or general population preference elicitation surveys. Examples of generic indexes are the EuroQol EQ-5D, the Health Utilities Index, the Quality of Well Being Scale, and the SF-6D.

Health-Adjusted Life Year (HALY): Summary measures of population health that describe morbidity and mortality with a single index value. Types of HALY measures include quality-adjusted life years, disability-adjusted life years, and healthy-year equivalents.

Health-Related Quality of Life (HRQL): A value that takes into account impairments, functional status, perceptions, and social opportunities during the lifetime of an individual as influenced by disease, injury, treatment, or policy.

Health State: An individual's general state of health, including aspects such as morbidity, functioning, and general well-being.

Health State Classification System: A classification system consisting of mutually exclusive and an exhaustive set of health states used to describe and measure HRQL. It consists of one or more concepts, domains, or indicators and is used to generate health states.

Healthy-Year Equivalent (HYE): A measurement of HRQL that incorporates two sets of preferences. The first set reflects individuals' preferences for life years. The second set reflects individuals' preferences for states of health.

Incidence: The number of new cases of disease.

Incremental Cost Effectiveness Ratio: The additional cost incurred by the next most effective strategy to produce an additional unit of health outcome. (See Cost-Effectiveness Ratio.)

Indicator, Health Status: A measure indicating the presence, absence, or degree of health-related quality of life.

Injury: A form of harm, damage, or loss that can either be physical or mental.

Instrumental Activities of Daily Living: An evaluation of independence that generally consists of performing six home management activities: preparing meals, shopping for personal items, managing money, using the telephone, doing light house work, and doing heavy housework.

Internal Consistency (of a measurement): The extent to which various components all measure the same thing.

Interobserver or Interrater Reliability: The correlation between responses to the same items obtained by different observers or raters.

Interval Scales: A scale in which the distance between adjacent numbers in one region is equal to the distance between adjacent numbers in another region of the scale.

League Table: A table, usually in ascending order of cost per unit of outcome, that is used to rank the cost-effectiveness or (less frequently) the net benefits of different policy or medical interventions. May also be referred to as a "scorecard."

Life Expectancy: The average number of years of life remaining for an individual of a certain age, based on statistical analysis of population death rates.

Monte Carlo Model: A simulation model used to assess uncertainty, that selects values from prespecified probability distributions for each parameter through repeated trials. Results are reported as probability distributions indicating the estimated likelihood of each outcome.

Meta-Analysis: Statistical methods for combining the results from different studies.

Morbidity: The conditions or qualities associated with illness or disease.

Multiattribute Assessment: An assessment that consists of a multidimensional preference-based health state classification system; an indirect method for obtaining utility scores.

Nominal Scale: Scales in which numbers are assigned arbitrarily with no inherent order, but only as a classification system.

Opportunity Cost: The value of the best alternative that must be forgone when scarce resources are used or invested for a particular purpose or policy alternative.

Ordinal Scale: A scale that implies a distinct order among categories, but without any prescription of the relative distance between adjacent values.

Outcome Measure: The final health consequence of an intervention.

Person Trade-Off (PTO): A choice-based elicitation method that determines the relative values of health states and interventions by asking questions about the equivalence of different-sized groups of people in different states of health.

Preferences: The exercise of choice, reflecting the desirability of a particular set of outcomes over another.

Prevalence: The number of cases of a given disease in a given population at a designated time.

Preventable Mortality: A decrease in the risk of death attributable to a particular intervention.

Proxy Respondent: A person who responds to a survey by providing information and details about another person who is in the survey sample.

Psychometrics: The branch of psychology dealing with the testing and measurement of psychological variables.

Psychophysics: The study of human perceptions and judgments about physical phenomena.

Quality-Adjusted Life Year (QALY): A health outcomes measure used in CEA that integrates the quality of life with length of life using a multiplicative formula, measured on a scale ranging from 0 to 1 that characterizes HRQL.

Quality of Life: The judgment or value of the experience of an individual or group that reflects their physical, emotional, and social well-being.

Rating Scale: A numerical scale that directly values preferences for health states under conditions of certainty.

Ratio Scale: An interval scale with a true zero point, so ratios between values are meaningful.

Rational Choice Theory: An economic theory based on three basic assumptions about how individuals make choices. The three basic assumptions are (1) ranking alternatives according to their preferences for the goods, (2) consistency of choices, and (3) the preference for more rather than less.

Reference Case: A set of rules or stipulated criteria that facilitates comparisons of alternatives. (See Gold et al., 1996b, for reference case criteria for health-related CEA.)

Reliability: The extent in which one gets the same or identical results with repeated measurement; the stability of measurement.

Response Shift: Changing internal standards or values regarding quality of life in a particular state of health based upon experience with that state.

Restricted-Activity Days: The number of days a person experiences restrictions in his or her normal activities due to impaired health.

Revealed Preference: Methods that use observable behavior or market data to determine the monetary value of nonmarket goods or services. For example, data on the wage differential associated with riskier jobs may be used to value the change in risk.

Risk Aversion: The preference for a certain rather than an uncertain outcome.

Sensitivity Analysis: A form of quantitative assessment that varies the value of key input parameters to determine the impact on the results, often used to characterize the uncertainty associated with the selected parameter estimates.

Social Discount Rate: The rate at which society is willing to trade off costs or benefits incurred in different time periods.

Social Welfare: The combined well-being of all members of society; the summation of all things that members of a society view as contributing to the quality of their lives.

Standard Gamble (SG): The determination of a utility of a particular outcome using a lottery-based approach. An SG score is obtained by discovering a point of indifference between a lottery consisting of a preferred outcome with a probability P and a less-preferred outcome with probability of 1–P, versus a guaranteed intermediately ranked certain outcome.

Stated Preference: Methods that ask individuals to state the monetary amount that they would be willing to pay to obtain a good or service; includes contingent valuation surveys and similar approaches.

Test–Retest Reliability: The reliability of results when the tests are repeated and in agreement to prior or earlier tests.

Time Preference: A characteristic of the utility function. A gain today is more valuable than the same gain in the future. The trade-off between current and future gains is reflected in the discount rate.

Time Trade-Off (TTO): A choice-based preference elicitation technique. The TTO score for a particular health state is the point of indifference between shorter period of time in perfect (or other desirable) health and a longer period in an impaired health state.

Utilitarianism: A theory of social justice that contends that the right policy is one that produces the greatest happiness or welfare for the greatest number of people.

Utility: A concept from welfare economics that refers to the level of satisfaction or well-being individuals achieve from the consumption of goods and services. May include goods that are not directly bought and sold in the market, such as good health.

Validity: A descriptive term meaning that a measure is well grounded and accurately reflects the concept that it is intended to measure.

Value: Sometimes used narrowly to refer solely to monetary worth or a numerical quantity; this report uses a broader definition that encompasses worth as measured by individual preferences, desirability, usefulness, or importance.

Value of a Statistical Life (VSL): A statistical life is the aggregation, across a population, of small reductions in the risk of preventable mortality. Estimates of willingness to pay for these risk reductions are then summed across the affected population to determine the value of a statistical life saved (or preventable death avoided) by a policy. For example, if each member of a population of 100,000 were willing to pay $50 for a 1/100,000 risk reduction, the corresponding value of a statistical life would be $5 million (i.e., $50 * 100,000).

Visual Analogue Scale (VAS): A format for preference measurement in which a subject marks a representation of a scale (e.g., a rule or thermometer) that indicates the intensity of response.

Von Neumann and Morgenstern Utility Function: A function that is based on a set of axioms, including transitivity and continuity, that represents one definition of rational choice in a risky environment.

Welfare Economics: The normative theory of economics that focuses on allocating resources so as to achieve the maximum or optimal level of well-being for members of society.

Well-Being: Subjective evaluation of one's mental, bodily, and emotional states.

Willingness to Accept (WTA): When used to value desirable benefits in BCA, the least amount of money that an individual would accept to forego the improvement.

Willingness to Pay (WTP): When used to value desirable benefits in BCA, the maximum amount of money that an individual would voluntarily exchange to obtain an improvement, given his or her budget constraints.

Years of Healthy Life (YHL): A duration of life that is discounted by a fraction between 0 and 1 that estimates the quality of life during a given period.

E

Biographical Sketches

COMMITTEE TO EVALUATE MEASURES OF HEALTH BENEFITS FOR ENVIRONMENTAL, HEALTH, AND SAFETY REGULATION

Robert S. Lawrence, M.D., *Chair*, is the Edyth Schoenrich Professor of Preventive Medicine, Associate Dean for Professional Practice and Programs, Director of the Center for a Livable Future, and Professor of Health Policy and Management at the Johns Hopkins Bloomberg School of Public Health, and Professor of Medicine at the Johns Hopkins School of Medicine. He is a founding member of Physicians for Human Rights and served as President of that organization from 1998 to 2003. Dr. Lawrence chaired the first U.S. Preventive Services Task Force (1984–1989) and served on the successor Task Force from 1990–1996. He currently consults for the Centers for Disease Control and Prevention (CDC) Task Force on Community Preventive Services. Dr. Lawrence graduated from Harvard Medical School, trained in Internal Medicine at the Massachusetts General Hospital in Boston, and served for three years as an Epidemic Intelligence Service Officer, CDC. Dr. Lawrence served as Chair of the Institute of Medicine (IOM) committees that investigated dioxin in the food supply, that considered extensions of Medicare benefits, and that set priorities for vaccine development.

Henry A. Anderson, M.D., is the Wisconsin State Environmental and Occupational Disease Epidemiologist and Chief Medical Officer. He holds adjunct professorships at the University of Wisconsin Medical School-Madison

Department of Population Health and Institute for Environmental Studies. His published work and research interests cover a broad spectrum of environmental, occupational, and public health topics, including disease surveillance, risk assessment, childhood asthma, lead poisoning, mercury and PCBs in fish, arsenic in drinking water, asbestos disease, and occupational fatalities and injuries. He was a founding member of the Agency for Toxic Substances and Disease Registry Board of Scientific Councilors (1988–1992) and the Director's Advisory Committee for the CDC National Center for Environmental Health (1999–2003). He currently chairs the National Institute of Occupational Safety and Health Science Advisory Board, serves on the Presidential Advisory Board on Radiation Worker Compensation, and the U.S. Environmental Protection Agency (EPA) Children's Health Protection Advisory Council. He is past chair of the Environmental Health Committee of the EPA Science Advisory Board and from 1997–2003 served on the EPA Science Advisory Board Executive Committee. He received his M.D. degree from the University of Wisconsin Medical School.

Richard Burnett, Ph.D., is a Senior Research Scientist with the Safe Environments Program at Health Canada, where he has worked since 1983 on issues related to the health effects of outdoor air pollution. He is also adjunct professor, Department of Epidemiology and Community Medicine, at the University of Ottawa. Dr. Burnett's work has focused on the use of administrative health and environmental information to determine the public health impacts of combustion-related pollution using nonlinear random effects models, time series, and spatial analytical techniques. He served on the 2001 National Research Council (NRC) Committee on Air Quality Management in the United States. His Ph.D. in mathematical statistics is from Queen's University.

Carl F. Cranor, Ph.D., is Professor of Philosophy at the University of California, Riverside, specializing in legal and moral philosophy. He has written widely on philosophic issues at the intersection of science and the law, including philosophic issues in risk assessment and the regulation of toxic substances, and analysis of the acceptability of risks. More recently his work concerns the use of science in the tort law and the precautionary principle. He wrote *Regulating Toxic Substances: A Philosophy of Science and the Law* and has just completed a book to be published by Cambridge University Press, tentatively entitled *Toxic Torts: Science, Law and the Possibility of Justice.* As a Congressional Fellow, he worked at the U.S. Congress' Office of Technology Assessment co-authoring *The Identification and Regulation of Carcinogens* (1987). He has served on science advisory panels for the State of California. An elected fellow of the American Association for the Advancement of Science and the Collegium Ramazzini,

Professor Cranor received his B.A degree from the University of Colorado, a Ph.D. from UCLA, and an M.S.L. from Yale Law School.

Maureen Cropper, Ph.D., is a Professor of Economics at the University of Maryland, a Lead Economist at the World Bank, and a University Fellow at Resources for the Future. Her research has focused on valuing environmental amenities (especially environmental health effects), on the discounting of future health benefits, and on the trade-offs implicit in environmental regulations. Her recent research focuses on factors affecting deforestation in developing countries and on the externalities associated with motorization. Dr. Cropper is past president of the Association of Environmental and Resource Economists and a former chair of the Advisory Council for Clean Air Act Compliance Analysis, a subcommittee of EPA's Science Advisory Board. She has served on the advisory boards of Resources for the Future, the Harvard Center for Risk Analysis, the Donald Bren School of the Environment, and the AEI-Brookings Center on Regulation. Dr. Cropper received a B.A. in Economics from Bryn Mawr College and a Ph.D. in Economics from Cornell University.

Norman Daniels, Ph.D., is Professor of Ethics and Population Health at the Harvard School of Public Health, formerly having served as Goldthwaite Professor and Chair of the Tufts Philosophy Department and Professor of Medical Ethics at Tufts Medical School. He has written widely in the philosophy of science, ethics, political and social philosophy, and medical ethics. His most recent books include *Seeking Fair Treatment: From the AIDS Epidemic to National Health Care Reform* (1995); *Benchmarks of Fairness for Health Care Reform* (co-authored, 1996); *From Chance to Choice: Genetics and Justice* (co-authored, 2000); *Is Inequality Bad for Our Health?* (co-authored, 2000); and (with James Sabin) *Setting Limits Fairly: Can We Learn to Share Medical Resources?* (2002). Professor Daniels is a fellow of the Hastings Center, a member of the IOM, and a founding member of the National Academy of Social Insurance and of the International Society for Equity in Health. He received his doctorate in philosophy from Harvard University.

Dennis G. Fryback, Ph.D., is a professor of Population Health Sciences and of Industrial Engineering at the University of Wisconsin-Madison. He joined the staff at the University of Wisconsin-Madison in 1974 and since 1984 has been a Professor of Preventive Medicine. Dr. Fryback has chaired the Health Care Technology Study Section for the U.S. Agency for Health Care Policy and Research. He was a member of the United States Preventive Services Task Force and served on the Panel on Cost Effectiveness in Health and Medicine convened by the Office of Disease Prevention and Health

Promotion of the Department of Health and Human Services (DHHS). In 1997–1998 he served as a member of the IOM's Committee on Summarizing Population Health and was appointed to the national advisory board for the U.S. Agency for Healthcare Research and Quality in 1997. Dr. Fryback is a founding member of the Society for Medical Decision Making (SMDM), has remained continuously active in SMDM activities since 1978, and has served as SMDM president. The SMDM named him a recipient of the SMDM Award for Career Achievement. He received an M.A. in mathematics and Ph.D. in mathematical psychology from the University of Michigan, where he trained in human decision making and decision analysis. He was elected to the IOM in 2000.

Alan M. Garber, M.D., Ph.D., is the Henry J. Kaiser Jr. Professor and a professor of medicine, of economics, of business, and of health research and policy at Stanford University. He has been the director of both the university's Center for Health Policy and the Center for Primary Care and Outcomes Research since their founding. He directs the health care program of the National Bureau of Economic Research and serves as a staff physician at the Veterans Affairs Palo Alto Health Care System, where he is the associate director of the VA Center for Health Care Evaluation. Dr. Garber's research is directed toward methods for improving health care delivery and financing, particularly for the elderly, in settings of limited resources. He has developed methods for determining the cost-effectiveness of health interventions, and studies ways to structure financial and organizational incentives to ensure that cost-effective care is delivered. He is Chair of the Medicare Coverage Advisory Committee, and is a member of the Blue Cross and Blue Shield Association's Medical Advisory Panel, the National Institutes of Health National Advisory Council on Aging, and the IOM, among other distinctions. Dr. Garber received his undergraduate degree summa cum laude and Ph.D. in economics from Harvard and an M.D. with research honors from Stanford.

Marthe R. Gold, M.D., M.P.H., has served as the Arthur C. Logan Professor and Chair of the Department of Community Health and Social Medicine at the City University of New York Medical School since 1997. She has served as a Senior Policy Adviser in the Office of the Assistant Secretary for Health, DHHS, and on the 1993 Task Force for Health Care Reform, where she worked on benefit design and protections for vulnerable populations. Dr. Gold directed the work of the Panel on Cost-Effectiveness in Health and Medicine, a nonfederal expert panel whose final report, issued by the DHHS in 1996, remains an influential guide to cost-effectiveness methodology for academic and policy uses. She co-edited the IOM 1998 report, *Summarizing Population Health*, and has participated in national and international groups seeking to standardize health status measures. Dr. Gold has published in the areas of socioeconomic predictors of and disparities in health, measurement of health outcomes, and the use of cost-effectiveness analysis in resource allocation. She has served on a number of advisory committees for agencies of the DHHS including the Agency for Healthcare Research and Quality, the CDC, and the National Center for Health Statistics, among other government and privately sponsored advisory groups. A family physician, she trained and subsequently served on the faculty of the Department of Community and Family Medicine at the University of Rochester Medical School.

James K. Hammitt, Ph.D., is Professor of Economics and Decision Sciences and Director of the Harvard Center for Risk Analysis at the Harvard School of Public Health. His research and teaching concern the development of decision analysis, benefit–cost analysis, game theory, and other quantitative methods and their application to health and environmental policy in the United States and internationally. He is particularly interested in the management of long-term environmental issues such as global climate change and stratospheric-ozone depletion, in comprehensive evaluation of risk-control measures (including ancillary benefits and countervailing risks), and in alternative methods for measuring the value of reducing health risks, including monetary and health-adjusted life-year metrics. Professor Hammitt serves as a member of the Environmental Economics Advisory Committee and the Advisory Council on Clear Air Compliance Analysis of the EPA Science Advisory Board. He recently concluded service as a member of the American Statistical Association Committee on Energy Statistics (Advisory Committee to the U.S. Energy Information Administration) and the NRC panel studying the implications of dioxin in the food supply. Professor Hammitt holds degrees in applied mathematics (A.B., Sc.M.) and public policy (M.P.P., Ph.D.) from Harvard University. He was previously Senior Mathematician at the RAND Corporation and a faculty member at the RAND Graduate School of Policy Studies.

Lisa I. Iezzoni, M.D., M.Sc., is Professor of Medicine at Harvard Medical School and Co-Director of Research in the Division of General Medicine and Primary Care, Department of Medicine, at Beth Israel Deaconess Medical Center in Boston. She received her degrees in medicine and health policy and management from Harvard University. Dr. Iezzoni has conducted numerous studies for the Agency for Healthcare Research and Quality, the Medicare agency, and private foundations on a variety of topics, including methods for predicting costs, clinical outcomes, and quality of care. She has published and spoken widely on risk adjustment and has edited *Risk Adjustment for Measuring Health Care Outcomes*, now in its third edition

(2003). A 1996 recipient of the Investigator Award in Health Policy Research from The Robert Wood Johnson Foundation, she is studying health care quality and policy issues relating to persons with disabilities. Her book *When Walking Fails* was published in the spring of 2003, and another book, *More Than Ramps: Improving Health Care Quality and Access for People with Disabilities*, co-authored with Bonnie L. O'Day, is scheduled for publication in late 2005. Dr. Iezzoni is a member of the IOM in the National Academy of Sciences.

Peter D. Jacobson, J.D., M.P.H., is Professor of Health Law and Policy in the Department of Health Management and Policy, University of Michigan School of Public Health, where he teaches courses on health law and law and public health. He is also Director of the Center for Law, Ethics, and Health. Before coming to the University of Michigan, he was Senior Behavioral Scientist at RAND from 1988 to 1996. In 1995, Professor Jacobson received an Investigator Award in Health Policy Research from The Robert Wood Johnson Foundation to examine the role of the courts in shaping health care policy. He has also published a series of articles on the development of legal doctrine in managed care litigation. He has written on the treatment of cost-effectiveness analysis by the courts for an IOM symposium. His most recent book is *Strangers in the Night: Law and Medicine in the Managed Care Era* (2002). Professor Jacobson is a member of the Board of Editors of the *Journal of Health Politics, Policy and Law*. He received his law degree from the University of Pittsburgh School of Law and his M.P.H. from UCLA.

Emmett Keeler, Ph.D., has been a senior mathematician with RAND since 1968. He is currently leading a large study of 40 organizations to evaluate interventions to improve care for chronic illness. He also leads a project that supplies cost-effectiveness analyses to a variety of UCLA geriatric interventions. Dr. Keeler teaches analytic methods at UCLA and at The Pardee RAND Graduate School and has taught at Harvard and the University of Chicago. In 2003 he received the distinguished investigator award from AcademyHealth. Dr. Keeler served on the NRC's Panel to Review the Scientific Evidence on the Polygraph and the IOM's Subcommittee on Economic Costs of Uninsured Populations. His Ph.D. in mathematics is from Harvard University.

Willard G. Manning, Ph.D., is Professor at the Harris School of Public Policy at The University of Chicago. His primary research focus has been the effects of health insurance and alternative delivery systems on the use of health services and health status. He has also the studied the economics of poor health habits. He is an expert in statistical issues related to health expenditures, and cost-effectiveness analysis. He has received article of the year awards for his work on the effects of managed care, on the costs of poor health habits, and on econometric methods for health expenditure data. He was a member of the Panel on Cost-Effectiveness in Health and Medicine. Dr. Manning has served on several IOM committees and is a member of the IOM. His Ph.D. in economics is from Stanford University.

Charles Poole, M.P.H., Sc.D., is an Associate Professor in the Department of Epidemiology at the University of North Carolina School of Public Health, where his work focuses on the development and application of epidemiologic research methods and principles. His areas of substantive research interest include environmental and occupational epidemiology. He served with the EPA, worked as an epidemiologic consultant, and taught at the Boston University School of Public Health. He has served on the editorial boards of several leading epidemiological journals. Dr. Poole has served on four previous NRC committees, including the Committee on Estimating the Health-Risk-Reduction Benefits of Proposed Air Pollution Regulations. He received his M.P.H. degree from the University of North Carolina and his Sc.D. degree from Harvard University.

David A. Schkade, M.B.A, Ph.D., is the Jerome S. Katzin Chair of the Rady School of Management at University of California, San Diego. Until 2004, he was the Herbert D. Kelleher/MCorp Regents Professor of Business at the University of Texas, Austin. He has been a visiting senior research scholar in the Woodrow Wilson School of Public Affairs at Princeton University, and on the faculties of the University of Chicago and Duke University. Professor Schkade has published on a variety of topics, including environmental resource valuation, the psychology of well-being, loss aversion, and jury decision making. His work has been supported by grants from public agencies, private foundations, and corporations. He currently serves on the editorial boards of three journals and has served on grant review and site visit panels of the National Science Foundation and the EPA. His work on punitive damages has been cited in several court cases, including opinions by the U.S. Supreme Court, the First U.S. District Court, and the California State Supreme Court. He received B.A. (Mathematics) and M.B.A. degrees from the University of Texas, Austin, and M.S. and Ph.D. degrees in Organizational Psychology from Carnegie Mellon University.

ADVISERS TO THE COMMITTEE

Alan Krupnick, Ph.D., is Senior Fellow and Director, Quality of the Environment at Resources for the Future in Washington, D.C. His research addresses the valuation of health and ecological improvements and also focuses on analyzing environmental issues, in particular, the benefits, costs, and design of air pollution policies, both in the United States and in developing countries. Dr. Krupnick has served as a consultant to state governments, federal agencies, private corporations, the Canadian government, the European Union, the World Health Organization, and the World Bank. He co-chaired an advisory committee that counseled the EPA on new ozone and particulate standards. Dr. Krupnick also served as senior economist on the President's Council of Economic Advisers, advising the Clinton Administration on environmental and natural resource policy issues. He is a regular member of expert committees from the National Academies.

Judith L. Wagner, Ph.D., is a Scholar-in-Residence at the IOM. She has more than 30 years' experience in health policy analysis and health technology economics. Most recently, as a Senior Analyst at the Congressional Budget Office, she specialized in prescription drug issues, including the design of a Medicare prescription drug benefit, Medicaid drug payment, and reform of current laws governing the entrance of generic drugs into the marketplace. Before joining CBO, she was a consultant at the Mayo Clinic in Rochester, MN, where she conducted cost and cost-effectiveness analyses of medical procedures and technologies. She also managed major assessments of the cost-effectiveness of preventive and diagnostic technologies at the U.S. Congress Office of Technology Assessment. Dr. Wagner holds a Ph.D. from Cornell University, where she studied economics and operations research with an emphasis on environmental applications. She also holds masters' degrees from the University of Michigan (in economics) and from Cornell (in environmental systems engineering).

Milton C. Weinstein, Ph.D., is the Henry J. Kaiser Professor of Health Policy and Management at the Harvard School of Public Health, Professor of Medicine at the Harvard Medical School, and Director of the Program on Economic Evaluation of Medical Technology. He is best known for his research on cost-effectiveness of medical practices and for developing methods of economic evaluation and decision analysis in health care. He is a co-developer of the Cost-Effectiveness of Preventing AIDS Complications computer simulation model and also of the Coronary Heart Disease Policy Model, which has been used to evaluate the cost-effectiveness of cardiovascular prevention and treatment. His current research relates to infectious disease treatment, screening, and vaccination. He was a member of both IOM committees on vaccine priorities and developed the methodology that was used to quantify the potential health and economic benefits of new vaccines. Dr. Weinstein has authored *Decision Making in Health and Medicine: Integrating Evidence and Values*; *Cost-Effectiveness in Health and Medicine*, the report of the Panel of Cost Effectiveness in Health and Medicine; *Clinical Decision Analysis*; and *Hypertension: A Policy Perspective.* He is a member of the IOM of the National Academies and a recipient of the Award for Career Achievement from the Society for Medical Decision Making. Dr. Weinstein received his A.B. and A.M. in Applied Mathematics (1970), his M.P.P. (1972), and his Ph.D. in Public Policy (1973) from Harvard University.

IOM STAFF AND CONSULTANT

Wilhelmine Miller, M.S., Ph.D., is a senior program officer at the IOM and staff director for the Committee. She has been at IOM for seven years, and co-directed the four-year, six-report IOM study on the consequences of uninsurance. Prior to joining IOM, Dr. Miller was an adjunct faculty member in the Departments of Philosophy at Georgetown University and Trinity College, Washington, DC, where she taught political philosophy, ethics, and public policy. She received her doctorate in philosophy from Georgetown in 1997. From 1976–1989 Dr. Miller served as a policy analyst and social scientist within the Department of Health and Human Services. She received her M.S. degree in health policy and management from Harvard University in 1976.

Ryan Palugod, B.A., is a research assistant in the IOM Division of Health Care Services. He has worked with several projects over his five-year tenure at IOM, including studies of uninsurance, immunization and vaccine finance, and the quality of mental health and substance abuse services. Prior to coming to IOM, Mr. Palugod worked as an administrative assistant with the American Association of Homes, Services for the Aging. He graduated from Towson University in 1999 with a degree in health care management and is pursuing a master's degree in public administration at George Mason University.

Lisa A. Robinson, M.P.P., is an independent consultant who specializes in the economic analysis of regulations. She was previously a Principal at Industrial Economics, Incorporated (IEc), where she directed numerous regulatory impact analyses for the EPA and other clients. Ms. Robinson also developed state-of-the-art methods for benefit–cost analysis and authored several guidance documents. Prior to her employment at IEc, she was the Director of Policy, Planning and Budget for a federal agency and an analyst at the U.S. Office of Management and Budget. She received her Master in Public Policy degree from the Kennedy School of Government at Harvard University in 1982.

References

Abbey, David E., Bessie L. Hwang, Raoul J. Burchette, Tony Vancuran, et al. 1995. Estimated Long-Term Ambient Concentrations of PM10 and Development of Respiratory Symptoms in a Nonsmoking Population. *Archives of Environmental Health* 50(2):139–152.

Adler, Matthew D. 2003. Risk, Death and Harm: The Normative Foundations of Risk Regulation. *Minnesota Law Review* 87:1293–1418.

Adler, Matthew D. 2005. *QALYs and Policy Evaluation: A New Perspective.* Working Paper 05-01. Washington, DC: AEI-Brookings Joint Center.

Agency for Healthcare Research and Quality (AHRQ). 2005. *The Guide to Clinical Preventive Services, 2005: Recommendations of the U.S. Preventive Services Task Force.* Rockville, MD: AHRQ.

Anderson, John R., Robert M. Kaplan, and Christopher F. Ake. 2004. Arthritis Impact on U.S. Life Quality: Morbidity and Mortality Effects From National Health Interview Survey Data 1986–1988 and 1994 Using QWBX1 Estimates of Well-Being. *Social Indicators Research* 69:67–91.

Anderson, Roger T., Mary McFarlane, Michelle J. Naughton, and Sally A. Shumaker. 1996. Conceptual Issues and Considerations in Cross-Cultural Validation of Generic Health-Related Quality of Life Instruments. In: Spilker, Bert, ed. *Quality of Life and Pharmacoeconomics in Clinical Trials.* Philadelphia: Lippincott-Raven Publishers. Pp. 605–612.

Andresen, Elena M., Barbara M. Rothenberg, and Robert M. Kaplan. 1998. Performance of a Self-Administered Mailed Version of the Quality of Well-Being (QWB-SA) Questionnaire Among Older Adults. *Medical Care* 36(9):1349–1360.

Arrow, Kenneth, P.R. Solow, E.E. Portney, R. Leamer, et al. 1993. Report of the NOAA Panel on Contingent Valuation. *Federal Register* 58(10):4601–4614.

Ashford, Nicholas A. 1980. The Limits of Cost–Benefit Analysis in Regulatory Decisions. *Technology Review* 82(6):70–72.

Bakker, C., M. Rutten, E. van Doorslaer, K. Bennett, et al. 1994. Feasibility of Utility Assessment by Rating Scale and Standard Gamble in Patients With Ankylosing Spondylitis and Fibromyalgia. *Journal of Rheumatology* 21:269–274.

Balaban, D.J., P.C. Sagi, N.I. Goldfarb, and S. Nettler. 1986. Weights for Scoring the Quality of Well-Being Instrument Among Rheumatoid Arthritics: A Comparison to the General Population Weights. *Medical Care* 24:973–980.

Bedford, Tim, and Roger M. Cooke. 2001. *Probabilistic Risk Analysis*. New York: Cambridge University Press.

Bell, Chaim M., Richard H. Chapman, Patricia W. Stone, Eileen A. Sandberg, and Peter J. Neumann. 2001. An Off-the-Shelf Help List: A Comprehensive Catalog of Preference Scores From Published Cost-Utility Analyses. *Medical Decision Making* 21(4):288–294.

Bleichrodt, Han, and Magnus Johannesson. 1997. Standard Gamble, Time Trade-Off and Rating Scale: Experimental Results on the Ranking Properties of QALYs. *Journal of Health Economics* 16(2):155–175.

Bleichrodt, Han, Jose L. Pinto, and Peter P. Wakker. 2001. Making Descriptive Use of Prospect Theory to Improve the Prescriptive Use of Expected Utility. *Management Science* 47(11):1498–1514.

Bleichrodt, Han, Jose L. Pinto, and Jose M. Abellan-Perpinan. 2003. A Consistency Test of the Time Trade-Off. *Journal of Health Economics* 22:1037–1052.

Boyle, M.H., G.W. Torrance, J.C. Sinclair, and S.P. Horwood. 1983. Economic Evaluation of Neonatal Intensive Care of Very Low-Birthweight Infants. *New England Journal of Medicine* 308(22):1330–1337.

Brauer, Carmen, and Peter Neumann. 2004. *A Catalogue of Preference Weights Used in Published Cost–Utility Analyses, 1998–2001*. Prepared for the Institute of Medicine Committee to Evaluate Measures of Health Benefits for Environmental, Health, and Safety Regulation.

———. 2005. *Using an Online Catalog of Utility Scores From Published Cost–Utility Analyses to Estimate Quality of Life Impacts in the EPA Case Study*. Prepared for the Institute of Medicine Committee to Evaluate Measures of Health Benefits for Environmental, Health, and Safety Regulation.

Brazier, John, Mark Deverill, C. Green, R. Harper, and A. Booth. 1999a. A Review of the Use of Health Status Measures in Economic Evaluation. *Health Technology Assessment* 3(9):1–164.

Brazier, John, Mark Deverill, and Colin Green. 1999b. A Review of the Use of Health Status Measures in Economic Evaluation. *Journal of Health Services Research and Policy* 4(3):174–184.

Brazier, John, Jennifer Roberts, and Mark Deverill. 2002. The Estimation of a Preference-Based Measure of Health From the SF-36. *Journal of Health Economics* 21:271–292.

Brazier, John E., and Jennifer Roberts. 2004. The Estimation of a Preference-Based Measure of Health From the SF-12. *Medical Care* 42(9):851–859.

Brazier, John E., T.P. Usherwood, R. Harper, and K. Thomas. 1998. Deriving a Preference Based Single Index From the UK SF-36 Health Survey. *Journal of Clinical Epidemiology* 51(11):1115–1129.

Briggs, Andrew. 2001. Handling Uncertainty in Economic Evaluation and Presenting the Results. In: Drummond, Michael, and McGuire, Alistair, eds. *Economic Evaluation in Health Care: Merging Theory with Practice*. Oxford: Oxford University Press. Pp. 172–214.

Briggs, Andrew H., Ron Goeree, Gord Blackhouse, and Bernie J. O'Brien. 2002. Probabilistic Analysis of Cost-Effectiveness Models: Choosing Between Treatment Strategies for Gastroesophageal Reflux Disease. *Medical Decision Making* 22(4):290–308.

Bush, J.W., M.M. Chen, and D.L. Patrick. 1973. Health Status Index in Cost Effectiveness: Analysis of PKU Program. In: Berg, Richard L., ed. *Health Status Indexes*. Chicago: Hospital Research and Educational Trust. Pp. 172–208.

Carter, Jimmy. 1978, March 23. *Improving Government Regulations, Executive Order 12044*. White House.

Centers for Disease Control and Prevention (CDC). 2002. United States Life Tables, 2000. *National Vital Statistics Reports* 51(3).

———. 2005. *2004 Behavioral Risk Factor Surveillance System Summary Data Quality Report*. [Online]. Available: http://www.cdc.gov/brfss/technical_infodata/surveydata/2004.htm [accessed September 5, 2005].

Chapman, Richard H., Patricia W. Stone, Eileen A. Sandberg, Chaim Bell, and Peter J. Neumann. 2000. A Comprehensive League Table of Cost-Utility Ratios and a Sub-Table of "Panel-Worthy" Studies. *Medical Decision Making* 20:451–467.

Chapman, Richard H., Marc Berger, Milton C. Weinstein, Jane C. Weeks, et al. 2004. When Does Quality-Adjusting Life-Years Matter in Cost-Effectiveness Analysis? *Health Economics* 13:429–436.

Chiang, C.L. 1965. An Index of Health: Mathematical Models. *Public Health Services Publication*. Washington, DC: National Center for Health Statistics.

Churchill, D.N., G.W. Torrance, D.W. Taylor, C.G. Barnes, et al. 1987. Measurement of Quality of Life in End-Stage Renal Disease: The Time Trade-Off Approach. *Clinical and Investigative Medicine* 10:14–20.

Claxton, Karl, Mark Sculpher, Chris McCabe, Andrew Briggs, et al. 2005. Probabilistic Sensitivity Analysis for NICE Technology Assessment: Not an Optional Extra. *Health Economics* 14(4):339–347.

Cranor, Carl F. 1995. The Use of Comparative Risk Judgments in Risk Management. In: Fan, A.M., and Chang, L.W., eds. *Toxicology and Risk Assessment: Principles, Methods, and Applications*. Marcel Dekker, Inc. Pp. 817–833.

Cropper, Maureen L., Sema K. Aydede, and Paul R. Portney. 1994. Preferences for Life Saving Programs: How the Public Discounts Time and Age. *Journal of Risk and Uncertainty* 8:243–265.

Culyer, A.J. 1991. The Normative Economics of Health Care Finance and Provision. In: McGuire, Alistair, Fenn, Paul, and Mayhew, Ken, eds. *Providing Health Care: The Economics of Alternative Systems of Finance and Delivery*. Oxford: Oxford University Press. Pp. 65–98.

Cutler, David M., and Elizabeth Richardson. 1997. Measuring the Health of the United States Population. *Brookings Papers on Economic Activity. Microeconomics* 217–271.

———. 1999. Your Money and Your Life; The Value of Health and What Affects It. In: Garber, Alan M., ed. *Frontiers in Health Policy Research 2*. Cambridge, MA: MIT Press. Pp. 99–132.

Daniels, Norman, and James E. Sabin. 1997. Limits to Health Care: Fair Procedures, Democratic Deliberation, and the Legitimacy Problem for Insurers. *Philosophy and Public Affairs* 4:303–350.

———. 2002. *Setting Limits Fairly: Can We Learn to Share Medical Resources?* Oxford: Oxford University Press.

de Hollander, Augustinus E.M., Johan M. Melse, Erik Lebret, and Pieter G.N. Kramers. 1999. An Aggregate Public Health Indicator to Represent the Impact of Multiple Environmental Exposures. *Epidemiology* 10(5):606–617.

Desvousges, William H., F. Reed Johnson, and H. Spencer Banzhaf. 1998. *Environmental Policy Analysis with Limited Information: Principles and Application of the Transfer Method*. Northampton, MA: Edward Elgar.

Dolan, Paul. 1997. Modeling Valuations for EuroQol Health States. *Medical Care* 35(11):1095–1108.
———. 2000. The Measurement of Health-Related Quality of Life for Use in Resource Allocation Decisions in Health Care. In: Culyer, Anthony J., and Newhouse, Joseph P., eds. *Handbook of Health Economics.* Vol. 1B. Amsterdam: Elsevier. Pp. 1724–1760.
Dolan, Paul, and Richard Edlin. 2002. Is It Really Possible to Build a Bridge Between Cost–Benefit Analysis and Cost-Effectiveness Analysis? *Journal of Health Economics* 21(5): 827–843.
Dolan, Paul, and Colin Green. 1998. Using the Person Trade-Off Approach to Examine Differences Between Individual and Social Values. *Health Economics* 7:307–312.
Dolan, Paul, and Claire Gudex. 1995. Time Preference, Duration and Health State Valuations. *Health Economics* 4:289–299.
Dolan, Paul, and Jennifer Roberts. 2002. Modelling Valuations for EQ-5D Health States: An Alternative Modeling Using Differences in Valuations. *Medical Care* 40(5):442–446.
Dolan, Paul, Claire Gudex, Paul Kind, and Alan Williams. 1996a. Valuing Health States: A Comparison of Methods. *Journal of Health Economics* 15(2):209–231.
———. 1996b. The Time Trade-Off Method: Results From A General Population Study. *Health Economics* 5:141–154.
Drummond, Michael F., Bernie J. O'Brien, Greg L. Stoddart, and George W. Torrance. 1997. *Methods for the Economic Evaluation of Health Programmes.* Oxford: Oxford University Press.
Eiser, C., and R. Morse. 2001a. Quality-of-Life Measures in Chronic Diseases of Childhood. *Health Technology Assessment* 5(4):1–157.
———. 2001b. A Review of Measures of Quality of Life for Children With Chronic Illness. *Archives of Disease in Childhood* 84(3):205–211.
Fanshel, S., and J. Bush. 1970. A Health Status Index and Its Application to Health Services Outcomes. *Operations Research* 18(6):1021–1066.
Feeny, David, William Furlong, Michael Boyle, and George W. Torrance. 1995. Multi-Attribute Health Status Classification Systems. *Pharmacoeconomics* 7(6):490–502.
Feeny, David, William Furlong, George W. Torrance, Charles H. Goldsmith, et al. 2002. Multiattribute and Single-Attribute Utility Functions for the Health Utilities Index Mark 3 System. *Medical Care* 40(2):113–128.
Feeny, David H., George W. Torrance, and William J. Furlong. 1996. Health Utilities Index. In: Spilker, B., ed. *Quality of Life and Pharmacoeconomics in Clinical Trials.* Philadelphia: Lippincott-Raven Publishers. Pp. 239–252.
Fenwick, Elisabeth, Bernie J. O'Brien, and Andrew Briggs. 2004. Cost-Effectiveness Acceptability Curves—Facts, Fallacies and Frequently Asked Questions. *Health Economics* 13:405–415.
Fischhoff, Baruch. 1991. Value Elicitation: Is There Anything in There? *American Psychologist* 46(8):835–847.
Fleishman, John, and William Lawrence. 2004 (December 1). *Health Status Measures in the Medical Expenditure Panel Survey.* Presentation to the Institute of Medicine Committee to Evaluate Measures of Health Benefits for Environmental, Health, and Safety Regulation.
Fox-Rushby, J.F., and K. Hanson. 2001. How to Do (Or Not to Do) . . . Calculating and Presenting Disability Adjusted Life Years (DALYs) in Cost-Effectiveness Analysis. *Health Policy and Planning* 16(3):326–331.
Frankel, H.L., J.R. Coll, S.W. Charlifue, G.C. Whiteneck, et al. 1998. Long-Term Survival in Spinal Cord Injury: A Fifty Year Investigation. *Spinal Cord* 36:266–274.

Franks, Peter. 2004 (November 30). *Towards Consistency in Cost-Effectiveness Analysis. Measuring Health Status: Tower of Babel or Glass Half Full . . . And Can We Do Better?* Presentation to the Institute of Medicine Committee to Evaluate Measures of Health Benefits for Environmental, Health, and Safety Regulation.

Franks, Peter, Erica I. Lubetkin, Marthe R. Gold, and Daniel J. Tancredi. 2003. Mapping the SF-12 to Preference-Based Instruments: Convergent Validity in a Low-Income Minority Population. *Medical Care* 41(11):1277–1283.

Franks, Peter, E.I. Lubetkin, M.R. Gold, D.J. Tancredi, and H. Jia. 2004. Mapping the SF-12 to the EuroQol EQ-5D Index in a National US Sample. *Medical Decision Making* 24(3):247–254.

Franks, Peter, Janel Hanmer, and Dennis Fryback. 2006. Relative Disutilities of 47 Risk Factors and Conditions Assessed With 7 Preference-Based Health Status Measures in a National U.S. Sample: Toward Consistency in Cost-Effectiveness Analysis. Forthcoming in *Medical Care.*

Freeman, A.M. 2003. *The Measurement of Environmental and Resource Value: Theory and Methods.* 2nd ed. Washington, DC: Resources for the Future.

Froberg, Debra G., and Robert L. Kane. 1989. Methodology for Measuring Health-State Preferences-II: Scaling Methods. *Journal of Clinical Epidemiology* 42(5):459–471.

Fryback, Dennis. 2003. *Understanding and Comparing Existing Summary Measures of Health and Health-Related Quality of Life.* Madison, WI: University of Wisconsin–Madison.

Fryback, Dennis G., and William F. Lawrence. 1997. Dollars May Not Buy as Many QALYs as We Think: A Problem with Defining Quality-of-Life Adjustments. *Medical Decision Making* 17:276–284.

Fryback, Dennis G., Erik J. Dasbach, Ronald Klein, Barbara E. Klein, et al. 1993. The Beaver Dam Health Outcomes Study: Initial Catalog of Health-State Quality Factors. *Medical Decision Making* 13(2):89–102.

Gabriel, S.E., M.E. Camion, and W.M. O'Fallon. 1993. Patient Preferences for Nonsteroidal Antiinflammatory Drug Related Gastrointestinal Complication and Their Prophylaxis. *Journal of Rheumatology* 20:358–361.

Gafni, Amiram. 2004 (November 30). *HYEs and QALYs: Spotting the Differences.* Presentation to the Institute of Medicine Committee to Evaluate Measures of Health Benefits for Environmental, Health, and Safety Regulation.

Gilbert, Daniel T., and Jane E.J. Ebert. 2002. Decisions and Revisions: The Affective Forecasting of Changeable Outcomes. *Journal of Personality and Social Psychology* 82(4): 503–514.

Gilliland, F.D., R. McConnell, J. Peters, and H. Gong, Jr. 1999. A Theoretical Basis for Investigating Ambient Air Pollution and Children's Respiratory Health. *Environmental Health Perspectives* 107(Suppl 3):403–407.

Gold, Marthe, Peter Franks, and Pennifer Erickson. 1996a. Assessing the Health of the Nation: The Predictive Validity of a Preference-Based Measure and Self-Rated Health. *Medical Care* 34(2):163–177.

Gold, Marthe R., Joanna E. Siegel, Louise B. Russell, and Milton C. Weinstein, eds. 1996b. *Cost-Effectiveness in Health and Medicine.* New York: Oxford University Press.

Gold, Marthe R., Peter Franks, Kristine I. McCoy, and Dennis G. Fryback. 1998. Towards Consistency in Cost-Utility Analyses: Using National Measures to Create Condition-Specific Values. *Medical Care* 36(6):778–792.

Gold, Marthe, David Stevenson, and Dennis G. Fryback. 2002. HALYs and QALYs and DALYs, Oh My: Similarities and Differences in Summary Measures of Population Health. *Annual Review of Public Health* 23:115–134.

Graham, John D. 2003a (May 30). *Memorandum to the President's Management Council: Benefit-Cost Methods and Life Saving Rules.* [Online]. Available: http://www.whitehouse.gov/OMB/inforeg/pmc_benefit_cost_memo.pdf [accessed January 3, 2006].

Graham, John D. 2003b. *Valuing Health: An OMB Perspective.* Remarks Prepared for Conference on Valuing Health Outcomes: An Assessment of Approaches. Washington, DC: Resources for the Future.

Graham, John D., and Jonathan B. Wiener. 1995. *Risk vs Risk.* Cambridge, MA: Harvard University Press.

Green, Colin. 2001. On the Societal Value of Health Care: What Do We Know About the Person Trade-Off Technique? *Health Economics* 10:233–243.

Greenberg, Dan, and Joseph S. Pliskin. 2002. Preference-Based Outcome Measures in Cost-Utility Analyses. *International Journal of Technology Assessment in Health Care* 18(3): 461–466.

Griebsch, Ingolf, Joanna Coast, and Jackie Brown. 2005. Quality-Adjusted Life-Years Lack Quality in Pediatric Care: A Critical Review of Published Cost-Utility in Child Health. *Pediatrics* 115(5):e600–e614.

Gudex, Claire, Paul Dolan, Paul Kind, and Alan Williams. 1996. Health State Valuations From the General Public Using the Visual Analogue Scale. *Quality of Life Research* 5(6):521–531.

Haffer, Samuel. 2004 (December 1). *Comparison of Major CMS Surveys Collecting Functional Status Information.* Presentation to the Institute of Medicine Committee to Evaluate Measures of Health Benefits for Environmental, Health, and Safety Regulation.

Hahn, Robert W. 2005. *In Defense of the Economic Analysis of Regulation.* Washington, DC: AEI-Brookings Joint Center for Regulatory Studies.

Hammitt, James K. 2002. QALYs Versus WTP. *Risk Analysis* 22(5):985–1001.

Hanmer, Janel, William F. Lawrence, John P. Anderson, Robert M. Kaplan, et al. 2006. Report of Nationally Representative Values for the Non-Institutionalized U.S. Adult Population for Seven Health Related Quality of Life Scores. Forthcoming in *Medical Decision Making.*

Harrington, Winston, Richard D. Morgenstern, and Peter Nelson. 2000. On the Accuracy of Regulatory Cost Estimates. *Journal of Policy Analysis and Management* 19(2):297–322.

Harris, John. 1987. QALYfying the Value of Life. *Journal of Medical Ethics* 13(3):117–123.

Harrison-Felix, Cynthia, Gale Whiteneck, Michael DeVivo, Flora M. Hammond, and Amitabh Jha. 2004. Mortality Following Rehabilitation in the Traumatic Brain Injury Model Systems of Care. *NeuroRehabilitation* 19:45–54.

Harvard Center for Risk Analysis. 2003. *The CEA Registry.* [Online]. Available: http://www.hsph.harvard.edu/cearegistry [accessed September 20, 2005].

Hausman, Daniel M. 2004 (November 30). *Evaluating Health Consequences: HALYs vs. WTP.* Presentation to the Institute of Medicine Committee to Evaluate Measures of Health Benefits for Environmental, Health, and Safety Regulation.

Hawthorne, Graeme, Jeff Richardson, and Neal A. Day. 2001. A Comparison of the Assessment of Quality of Life (AQoL) With Four Other Generic Utility Instruments. *Annals of Medicine* 33(5):358–370.

Heitjan, Daniel F. 2000. Fieller's Method and Net Health Benefits. *Health Economics* 9:327–335.

Hennessy, Sue, and Paul Kind. 2002. *Measuring Health Status in Children: Developing and Testing a Child-Friendly Version of EQ-5D.* [Online]. Available: http://www.euroqol.org/meetings/meeting2002/Chap21.pdf [accessed August 15, 2005].

Hicks, John R. 1939. *Value and Capital: An Inquiry to Some Fundamental Principles of Economic Theory.* Oxford: Oxford University Press.

Hirth, Richard A., Michael E. Chernew, Edward Miller, A.M. Fendrick, and William G. Weissert. 2000. Willingness to Pay for a Quality-Adjusted Life Year: In Search of a Standard. *Medical Decision Making* 20:332–342.

Holbrook, Troy L., John P. Anderson, William J. Sieber, Deirdre Browner, and David B. Hoyt. 1999. Outcome After Major Trauma: 12-Month and 18-Month Follow-Up Results From the Trauma Recovery Project. *Journal of Trauma Injury, Infection, and Critical Care* 46(5):765–773.

Houle, Christian, and Jean-Marie Berthelot. 2000. A Head-to-Head Comparison of the Health Utilities Index Mark 3 and the EQ-5D for the Population Living in Private Households in Canada. *Quality of Life Newsletter* 24:5–6.

Hubbell, Bryan J. 2004. *Health Based Cost Effectiveness of Ambient PM Reductions.* Unpublished draft paper. Raleigh-Durham, NC: Environmental Protection Agency.

Hubbell, Bryan J., Aaron Hallberg, Donald R. McCubbin, and Ellen Post. 2005. Health-Related Benefits of Attaining the 8-Hour Ozone Standard. *Environmental Health Perspectives* 113(1):73–82.

Hunink, Myriam, Paul P. Glasziou, Joanna E. Siegel, Jane C. Weeks, et al. 2001. *Decision Making in Health and Medicine: Integrating Evidence and Values.* Cambridge: Cambridge University Press.

Hurley, Jeremiah. 2000. An Overview of the Normative Economics of the Health Sector. In: Culyer, A.J., and Newhouse, Joseph P., eds. *Handbook of Health Economics.* New York: Elsevier Science. Pp. 56–110.

Institute of Medicine. 1997. *Enabling America: Assessing the Role of Rehabilitation Science and Engineering.* Washington, DC: National Academy Press.

———. 1998. *Summarizing Population Health: Directions for the Development and Application of Population Metrics.* Washington, DC: National Academy Press.

———. 2005. *Estimating the Contributions of Lifestyle-Related Factors to Preventable Death: A Workshop Summary.* Washington, DC: National Academies Press.

Jacobson, Peter D., and Richard E. Hoffman. 2003. Regulating Public Health: Principles and Applications of Administrative Law. In: Goodman, Richard A., et al., eds. *Law in Public Health Practice.* New York: Oxford University Press. Pp. 23–42.

Jacobson, Peter D., and Matthew L. Kanna. 2001. Cost-Effectiveness Analysis in the Courts: Recent Trends and Future Prospects. *Journal of Health Politics, Policy and Law* 26:291–326.

Johannesson, Magnus. 2001. Should We Aggregate Relative or Absolute Changes in QALYs? *Health Economics* 10:537–577.

Johannesson, Magnus, Joseph S. Pliskin, and Milton C. Weinstein. 1994. A Note on QALYs, Time Tradeoff, and Discounting. *Medical Decision Making* 14:189–193.

Johnson, F. Reed, Erin E. Fries, and H. Spencer Banzhaf. 1997. Valuing Morbidity: An Integration of the Willingness-to-Pay and Health-Status Index Literatures. *Journal of Health Economics* 16:641–665.

Johnson, F. Reed, H. Spencer Banzhaf, William H. Desvousges. 2000. Willingness to pay for improved respiratory and cardiovascular health: A multiple-format stated-preference approach. *Health Economics* 9:295–317.

Johnson, Jeffrey A., Nan Luo, James W. Shaw, Paul Kind, et al. 2005. Valuations of EQ-5D Health States: Are the United States and United Kingdom Different? *Medical Care* 43(3):221–228.

Jones-Lee, M.W., ed. 1992. Paternalistic Altruism and the Value of Statistical Life. *Economic Journal* 102:80–90.

Juniper, E.F., G.H. Guyatt, D.H. Feeny, L.E. Griffith, et al. 1997. Minimum Skills Required by Children to Complete Health-Related Quality of Life Instruments for Asthma: Comparison of Measurement Properties. *European Respiratory Journal* 10(10):2285–2294.

Just, Richard E., Darrell L. Hueth, and Andrew Schmitz. 2004. *The Welfare Economics of Public Policy: A Practical Approach to Project and Policy Evaluation*. Northhampton, MA: Edward Elgar.

Kahneman, Daniel, and Amos Tversky, eds. 1979. Prospect Theory: An Analysis of Decision Under Risk. *Econometrica* 47(2):263–292.

———. 2000. *Choices, Values and Frames*. Cambridge: Cambridge University Press.

Kahneman, Daniel, Peter P. Wakker, and Rakesh Sarin. 1997. Back to Bentham? Explorations of Experienced Utility. *Quarterly Journal of Economics* 112(2):375–405.

Kaldor, Nicholas. 1939. Welfare Propositions of Economics and Interpersonal Comparisons of Utility. *Economic Journal* 49(196):549–552.

Kaplan, Robert M., and John P. Anderson. 1988. A General Health Policy Model: Update and Applications. *Health Service Research* 23(2):203–235.

———. 1996. The General Health Policy Model: An Integrated Approach. In: Spilker, Bert, ed. *Quality of Life and Pharmacoeconomics in Clinical Trials*. Philadelphia: Lippincott-Raven Publishers. Pp. 309–322.

Kaplan, Robert M., and James W. Bush. 1982. Health-Related Quality of Life Measurement for Evaluation Research and Policy Analysis. *Health Psychology* 1(1):61–80.

Kaplan, Robert M., J.W. Bush, and Charles C. Berry. 1976. Health Status: Types of Validity and the Index of Well-Being. *Health Services Research* 11(4):478–507.

Kaplan, Robert M., D. Feeny, and D.A. Revicki. 1993. Methods for Assessing Relative Importance in Preference Based Outcome Measures. *Quality of Life Research* 2:467–475.

Kaplan, Robert M., William J. Sieber, and Theodore G. Ganiatas. 1997. The Quality of Well-Being Scale: Comparison of the Interviewer-Administered Version With a Self-Administered Questionnaire. *Psychology and Health* 12:783–791.

Keeler, Emmett B., and Shan Cretin. 1983. Discounting of Life-Saving and Other Nonmonetary Effects. *Management Science* 29(3):300–306.

Keeney, Ralph L., and Howard Raiffa. 1976. *Decision With Multiple Objectives: Preferences and Value Tradeoffs*. New York: John Wiley and Sons.

Keeney, Ralph L., and Detlof von Winterfeldt. 1991. Eliciting Probabilities From Experts in Complex Technical Problems. *IEEE Transactions on Engineering Management* 38:191–201.

Kind, Paul. 2004 (November 30). *Issues in the Measurement and Valuation of Health*. Presentation to the Institute of Medicine Committee to Evaluate Measures of Health Benefits for Environmental, Health, and Safety Regulation.

Kind, Paul, Paul Dolan, Clair Gudex, and Alan Williams. 1998. Variations in Population Health Status: Results from a United Kingdom National Questionnaire Survey. *British Medical Journal* 316(7133):736–741.

Kopec, Jacek A., and Kevin D. Willison. 2003. A Comparative Review of Four Preference-Weighted Measures of Health-Related Quality of Life. *Journal of Clinical Epidemiology* 56:317–325.

Kopp, Raymond, Alan J. Krupnick, and Michael Toman. 1997. Cost Benefit Analysis and Regulatory Reform: An Assessment of the Science and the Art. *Human and Ecological Risk Assessment* 3(5):787–852.

Krabbe, Paul F.M., Marie-Louise Essink-Bot, and Gouke J. Bonsel. 1997. The Comparability and Reliability of Five Health-State Valuation Methods. *Social Science and Medicine* 45(11):1641–1652.

Krupnick, Alan K. 2004. *Valuing Health Outcomes: Policy Choices and Technical Issues*. Washington, DC: Resources for the Future.

Landgraf, Jeanne M., and Linda N. Abetz. 1996. Measuring Health Outcomes in Pediatric Populations: Issues in Psychometrics and Application. In: Spilker, Bert, ed. *Quality of Life and Pharmacoeconomics in Clinical Trials*. Philadelphia: Lippincott-Raven Publishers. Pp. 793–802.

Laufer, Franklin. 2005. Thresholds in Cost-Effectiveness Analysis—More of the Story. *Value in Health* 8(1):86–87.

Lave, L.B. 1996. Benefit–Cost Analysis: Do the Benefits Exceed the Costs? In: Hahn, R.W., ed. *Risks, Costs, and Lives Saved*. New York: Oxford University Press. Pp. 104–134.

Lawrence, William F., and John A. Fleishman. 2004. Predicting EuroQol EQ-5D Preference Scores From the SF-12 Health Survey in a Nationally Representative Sample. *Medical Decision Making* 24:160–169.

Lenert, Leslie, and Robert M. Kaplan. 2000. Validity and Interpretation of Preference-Based Measures of Health-Related Quality of Life. *Medical Care* 38(9 Suppl II):II-138–II-150.

Lind, Richard C. 1982. A Primer on the Major Issues Relating to the Discount Rate for Evaluating National Energy Options. In: Lind, Richard C., et al. *Discounting for Time and Risks in Energy Policy*. Washington, DC: Resources for the Future.

Llewellyn-Thomas, Hilary A., Heather J. Sutherland, R. Tibshirani, A. Ciampi, et al. 1982. The Measurement of Patients' Value in Medicine. *Medical Decision Making* 2(4):449–462.

Llewellyn-Thomas, Hilary A., Heather J. Sutherland, and Elaine C. Thiel. 1993. Do Patients' Evaluations of a Future Health State Change When They Actually Enter That State? *Medical Care* 31(11):1002–1012.

Lohr, Kathleen N., Neil K. Aaronson, Jordi Alonso, Audrey Burnam, et al. 1996. Evaluating Quality-of-Life and Health Status Instruments: Development of Scientific Review Criteria. *Clinical Therapeutics* 18(5):979–992.

Loomes, Graham, and Lynda McKenzie. 1989. The Use of QALYs in Health Care Decision Making. *Social Science and Medicine* 28(4):299–308.

Luo, Nan, Jeffrey A. Johnson, James W. Shaw, David Feeny, et al. 2005. Self-Reported Health Status of the General Adult U.S. Population As Assessed by the EQ-5D and Health Utilities Index. *Medical Care* 43(11):1078–1086.

MacKenzie, Ellen J., Anne Damiano, Ted Miller, and Steve Luchter. 1996. The Development of the Functional Capacity Index. *Journal of Trauma* 41(5):799–807.

MacKenzie, Ellen J., Maria Segui-Gomez, Ted Miller, Anne Damiano, et al. 2004. *The Functional Capacity Index*. Presentation prepared for the Institute of Medicine Committee to Evaluate Measures of Health Benefits for Environmental, Health, and Safety Regulation.

Magaziner, Jay, Eleanor Simonsick, T.M. Kashner, and J.R. Hebel. 1988. Patient-Proxy Response Comparability on Measures of Patient Health and Functional Status. *Journal of Clinical Epidemiology* 41(11):1065–1074.

Manning, Willard G., D.G. Fryback, and M.C. Weinstein. 1996. Reflecting Uncertainty in Cost-Effectiveness Analysis. In: Gold, Marthe R., Siegel, Joanna E., Russell, Louise B., and Weinstein, Milton C., eds. *Cost-Effectiveness in Health and Medicine*. New York: Oxford University Press. Pp. 247–275.

Margolis, Howard. 1996. *Dealing with Risk: Why the Public and the Experts Disagree on Environmental Issues*. Chicago: University of Chicago Press.

Mason, Bryce. 2005. *Statistical Analysis of Expert Ratings on Health-Related Quality of Life (HRQL) Metrics*. Memorandum prepared for the Institute of Medicine Committee to Evaluate Measures of Health Benefits for Environmental, Health, and Safety Regulation.

Mathers, Colin D., Christina Bernard, Kim M. Iburg, Mie Inoue, et al. 2003. *The Global Burden of Disease in 2002: Data Sources, Methods and Results*. Geneva, World Health Organization (GPE Discussion Paper No. 54). [Online]. Available: http://www.who.org/int/evidence [accessed August 10, 2005].

Matza, Louis S., Andrine R. Swensen, Emuella M. Flood, Kristina Secnik, et al. 2004. Assessment of Health-Related Quality of Life in Children: A Review of Conceptual, Methodological, and Regulatory Issues. *Value in Health* 7(1):79–92.

McDowell, Ian, and Claire Newell. 1996. *Measuring Health: A Guide to Rating Scales and Questionnaires*. New York: Oxford University Press.

McNeil, Barbara J., Ralph Weichselbaum, and Stephen G. Pauker. 1978. Fallacy of the Five-Year Survival in Lung Cancer. *New England Journal of Medicine* 299:1397–1401.

———. 1981. Speech and Survival: Tradeoffs Between Quality and Quantity of Life in Laryngeal Cancer. *New England Journal of Medicine* 305:982–987.

Mehrez, Abraham, and Amiriam Gafni. 1990. Evaluating Health Related Quality of Life: An Indifference Curve Interpretation for the Time Trade-Off Technique. *Social Science and Medicine* 31:1281–1283.

———. 1991. The Healthy-Years Equivalents: How to Measure Them Using the Standard Gamble Approach. *Medical Decision Making* 11:140–146.

Menzel, Paul. 1999. How Should What Economists Call "Social Values" Be Measured? *Journal of Ethics* 3:249–273.

Menzel, Paul, Marthe R. Gold, Erik Nord, Jose-Louis Pinto-Prades, et al. 1999. Toward A Broader View of Values in Cost-Effectiveness Analysis of Health. *Hastings Center Report* 29(3):7–15.

Meyers, Allan R., and Elena M. Andresen. 2000. Enabling Our Instruments: Accomodation, Universal Design, and Access to Participation in Research. *Archives of Physical Medicine and Rehabilitation* 81(Suppl 2):S5–S9.

Miller, Ted, J. Viner, S. Rossman, N. Pindus, et al. 1991. *The Cost of Highway Crashes.* Washington, DC: Urban Institute.

Mishan, E.J. 1971. *Cost–Benefit Analysis: An Informal Introduction.* London: Allen and Unwin.

———. 1988. *Cost–Benefit Analysis.* 4th ed. London: Unwin Hyman.

Mitchell, Robert C., and Richard T. Carson. 1989. *Using Surveys to Value Public Goods: The Contingent Valuation Method.* Washington, DC: Resources for the Future.

Miyamoto, John M., and Stephen A. Eraker. 1985. Parameter Estimates for a QALY Utility Model. *Medical Decision Making* 5(2):191–213.

———. 1988. A Multiplicative Model of the Utility of Survival Duration and Health Quality. *Journal of Experimental Psychology: General* 117(1):3–20.

Molzahn, A.E., H.C. Northcott, and L. Hayduk. 1996. Quality of Life of Patients With End Stage Renal Disease: A Structural Equation Model. *Quality of Life Research* 5:426–432.

Morgan, M. Granger, and Max Henrion. 1990. *Uncertainty: A Guide to Dealing With Uncertainty in Quantitative Risk and Policy Analysis.* New York: Cambridge University Press.

Moriarty, David. 2004 (December 1). *Tracking Health-Related Quality of Life in the United States, 1993–2004.* Presentation to the Institute of Medicine Committee to Evaluate Measures of Health Benefits for Environmental, Health, and Safety Regulation.

Morrall, John, III. 1986. A Review of the Record. *Regulation* 10:25–34.

———. 2003. *Saving Lives: A Review of the Record.* Working Paper 03-06. Washington, DC: AEI-Brookings Joint Center for Regulatory Studies.

Murray, Christopher J.L., and Arnab K. Acharya. 1997. Understanding DALYs. *Journal of Health Economics* 16:703–730.

Murray, Christopher J.L., and Alan D. Lopez, eds. 1996. *The Global Burden of Disease.* Washington, DC: World Health Organization.

Najman, J.M., and S. Levine. 1981. Evaluating the Impact of Medical Care and Technologies on the Quality of Life: A Review and Critique. *Social Science and Medicine* 15:107–115.

National Center for Health Statistics (NCHS). 2004. *Health, United States, 2004: With Chartbook on Trends in the Health of Americans.* Hyattsville, MD: U.S. Government Printing Office. Department of Health and Human Services.

———. 2005. *2004 National Health Interview Survey (NHIS) Public Use Data Release: NHIS Survey Description.* Hyattsville, MD: NCHS and Centers for Disease Control and Prevention. Department of Health and Human Services.

National Highway Traffic Safety Administration (NHTSA). 1996. *The Economic Cost of Motor Vehicle Crashes, 1994.* DOT-HS-808-425. Washington, DC: National Highway Traffic Safety Administration.

―――. 1999a. *Final Economic Assessment: FMVCSS No. 213, FMVSS No. 225, Child Restraint Systems; Child Restraint Anchorage Systems.* Washington, DC: Office of Regulatory Analysis.

―――. 1999b. Federal Motor Vehicle Safety Standards; Child Restraint Anchorage Systems; Final Rule. *Federal Register* 64(43):10786–10850.

―――. 2002a. *The Economic Impact of Motor Vehicle Crashes, 2000.* DOT-HS-809-446. Washington, DC: National Highway Traffic Safety Administration.

―――. 2002b. *National Automotive Sampling System (NASS) Crashworthiness Data System, Analytical User's Manual, 2002 File.* Washington, DC: National Center for Statistics and Analysis.

National Research Council (NRC). 2002. *Estimating the Public Health Benefits of Proposed Air Pollution Regulations.* Washington, DC: National Academy Press.

Neumann, Peter J. 2005. *Using Cost-Effectiveness Analysis to Improve Health Care: Opportunities and Barriers.* New York: Oxford University Press.

Neumann, Peter J., Patricia W. Stone, Richard H. Chapman, Eileen A. Sandberg, and Chaim M. Bell. 2000. The Quality of Reporting in Published Cost-Utility Analyses, 1976–1997. *Annals of Internal Medicine* 132(12):964–972.

Nichol, Michael B., Nishan Sengupta, and Denise R. Globe. 2001. Evaluating Quality-Adjusted Life Years: Estimation of the Health Utility Index (HUI2) From the SF-36. *Medical Decision Making* 21(2):105–112.

Nord, Erik. 1992. An Alternative to QALYs: The Saved Young Life Equivalent (SAVE). *British Medical Journal* 305:875–877.

―――. 1999. *Cost-Value Analysis in Health Care: Making Sense Out of QALYs.* Cambridge: Cambridge University Press.

―――. 2001. The Desirability of a Condition Versus the Well Being and Worth of a Person. *Health Economics* 10:579–581.

Nord, Erik, Jose L. Pinto, Jeff Richardson, Paul Menzel, and Peter Ubel. 1999. Incorporating Societal Concerns for Fairness in Numerical Valuations of Health Programmes. *Health Economics* 8:25–39.

O'Brien, Bernie, and J.L. Viramontes. 1994. Willingness to Pay: A Valid and Reliable Measure of Health State Preference? *Medical Decision Making* 14(3):289–297.

O'Connor, A.M., and R.A. Pennie. 1995. Reliability and Validity of Measures Used to Elicit Health Expectations, Values, Tradeoffs and Intentions to be Immunized for Hepatitis B. *Journal of Clinical Epidemiology* 48(2):255–262.

Oostenbrink, Jan B., Marco J.D. Tangelder, Jan J.V. Busschbach, et al. 2001. Cost-Effectiveness of Oral Anticoagulants Versus Aspirin in Patients After Infrainguinal Pass Grafting Surgery. *Journal of Vascular Surgery* 34:254–262.

Parker, Richard W. 2003. Grading the Government. *University of Chicago Law Review* 70:1345–1373.

Patrick, Donald L., and Yen-Pin Chiang. 2000. Measurement of Health Outcomes in Treatment Effectiveness Evaluations. *Medical Care* 38(9 Suppl II):II-14–II-25.

Patrick, Donald L., and Pennifer Erickson. 1993. *Health Status and Health Policy: Allocating Resources to Health Care.* New York: Oxford University Press.

Patrick, Donald L., J.W. Bush, and M.M. Chen. 1973. Methods for Measuring Levels of Well-Being for a Health Status Index. *Health Services Research* 8:228–245.

Payne, John W., James R. Bettman, and David A. Schkade. 1999. Measuring Constructed Preferences: Towards a Building Code. *Journal of Risk and Uncertainty* 19(1–3):243–270.

Peters, Annette, Douglas W. Dockery, James E. Muller, and Murray A. Mittleman. 2001. Increased Particulate Air Pollution and the Triggering of Myocardial Infarction. *Circulation* 103:2810–2815.

Petrou, Stavros. 2003. Methodological Issues Raised by Preference-Based Approaches to Measuring the Health Status of Children. *Health Economics* 12:697–702.

Phelps, Charles E., and Alvin J. Mushlin. 1991. On the (Near) Equivalence of Cost-Effectiveness and Cost-Benefit Analysis. *International Journal of Technology Assessment in Health Care* 7(1):12–21.

Pickard, A.S., and Sara J. Knight. 2005. Proxy Evaluation of Health-Related Quality of Life: A Conceptual Framework for Understanding Multiple Proxy Perspectives. *Medical Care* 43(5):493–499.

Pliskin, Joseph S., Donald Shepard, and Milton C. Weinstein. 1980. Utility Functions for Life Years and Health Status. *Operations Research* 28:206–224.

Pope, C. Arden, III, Richard T. Burnett, Richard J. Thun, Eugenia E. Calle, et al. 2002. Lung Cancer, Cardiopulmonary Mortality, and Long-Term Exposure to Fine Particulate Air Pollution. *Journal of the American Medical Association* 287(9):1137–1141.

Portney, Paul R., and John P. Weyant, eds. 1999. *Discounting and Intergenerational Equity.* Washington, DC: Resources for the Future.

Rawls, John. 1971. *A Theory of Justice.* Cambridge, MA: Harvard University Press.

———. 1993. *Political Liberalism.* New York: Columbia University Press.

Reagan, Ronald. 1981 (February 17). *Federal Regulation, Executive Order 12291.* White House.

Reed, W.W., J.E. Herbers, and G.L. Noel. 1993. Cholesterol Lowering Therapy: What Patients Expect in Return. *Journal of General Internal Medicine* 8:591–596.

Revesz, Richard L. 1999. Environmental Regulation, Cost-Benefit Analysis, and the Discounting of Human Lives. *Columbia Law Review* 99(4):941–1017.

Revicki, Dennis A. 1992. Relationship Between Health Utility and Psychometric Health Status Measures. *Medical Care* 30(5 Suppl):MS274–MS282.

Richardson, Jeff, and Erik Nord. 1997. The Importance of Perspective in the Measurement of Quality-Adjusted Life Years. *Medical Decision Making* 17:33–41.

Riis, Jason, George Loewenstein, Jonathan Baron, Christopher Jepson, et al. 2005. Ignorance of Hedonic Adaptation to Hemo-Dialysis: A Study Using Ecological Momentary Assessment. *Journal of Experimental Psychology: General* 134(1):3–9.

Rizzo, J.A., S. Pashko, R. Friedkin, J. Mullahy, and J.L. Sindelar. 1998. Linking the Health Utilities Index to National Medical Expenditure Survey Data. *Pharmacoeconomics* 13(5):531–541.

Rizzo, John A., and Jody L. Sindelar. 1999. Linking Health-Related Quality-of-Life Indicators to Large National Data Sets. *Pharmacoeconomics* 16(5 Pt 1):473–482.

Robinson, Lisa A. 2004. *Current Federal Agency Practices for Valuing the Impact of Regulations on Human Health and Safety.* Prepared for the Institute of Medicine Committee to Evaluate Measures of Health Benefits for Environmental, Health, and Safety Regulation.

Robinson, Lisa A., Phaedra Corso, Xiangming Fang, Robert Black, and Wilhelmine Miller. 2005a. *Alternative Approaches for Estimating Health-Related Quality of Life Impact: Child Restraints Case Study.* Prepared for the Institute of Medicine Committee to Evaluate Measures of Health Benefits for Environmental, Health, and Safety Regulation.

Robinson, Lisa A., Wilhelmine Miller, and Robert Black. 2005b. *Alternative Approaches for Estimating Health-Related Quality of Life Impact: Juice Processing Regulation Case Study.* Prepared for the Institute of Medicine Committee to Evaluate Measures of Health Benefits for Environmental, Health, and Safety Regulation.

———. 2005c. *Alternative Approaches for Estimating Health-Related Quality of Life Impact: Nonroad Engine Air Emissions Regulation Case Study.* Prepared for the Institute of Medicine Committee to Evaluate Measures of Health Benefits for Environmental, Health, and Safety Regulation.

Rothman, Margaret L., Susan C. Hedrick, Kris A. Bulcroft, et al. 1991. The Validity of Proxy-Generated Scores as Measures of Patient Health Status. *Medical Care* 29(2):115–124.

Sackett, David L., and George W. Torrance. 1978. The Utility of Different Health States as Perceived by the General Public. *Journal of Chronic Diseases* 31:697–704.

Salomon, Joshua A. 2003. Reconsidering the Use of Rankings in the Valuation of Health States: A Model for Estimating Cardinal Values From Ordinal Data. *Population Health Metrics* 1:1–12.

Salomon, Joshua A., and Christopher C.L. Murray. 2004. A Multi-Method Approach to Measuring Health-State Valuations. *Health Economics* 13:281–290.

Scharff, Robert L., and Amber Jessup. 2001. *Valuing Chronic Disease for Heterogeneous Populations: The Case of Arthritis.* Unpublished manuscript. College Park, MD: FDA.

Schelling, Thomas. 1968. The Life You Save May Be Your Own. In: Chase, S., Jr., ed. *Problems in Public Expenditure Analysis.* Washington, DC: Brookings Institution.

Shaw, James W., Jeffrey A. Johnson, and Stephen J. Coons. 2005. U.S. Valuation of the EQ-5D Health States: Development and Testing of the D1 Valuation Model. *Medical Care* 43(3):203–220.

Silvers, Anita. 1996. (In) Equality, (Ab) Normality and the Americans With Disabilities Act. *Journal of Medicine and Philosophy* 21:209–224.

Skrzycki, Cindy. 2003. *Under Fire, EPA Drops the "Senior Death Discount."* [Online]. Available: http://www.rff.org/rff/news/coverage/2003/may/under-fire-epa-drops-the-senior death-discount.cfm [accessed July 28, 2005].

Slevin, M.L., L. Stubbs, H.J. Plant, et al. 1990. Attitudes to Chemotherapy: Comparing the Views of Patients With Cancer With Those of Doctors, Nurses and the General Public. *British Medical Journal* 300:1458–1460.

Slovic, Paul. 2000. *The Perception of Risk.* London: Earthscan Publications.

Slovic, Paul, Baruch Fischhoff, and Sarah Lichtenstein. 2000. Facts and Fears: Understanding Perceived Risk. In: Slovic, Paul. *The Perception of Risk.* London: Earthscan Publications. Pp. 137–153.

Slovic, Paul, Melissa L. Finucane, Ellen Peters, and Donald G. MacGregor. 2004. Risk as Analysis and Risk as Feelings: Some Thoughts about Affect, Reason, Risk, and Rationality. *Risk Analysis* 24(2): 311–322.

Smith, Noel, Sue Middleton, Kate Ashton-Brooks, et al. 2004. *Disabled People's Cost of Living: More Than You Would Think.* York, UK: Joseph Rowntree Foundation.

Smith, V. Kerry, George V. Houtven, and Subhrendu K. Pattanayak. 2002. Benefit Transfer Via Preference Calibration: "Prudential Algebra" for Policy. *Land Economics* 78(1):132–152.

Smith, V. Kerry, Subhrendu K. Pattanayak, and George L. Van Houtven. 2003. *Preference Calibration With QALYs.* [Online]. Available: http://pubdevelopment.rti.org/www/pubs/pref_calib_QALYs.pdf [accessed August 15, 2005].

Stewart, Susan T., Rebecca M. Woodward, and David M. Cutler. 2005. *A Proposed Method for Monitoring U.S. Population Health: Linking Symptoms, Impairments, Chronic Conditions, and Health Ratings.* NBER Working Paper 11358. Cambridge, MA: National Bureau of Economic Research.

Sullivan, Patrick W., William F. Lawrence, and Vahram Ghushchyan. 2005. A National Catalog of Preference-Based Scores for Chronic Conditions in the United States. *Medical Care* 43(7):736–749.

Sunstein, Cass R. 1996. Health-Health Tradeoffs. *University of Chicago Law Review* 63: 1533–1571.

Sunstein, Cass R., and Arden Rowell. 2005. *On Discounting Regulatory Benefits: Risk, Money, and Intergenerational Equity.* Working Paper 05-08. Washington, DC: AEI-Brookings Joint Center for Regulatory Studies.

Tengs, Tammy O. 2004. Cost-Effectiveness Versus Cost-Utility Analysis of Interventions for Cancer: Does Adjusting for Health-Related Quality of Life Really Matter? *Value in Health* 7(1):70–78.

Tengs, Tammy O., and Ting H. Lin. 2003. A Meta-Analysis of Quality-of-Life Estimates for Stroke. *Pharmacoeconomics* 21(3):191–200.

Tengs, Tammy O., Miriam E. Adams, Joseph S. Pliskin, Dana G. Safran, Joanna E. Siegel, et al. 1995. Five-Hundred Life-Saving Interventions and Their Cost-Effectiveness. *Risk Analysis* 15(3):369–390.

Tengs, Tammy O., Michelle Yu, and Elvina Luistro. 2001. Health-Related Quality of Life After Stroke: A Comprehensive Review. *Stroke* 32:964–972.

Torrance, George, Valery Walker, Ronald Grossman, and Jayanti Mukherjee. 1999. Economic Evaluation of Ciprofloxcin Compared With Usual Antibacterial Care for the Treatment of Acute Exacerbations of Chronic Bronchitis in Patients Followed for 1 year. *Pharmacoeconomics* 16(5 Pt 1):499–520.

Torrance, George W. 1976. Social Preferences for Health States: An Empirical Evaluation of Three Measurement Techniques. *Socio-Economic Planning Sciences* 10:129–136.

Torrance, George W., David L. Sackett, and Warren H. Thomas. 1973. Utility Maximization Model for Program Evaluation: A Demonstration Application. In: Berg, Richard L., ed. *Health Status Indexes.* Chicago: Hospital Research and Educational Trust. Pp. 156–164.

Torrance, George W., Michael H. Boyle, and Sargent P. Horwood. 1982. Applications of Multi-Attribute Theory to Measure Social Preferences for Health States. *Operations Research* 30(6):1043–1069.

Torrance, George W., William Furlong, David Feeny, and Michael Boyle. 1995. Multi-Attribute Preference Functions: Health Utilities Index. *Pharmacoeconomics* 7(6):503–520.

Torrance, George W., David H. Feeny, William J. Furlong, Ronald D. Barr, et al. 1996. Multiattribute Utility Function for a Comprehensive Health Status Classification System: Health Utilities Index Mark 2. *Medical Care* 34(7):702–722.

Treasury, H.M. 2005. *Managing Risks to the Public: Appraisal Guidance.* London: Controller of Her Majesty's Stationery Office.

Ubel, Peter A., Michael L. DeKay, Jonathan Baron, and David A. Asch. 1996. Cost-Effectiveness Analysis in a Setting of Budget Constraints. *New England Journal of Medicine* 334(18):1174–1177.

Ubel, Peter A., George Loewenstein, Dennis Scanlon, and Mark Kamlet. 1998. Value Measurement in Cost-Utility Analysis: Explaining the Discrepancy Rating Scale and Person Trade-Off Elicitations. *Health Policy* 43:33–44.

Ubel, Peter A., Jeff Richardson, and Paul Menzel. 2000. Societal Value, The Person Trade-Off, and the Dilemma of Whose Values to Measure for Cost-Effectiveness Analysis. *Health Economics* 9:127–136.

U.S. Environmental Protection Agency (EPA). 1997. *Final Report to Congress on the Benefits and Costs of the Clean Air Act, 1970 to 1990.* EPA-410-R-97-002. Washington, DC: EPA.

———. 1999. *Final Report to Congress on the Benefits and Costs of the Clean Air Act, 1990 to 2010.* EPA-410-R-99-00. Washington, DC: EPA.

———. 2000a. *Guidelines for Preparing Economic Analyses.* EPA 240-R-00-003. Washington, DC: EPA.

———. 2000b. *Valuing Fatal Cancer Risk Reductions.* Washington, DC: EPA.

————. 2003. *Regulations: A Vital Tool for Protecting Public Health and the Environment.* Washington, DC: EPA.

————. 2004a. Control of Emissions of Air Pollution From Nonroad Diesel Engines and Fuel: Final Rule. *Federal Register* 69(124):38957–39273.

————. 2004b. *Final Regulatory Impact Analysis: Control of Emissions From Nonroad Diesel Engines.* EPA 420-R-04-07. Washington, DC: EPA.

————. 2005a. *Regulatory Impact Analysis for the Final Clean Air Interstate Rule.* EPA-452/R-05-002. Washington, DC: EPA.

————. 2005b. *Valuing Time Losses Due to Illness.* EPA 815-R-05-003. Washington, DC: EPA.

U.S. Executive Office of the President (EOP). 1993. *Executive Order 12866. Regulatory Planning and Review.* As amended by *Executive Order 13258* (2002).

————. 1994. *Executive Order 12898. Federal Actions to Address Environmental Justice in Minority Populations and Low-Income Populations.* As amended by *Executive Order 12948* (1995).

————. 1997. *Executive Order 13045. Protection of Children From Environmental Risks and Safety Risks.* As amended by *Executive Order 13299* (2001) and *Executive Order 13296* (2003).

————. 2002. Ranking Regulatory Investments in Public Health. In: *Fiscal Year 2003 Analytical Perspectives, Budget of the United States Government.* Washington, DC: U.S. Government Printing Office. Pp. 419–421.

U.S. Food and Drug Administration (FDA). 1998. Preliminary Regulatory Impact Analysis and Initial Regulatory Flexibility Analysis of the Proposed Rules to Ensure the Safety of Juice and Juice Products; Proposed Rule. *Federal Register* 63(84):24253–24378.

————. 2001. Hazard Analysis and Critical Control Point (HAACP); Procedures for the Safe and Sanitary Processing of Juice; Final Rule. *Federal Register* 66(13):6138–6202.

U.S. Office of Management and Budget (OMB). 1997. *Report to Congress on the Costs and Benefits of Federal Regulations.*

————. 2000. *Guidelines to Standardize Measures of Costs and Benefits and the Format of Accounting Statements (Memorandum M-00-08).* Washington, DC: Office of Management and Budget.

————. 2003a. Circular A-4, *Regulatory Analysis.* Washington, DC: Office of Management and Budget.

————. 2003b. *Informing Regulatory Decisions: 2003 Report to Congress on the Costs and Benefits of Federal Regulations and Unfunded Mandates on State, Local, and Tribal Entities.* Washington, DC: U.S. Office of Management and Budget.

————. 2004. *Informing Regulatory Decisions: 2004 Draft Report to Congress on the Costs and Benefits of Regulations and Unfunded Mandates on State, Local, and Tribal Entities.* Washington, DC: U.S. Office of Management and Budget.

Viscusi, W. Kip, ed. 1994. The Mortality Costs of Regulatory Expenditures. *Journal of Risk and Uncertainty* 8(1):5–122.

Viscusi, W. Kip, W.A. Magat, and A. Forrest. 1988. Altruistics and Private Values of Risk Reduction. *Journal of Policy Analysis and Management* 7(2):227–245.

von Neumann, John, and Oscar Morgenstern. 1947. *Theories of Games and Economic Behavior.* Princeton, NJ: Princeton University Press.

Walker, Rebecca L., and Andrew W. Siegel. 2002. Morality and the Limits of Societal Values in Health Care Allocation. *Health Economics* 11:265–273.

Wang, Caroline. 1992. Culture, Meaning and Disability: Injury Prevention Campaigns and the Production of Stigma. *Social Science and Medicine* 35(9):1093–1102.

Ware, John E., Jr. 2000. SF-36 Health Survey Update. *Spine* 25(24):3130–3139.

Wasserman, David, and Arlene Asch. 2004 (November 30). *Mending, Not Ending CEA.* Presentation to the Institute of Medicine Committee to Evaluate Measures of Health Benefits for Environmental, Health, and Safety Regulation.

Weinstein, Milton C., and William B. Stason. 1977. Foundations of Cost-Effectiveness Analysis for Health and Medical Practices. *New England Journal of Medicine* 296(13):716–721.

Weinstein, Milton C., Pamela G. Coxson, Lawrence W. Williams, Theodore M. Pass, et al. 1987. Forecasting Coronary Heart Disease Incidence, Mortality, and Cost: The Coronary Heart Disease Policy Model. *American Journal of Public Health* 77(11):1417–1426.

Weitzman, Martin L. 1999. Just Keep Discounting, But . . . In: Portney, Paul R., and Weyant, John P., eds. *Discounting and Intergeneration Equity.* Washington, DC: Resources of the Future. Pp. 23–29.

Wildavsky, Aaron. 1980. Richer is Safer. *The Public Interest* 60:23–39.

Willan, Andrew R., and Bernie J. O'Brien. 1996. Confidence Intervals for Cost-Effectiveness Ratios: An Application of Fieller's Theorem. *Health Economics* 5(4):297–305.

Williams, Alan. 1995. *The Role of the EuroQoL Instrument in QALY Calculations.* York, England: Centre for Health Economics.

———. 1997. Intergenerational Equity: An Exploration of the "Fair Innings" Argument. *Health Economics* 6:117–132.

Wilson, Timothy D., Jay Meyers, and Daniel T. Gilbert. 2001. Lessons From the Past: Do People Learn From Experience That Emotional Reactions Are Short-Lived? *Personality and Social Psychology Bulletin* 27(12):1648–1661.

Index